Essentials of Clinical Psychology

Essentials of Clinical Psychology: An Indian Perspective offers a comprehensive, user-friendly introduction to the theory and practice of clinical psychology within an Indian cultural, social, and educational context.

The book starts with an introduction of what Clinical Psychology is and what it looks like in practice, giving a review of its history and contemporary traditions with an essential emphasis on its development from both a global as well as the Indian perspective. The following chapters cover a range of topics such as research methods, mental health and hygiene, and clinical psychology functions and training. The second half of the book then focuses on the classification of mental disorders for knowledge in diagnosing and treating patients, with chapters devoted to the description of various types of behavioral and mental disorders appearing in the Diagnostic and Statistical Manual of Mental Disorders (DSM) and the International Classification of Diseases (ICD). Disorders examined include eating disorders, sleep disorders, degenerative disorders, psychotic disorders, and neurodevelopmental disorders. Each chapter ends with chapter summaries, review questions, and recommended readings. Each chapter has its section-wise summaries and ends with review questions and cited references.

This textbook will serve as a must-have reference for all undergraduate and postgraduate students interested in Clinical Psychology, as well as for candidates selecting Psychology as their optional paper in competitive examinations. The book is designed according to Indian university course syllabi but also provides a guide to anyone looking to understand the current state of study and practice within Indian Clinical Psychology.

S. K. Mangal, PhD (Education), has authored several books including: *Advanced Educational Psychology, Emotional Intelligence: Managing Emotions to Win in Life, Research Methodology in Behavioural Sciences, Statistics in Psychology and Education, General Psychology, Abnormal Psychology, Child Psychology & Development, Sports Psychology,* and *Essentials of Social Psychology: An Indian Perspective.* He has devised a few psychology tools including the Emotional Intelligence Inventory and the Teacher Adjustment Inventory. The areas of his research interest are emotional intelligence and teacher adjustment.

Shubhra Mangal, PhD (Education), has co-authored and written a number of books related to the pure and applied aspect of the subject of psychology which includes *An Introduction to Psychology, Our Life and Psychology, Emotional Intelligence: Managing Emotions to Win in Life, Research Methodology in Behavioural Sciences, Sports Psychology, Child Psychology & Development,* and *Essentials of Social Psychology.* She has devised an emotional intelligence inventory for the measurement of emotional intelligence of schoolteachers. The areas of her research interest are emotional intelligence and teacher education.

Essentials of Clinical Psychology

An Indian Perspective

S. K. Mangal
Shubhra Mangal

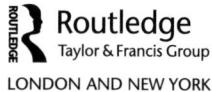
Routledge
Taylor & Francis Group

LONDON AND NEW YORK

Designed cover image: Carol Yepes as rendered the owner of the image on Getty Images.

First published 2024
by Routledge
4 Park Square, Milton Park, Abingdon, Oxon OX14 4RN

and by Routledge
605 Third Avenue, New York, NY 10158

Routledge is an imprint of the Taylor & Francis Group, an informa business

British Library Cataloguing-in-Publication Data
A catalogue record for this book is available from the British Library

Library of Congress Cataloging-in-Publication Data
Names: Mangal, S. K., 1940– author. | Mangal, Shubhra, author.
Title: Essentials of clinical psychology : an Indian perspective /
    S.K. Mangal, Shubhra Mangal.
Description: Abingdon, Oxon ; New York, NY : Routledge, 2023. |
    Includes bibliographical references and index.
Identifiers: LCCN 2023004811 (print) | LCCN 2023004812 (ebook) |
    ISBN 9781032504001 (hardback) | ISBN 9781032503998 (paperback) |
    ISBN 9781003398325 (ebook)
Subjects: LCSH: Clinical psychology—Textbooks. | Clinical psychology—
    India—Textbooks.
Classification: LCC RC467 .M28 2023 (print) | LCC RC467 (ebook) |
    DDC 616.8900954—dc23/eng/20230508
LC record available at https://lccn.loc.gov/2023004811
LC ebook record available at https://lccn.loc.gov/2023004812

ISBN: 978-1-032-50400-1 (hbk)
ISBN: 978-1-032-50399-8 (pbk)
ISBN: 978-1-003-39832-5 (ebk)

DOI: 10.4324/9781003398325

Typeset in Bembo
by Apex CoVantage, LLC

Contents

18 Clinical Assessment (Non-Testing Devices)   343

19 Clinical Assessment—Psychological and Neurological Testing 358

20 Clinical Intervention or Therapeutic Approaches 387

Preface

What is most valuable to us in terms of our existence, survival, development, and progress, is to remain essentially physically and mentally healthy in our living and functioning. It is not unusual for us to witness this naked truth in our lifetime in one form or another, be it falling victim to some dreaded disease, accidents, catastrophes, facing acute physical health problems, or getting trapped in a number of mental health issues. In general, the changing life patterns and increasingly stressful situations in one's living and functioning are compelling the societies and nations of the world to consider the substantial expansion of clinical facilities and availability of the trained clinical psychologists. The focus is now to have a sufficient number of qualified and licensed health professionals who are equipped with adequate knowledge of the theory and practice of clinical psychology for the assessment, diagnosis, and psychological treatment of mental, behavioral, and emotional issues and disorders with a broader view of supporting their overall adjustment, happiness, and well-being in their personal, social, and professional life. This mission requires the proper provision of suitable study courses on the subject of clinical psychology in a good number of institutions and universities, which is happening now on a global basis, including our own country. We see that more and more universities and institutions in our country are making provision for the study of the subject of clinical psychology in their prescribed undergraduate programs (BA and BA Hons. Clinical Psychology) and PG (MA and MPhil Psychology and Clinical Psychology), courses in the manner as needed to equip the students and trainees with the essentials of the theory and practice of the discipline of clinical psychology, with an eye on preparing them for playing the role of a trained clinical psychology professional. The knowledge and skills related to the use and applications of clinical psychology are required not only for working as a clinical psychologist, but also on the part of other health professionals and workers such as guidance and counseling personnel, social workers, school psychologists, forensic experts, psychiatrists, and practitioners of medicines.

It is this multifaceted use and application of the subject of clinical psychology that has resulted in its popularity as one of the demanding courses at the undergraduate and postgraduate levels of college and university studies. The present text is aimed to serve the needs of these courses in a comprehensive and understandable way. To this end, the subject matter has been presented in 20 properly sequenced and well-knitted chapters.

We know well that a text aimed to present the subject matter of clinical psychology must make its readers acquainted with its true meaning, nature, and scope from the outset, a task that has been carried out successfully through the discussion in Chapter 1. Moreover, here an attempt has also been made to distinguish clinical psychology from other related disciplines and fields such as Psychiatry, Guidance and counseling, School psychology and Social work.

In Chapter 2, a useful discussion has been carried out of all the essentials related to the role of clinical psychologists and their preparation as trained professionals by focusing on aspects such as what they do and how they differ from other mental health professionals such as psychiatrists, guidance and counseling personnel, school psychologists and social workers, as well as what is needed in terms of proper training and becoming a licensed clinical psychologist.

The knowledge regarding the derivation, origin, and history of a subject is regarded as essential to connect with the ideas, principles, and theoretical notions of the subject for application in the field of its operation. With this objective, a detailed account of the history of clinical psychology has been presented in Chapter 3 with an essential emphasis on its development from a global as well as the Indian perspective. Information regarding the existence of the major clinical psychology associations and the publication of journals in the field of clinical psychology has also been provided.

The study of clinical psychology related to the causation, diagnosis, assessment, and treatment of mental and behavioral problems and disorders requires from clinical psychologists and investigators the usage of appropriate methods of research and investigation sufficiently scientific, objective as well as relevant for carrying out such study. Chapter 4 endeavors to acquaint students of clinical psychology with the use of these research methods, along with the ways of analyzing data and consideration of ethical issues.

Chapter 5 deals with concepts related to one's mental health and hygiene, the characteristics of mentally healthy and unhealthy people, the need and importance of remaining mentally healthy on our part, and the role of clinical psychologists in helping people with the maintenance of their mental health. People who grapple with mental health problems demonstrate unique characteristics of abnormality in their behavior. What are these behavioral abnormalities? What criteria can be laid down for deciding the abnormality or normality of one's behavior? What causes abnormality in one's behavior? Discussion on these aspects has been carried out in Chapter 6.

Chapter 7 deals with an important topic in the subject of clinical psychology—the Classification of Mental Disorders. Such classification is essential for the diagnosis of a disorder, as well as its summarized communication to the professionals concerned for treatment. The importance of such classification along with descriptions of a number of classification systems, such as the DSM and ICD, published from time to time by the American Psychiatric Association and World Health Organization, have been highlighted in this chapter.

The next ten chapters from 8 to 17 are devoted to the description of various types of behavioral and mental disorders appearing in the DSM and ICD, discussed in Chapter 7. For this purpose, Chapter 8 begins with a discussion of the nature, causes, prevention and treatment of various types of psycho-physiological or Psychosomatic disorders.

Next, in Chapter 9, a fruitful discussion has been carried out regarding the nature, causes, symptoms, and treatment of various types of Neuroses or Psychoneurotic Disorders such as Anxiety Disorders, Trauma-and Stressor-Related Disorders, Obsessive-Compulsive and Related Disorders, Depressive Disorders, Conversion Disorders, and Dissociative Disorders. Chapter 10 then focuses on the nature, symptoms, causes and treatment of various types of Psychoses or Psychotic disorders classified as Schizophrenia Spectrum and other Related Disorders, and Bipolar and Related Disorders (Mood or Affective disorders).

In Chapter 11, there is a detailed description of the various types of Neurodevelopmental disorders such as Mental Retardation, Attention-Deficit/Hyperactivity Disorder (ADHD), and Autism and Learning Disorders or Disabilities. Chapter 12 discusses disruptive, impulse-control and conduct disorders such as Oppositional Defiant Disorder, Intermittent Explosive Disorder, and Conduct disorders (described in the form of delinquent and criminal behavior).

The usage of substances like alcohol and various types of drugs gives birth to a number of problems including the causation of various types of Substance-related addictive disorders. In this concern, a discussion related to the criteria for the diagnosis, causation, harmful effects, prevention, and treatment of alcoholics and drug addicts has been made in Chapter 13.

Chapter 14 deals with the various types of Sexual Deviations and Sexual disorders including their nature, causation, prevention, and treatment. In sequence: Chapter 15 presents a detailed description of the nature, identification, causes, and treatment of the various types of elimination disorders (such as Enuresis and Encopresis) and eating Disorders (such as Anorexia Nervosa, Bulimia Nervosa, and Binge Eating Disorder); Chapter 16 discusses the nature, identification, causation, and treatment of the various types of sleep disorders, broadly classified as Dyssomnias and Parasomnias; and Chapter 17 carries out a useful discussion of the nature, identification, causation, and treatment of the various types of old age or degenerative disorders named as Delirium, Dementia, Alzheimer's disease, Vascular Dementia, Pick's disease, Parkinson's disease, and Huntington's disease.

Afterwards, the discussion carried out in Chapters 18 and 19 offers a valuable contribution to clinical psychology students and health professionals for getting them equipped with the essentials of the clinical assessment and treatment of mental disorders and other related emotional and behavioral problems. For this purpose, Chapter 18 details the methods of clinical assessment like Observation, Case history, and Interviewing (falling in the category of non-testing devices). A discussion related to Psychological testing (involving the use of Achievement Tests, Intelligence Tests, Personality tests, etc.) and Neuro-psychological testing has been carried out in Chapter 19. Chapter 20 discusses the required activities on the part of clinical psychologists and mental health professionals for providing clinical intervention and therapeutic treatment to affected individuals with the help of various therapeutic approaches classified as medical therapies and Psychotherapies. In the end, it also acquaints the reader with the ways and means for the Rehabilitation of the mentally ill.

Thus, the coverage of the subject matter of clinical psychology is quite wide and exhaustive for serving the needs of the syllabi of Indian universities, meant for undergraduate and postgraduate courses of BA, BA (Hons.), MA and MPhil courses of the academic disciplines of Psychology and Clinical psychology, including MPhil Clinical psychology and PsyD Clinical psychology courses prescribed by the Rehabilitation Council of India. It is also able to meet the requirements of clinical psychology courses of the related disciplines such as MSW (Master of Social Work), Social Neuroscience, Psychiatry, Medicine, and Public Health. Besides this, the text also provides the requisite information and knowledge to persons who are offering their services as administrators, policymakers, Public Relation Officers, Social workers, and even parents and teachers, for equipping them to help the persons and groups they lead in their social and professional functioning in dealing with their mental health problems.

The text has been adequately illustrated with examples, figures, tables, and box material for the clarity of important terms and concepts as well as summing up what has been discussed in the corresponding paragraphs, which will surely assist readers in their understanding of the concepts and topics discussed. Moreover, the style, language, and presentation have been kept simple, engaging, and lively for facilitating readers in their understanding of the concepts and facts of clinical psychology with a proper synthesis of theory with its practical applications in clinical settings. Care has also been taken to lay down the learning objectives at the beginning of each chapter for setting clear directions to the concepts discussed and the content provided. In addition, with an aim to help the students in their self-evaluation as well as preparation for the final examination, review questions have been given at the end of each chapter. Moreover, for helping the readers delve deep into the subject, all the related references have been given at the tail of each chapter, as well as a detailed Bibliography at the end of the text.

The authors are very much indebted to the various authors, researchers and authorities related to the subject of clinical psychology whose views and opinions have been incorporated in the text. The authors are indebted to all of them for their direct and indirect impact in setting the direction and evolution of the ideas for the text material. The authors are also obliged to the publisher Routledge Imprint (Taylor & Francis Group), especially the editorial and production teams, for their praiseworthy efforts in presenting this text in such a useful form.

With this submission, it is earnestly hoped that the text will be widely read and appreciated by all those for whose interests it has been written. However, nothing is ever perfect and complete, and therefore, suggestions for bringing any improvements to the text will be highly appreciated and thankfully acknowledged by the authors and the publisher.

S.K. Mangal
Shubhra Mangal

About the Authors

S. K. Mangal, PhD (Education), was the principal, professor, and the head of the Department of Post Graduate Studies at C. R. College of Education, Rohtak, Haryana. He has authored several books associated with the pure and applied aspect of the subject psychology, including, *Essentials of Educational Psychology, Advanced Educational Psychology, Emotional Intelligence: Managing Emotions to Win in Life, Research Methodology in Behavioural Sciences, Statistics in Psychology and Education, Psychology for Nursing, Psychology for Physiotherapy, General Psychology, Abnormal Psychology, Child Psychology and Development, Psychology of Learning and Development, Sports Psychology,* and *Essentials of Social Psychology: An Indian Perspective.* Mangal has been a distinguished administrator and researcher. He has devised various educational and psychological tests and has published in reputed journals. The areas of his interest are emotional intelligence and teacher adjustment.

Shubhra Mangal, PhD (Education), was the principal, professor and the head of the Department of Post Graduate Studies, C. R. S. College of Education, Noida. She has devised an emotional intelligence inventory for the measurement of emotional intelligence of schoolteachers. She has co-authored and also written a number of books related to the pure and applied aspect of the subject of psychology which include *Introductory Psychology, Our Life and Psychology, Emotional Intelligence: Managing Emotions to Win in Life, Research Methodology in Behavioral Sciences, Psychology of Learning and Development, Child Psychology and Development, Sports Psychology,* and *Essentials of Social Psychology: An Indian Perspective.* The areas of her research interest are emotional intelligence and teacher education.

Chapter 1

Clinical Psychology—Meaning, Nature, and Scope

Learning Objectives

After going through this chapter, you will be able to:

- Explain the meaning and define the term Clinical psychology.
- Throw light on the nature of Clinical psychology.
- Provide your views about the scope of Clinical psychology.
- Describe what is included in the study of the subject of Clinical psychology.
- Name some of the important specializations available for study in the field of Clinical psychology.
- Discuss the uses and applications of Clinical psychology.

Clinical Psychology: Meaning and Definition

Much like other sciences, Psychology, defined as the science of behavior, has two aspects: pure and applied. Pure psychology formulates broad principles, brings out theories and suggests techniques for the study of human behavior, which finds practical shape in its applied aspect—branches of applied psychology like occupational psychology, clinical psychology, crime psychology, industrial psychology, educational psychology, child psychology, sports psychology, and so on.

In pictorial form, the pure and applied aspects of the subject of psychology, along with its branches, can be represented as shown in Figure 1.1.

Like its parent discipline psychology, all of the branches of clinical psychology also perform the function of studying the behavior of people in their unique environment. Likewise, where in educational psychology we study the behavior of the learners or students in the educational environment for helping them improve learning and overall welfare, in clinical psychology we study the behavior of people suffering from abnormalities, maladjustments, mental illnesses or disorders in a clinical setup or environment for helping them to overcome their problems and enjoy better health and well-being. In this way, clinical psychology may be seen to represent one of the branches or offshoots of its parent subject psychology, which helps us in studying the behavior of the abnormal and mentally ill aimed to help them in assessing and diagnosing their illness-related psychological problem for seeking its proper treatment. This is a simple meaning and explanation for the term clinical psychology. However, for understanding its meaning and nature in a more clear

DOI: 10.4324/9781003398325-1

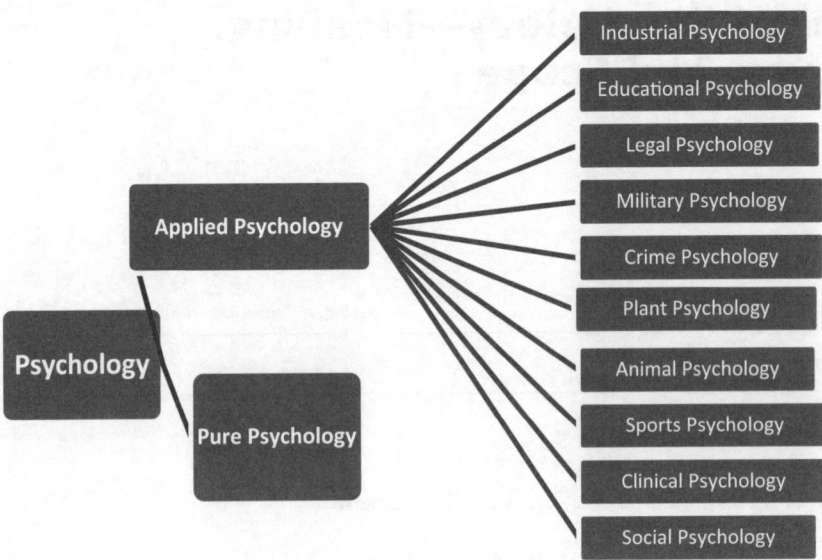

Figure 1.1 Psychology and its branches.

and comprehensive way let us seek help from the definitions provided in some of the well-known dictionaries and writings of the authors.

Collins English Dictionary: Clinical psychology is "the branch of psychology dealing with the diagnosis and treatment of personality and behavioral disorders."[1]

Merriam-Webster Dictionary: Clinical psychology is "a branch of psychology concerned with researching, diagnosing, assessing, and treating mental, emotional, and behavioral issues."[2]

Encyclopedia Britannica: Clinical psychology is "a branch of psychology concerned with the practical application of research methodologies and findings in the diagnosis and treatment of mental disorders."[3]

N., Sam M. S.: "Clinical psychology represents a field of psychology devoted to psychological methods of diagnosing and treating mental and emotional disorders, as well as research into the causes of these disorders and the effects of therapy."[4]

Canadian Psychological Association: "Clinical psychology is a broad field of practice and research within the discipline of psychology applying psychological principles to the assessment, prevention, amelioration, and rehabilitation of psychological distress, disability, dysfunctional behavior, and health-risk behavior, and to the enhancement of psychological and physical well-being."[5]

American Psychological Association: "Clinical psychology is the psychological specialty that provides continuing and comprehensive mental and behavioral health care for individuals and families; consultation to agencies and communities; training, education and supervision; and research-based practice."[6]

American Psychological Association (APA) (2012): "The field of Clinical Psychology integrates science, theory, and practice to understand, predict, and alleviate maladjustment, disability, and discomfort as well as to promote human adaptation, adjustment, and personal development. Clinical Psychology focuses on the intellectual, emotional, biological, psychological, social, and behavioral aspects of human functioning across the life span, in varying cultures, and at all socioeconomic levels."

Korchin (1986), "Clinical Psychology is most distinctly defined by the clinical attitude, that is, a concern with understanding and helping individuals in psychological distress."

Sexton and Hogan (1992): "Clinical psychology is a broad discipline concerned with the scientific study of psychopathology and with the assessment and treatment of persons with emotional, cognitive, and behavioral problems."

Myers (2013): "Clinical psychology is essentially the branch of psychology that studies, assesses, and treats people with psychological problems or disorders."

A proper analysis of what has been said about the meaning of the term clinical psychology may help us in concluding about the following characteristics of clinical psychology.

- Clinical psychology is a subfield or branch of the larger discipline of psychology. Like all other branches of psychology, it is concerned with the study of human behavior and mental processes, but for this purpose the subjects chosen are the persons suffering from maladjustment, mental illness, and disorders.
- It is mainly concerned with the assessment, diagnosis and treatment of mental illness, and disorders.
- It believes in the use of science and research-based methods and techniques for helping people overcome the distress caused by mental, emotional, and behavioral problems through their proper assessment, diagnosis, and the employment of suitable therapy or treatment measures.
- Clinical psychology represents a unique specialty area within psychology that is found to provide knowledge, understanding, and skills necessary for (i) understanding the abnormality, maladjustment and malfunctioning of people's behavior, (ii) knowing about the possible causes and factors responsible for such behavior, and (iii) suggesting possible treatment and follow up based on such diagnosis.
- Clinical psychology generates research for the etiology of mental illness and disorders, their proper diagnosis, therapeutic measures and their outcomes to optimize the help provided to the individuals concerned. For this purpose, it emphasizes conducting research and using research-based practices on the part of the scholars and practitioners of clinical psychology.
- Clinical psychology is fully devoted to helping individuals in the task of seeking adjustment to the self and their environment, and bringing out necessary changes in their ways of thinking and functioning for solving their mental, emotional, and behavioral problems and helping them to achieve their highest potential.
- Clinical psychology stands for executing its multidimensional functions in the area of mental health including the prevention, control and treatment of mental disorders and illness and adjustment problems prevalent among individuals, families, and communities of a diverse population.
- Clinical psychology has a broad vision of seeking the overall welfare of people belonging to diverse human populations with the purpose of alleviating their psychological distress, disability, dysfunctional and health-risk behavior and promoting their physical, mental, and social well-being as much as possible.
- With the study and practice of clinical psychology, one is benefitted in terms of acquiring a sense of clinical attitude—a sincere passion for helping the people in overcoming their psychological distress.
- Its study, research, and practice aims to equip professionals for their multidimensional services such as providing continuing and comprehensive mental and behavioral healthcare for individuals and families; engaging in research-based practice; providing consultation to agencies and communities; and training, education and supervision in a clinical setup for newcomers.

With this understanding about the meaning and characteristic features of the term clinical psychology we may be now in a position to define clinical psychology as: a specialized branch or field of the discipline psychology helpful in studying the behavior of individuals in a clinical environment and applying research-based psychological theory and practice for the purpose of understanding, diagnosing, preventing, and treating mental, emotional, and behavioral problems and disorders, as well as for promoting overall physical, mental, and social well-being of individuals, families, and communities belonging to a diverse population.

Nature of Clinical Psychology

One question often put forward is "What is the nature of clinical psychology?" The answer is quite straightforward: "The nature of the subject of clinical psychology is sufficiently scientific." The arguments provided by thinkers in this area may be summarized as such:

> ### Clinical Psychology
>
> An applied branch of the subject of psychology related to the study of the behavior of individuals in a clinical setup for the purpose of diagnosing, assessing, and treating their mental health problems and also to help them in their adequate adjustment to achieve their highest potential.

1. Clinical psychology is an applied branch of the subject of psychology. By applying the principles and techniques of psychology, it tries to study the behavior (cognitive, conative, and affective) of individuals in the context of a clinical setup or environment. The work and functioning of the subject of clinical psychology is quite similar to its parent subject, psychology. The only difference is that where in psychology we deal with the behavior of the individuals in general functioning in all walks of life, clinical psychology limits its study to the behavior of individuals in a clinical or medical setup or environment for helping them in overcoming their emotional, mental and behavior problems, abnormalities, illness and disorders, leading to their overall well-being. Hence, in their functioning and purposes both may be seen to carry out the work of a similar nature—the study of behavior. There is no secret that psychology is defined and accepted as the science of behavior, and as a behavioral science its nature is also regarded as sufficiently scientific. If it is so, then, how can we deny the fact that clinical psychology (one of the major components of the subject psychology) is a science, and its nature is scientific?

2. Generally, we accept and include a subject in the category of sciences if it is found (i) to employ the scientific method and approach for its study, (ii) to be capable of describing and explaining the what, why and how of things studied by it, (iii) to predict the future of things or events on the basis of their present status and functioning, and (iv) to challenge and re-verify the results of research.

Let us try to weigh the nature of clinical psychology on the above criterion.

- Clinical psychology employs scientific methods and the scientific approach to study the emotional, mental, and behavioral functioning of individuals, particularly related to their abnormalities, maladjustment, illness or disorders for the purpose of their proper diagnosis, inherent causes, and treatment. See, here, our emphasis on the suffix "scientific"; it is here for distinguishing clinical psychology from other more subjective ways of looking into the behavior and mental processes of the individuals in the context of clinical settings or situations. The clinical psychologists and researchers often, in general, are found to base their research findings on the solid grounds of objective observations and valid studies involving sufficiently scientific approach instead of guesswork, hearsay, vague impressions and armchair theorizing. The methods used in this concern, such as the Experimental method (carried out in clinical laboratory as well as in field settings) and the Naturalistic observation method, allow them to set hypotheses, collect the relevant data, then reach valid conclusions for arriving at one of the set hypotheses, and lastly, place the hypothesis under the hammer of objective validity and reliability. In this way, the approach adopted in the studies conducted in clinical psychology is also found to be sufficiently objective, reliable, and valid, and also found to be true in the repeated similar clinical conditions much like the other disciplines accepted and recognized as sciences. Like sciences, the studies conducted in clinical psychology also help in establishing cause-and-effect relationships, and possess the predictive value as emphasized later.

- Clinical psychology tries to describe and explain the what, when, where, how and why of emotional, mental, and behavioral functioning, particularly related to their maladjustment, abnormalities, illness, and disorders.
- Its ability to carry out the study in experimental conditions by controlling the involved variables, conducting systematic observations in an objective way by using the developed observation devices, and searching for the common features or general trends of behaving and performing on the part of the individuals affected from various types of maladjustment, mental, emotional, and behavioral problems, illness or disorders, may help well in the prediction of the future behavior of afflicted individuals, before and after getting treatment for their problems and ailments.
- The results or findings of the studies carried out in clinical psychology, the rules and principles established, and the theories drawn out of these findings are always open for being re-examined and challenged for the emergence of new rules, principles, and theories at the hands of future researchers. This flexibility and scope for bringing needed change helps clinical psychology to remain scientific in its approach as well as in application, much like the natural sciences.

The contemporary trend in Clinical psychology fully recognizes and accepts the study and application of clinical psychology as a full-fledged scientific discipline. The truth of this trend may be demonstrated by going through the following argument put forward by Richard McFall (1991), professor of psychology at Indiana University, in the following words:

Scientific clinical psychology is the only legitimate and acceptable form of clinical psychology . . . after all, what is the alternative? . . .. Does anyone seriously believe that a reliance on intuition and other unscientific methods is going to hasten advances in knowledge?

McFall (1991: 76–77)

Expanding on the scientific nature of Clinical psychology, specifically with its application in behavior therapy, Truax (2002) explains that "the endeavor of developing and testing hypotheses in the real clinical setting is much like that of a scientist."

In spite of all this, however, we can't term clinical psychology a perfect science. It falls in the category of behavioral sciences and hence has its own limitations. Human behavior—normal or abnormal—is unpredictable. It is highly variable and unreliable. Therefore, clinical psychology, the applied behavioral science, cannot claim objectivity, exactness, and validity as claimed by natural sciences such as physics, chemistry, and biology, or even applied sciences like medicine and engineering.

To Sum Up

The nature of the subject of clinical psychology is considered sufficiently scientific because:

- It is one of the branches or components of the subject psychology being defined as a scientific study of the social behavior of individuals.
- It makes use of scientific methods and approaches to study the social behavior of individuals in clinical situations. Here, we can carry out the study in experimental conditions by controlling the involved variables or conducting the systematic observations in an objective way.
- It is capable of describing and explaining the what, when, where, how, and why of the behavior of people affected by mental, emotional, and behavioral problems.
- Like sciences, the studies conducted in clinical psychology also help in establishing cause-and-effect relationships and possess the predictive value to help in the foretelling of future behavior of individuals affected with emotional, mental, and behavioral problems before and after receiving proper treatment.

Relationship of Clinical Psychology to Other Related Fields or Disciplines

Clinical psychology is an applied branch of psychology that is used for serving clinical purposes, such as assessing, diagnosing, preventing, and treating emotional, mental, and behavioral problems, ailments, and disorders of people with the objective of supporting their improved mental health and overall well-being. Such clinical purposes in their varying forms are also served by other disciplines such as psychiatry, counseling psychology, school psychology, and social work; for this reason these disciplines are also referred to as the disciplines or fields related to clinical psychology. What type of relationship do they have with clinical psychology or in what ways are these related fields or disciplines similar or dissimilar to clinical psychology? Knowledge about this may very well help us in knowing more about the nature of the subject of clinical psychology. Let us venture in this direction.

Clinical Psychology and Psychiatry

Similarities: Clinical Psychology and Psychiatry may be found alike with regard to the following.

1. Psychiatry and clinical psychology are both regarded as scientific disciplines as they both make use of scientific methods for understanding and helping emotionally and intellectually disturbed individuals in overcoming their problems.
2. Both share a common broader goal—helping people live a healthy and well-functioning life.
3. Both are meant to provide education and training for the requisite understanding, assessment, diagnosis, and therapy for mental health disorders.
4. Both advocate for the use of information and guidance of researched sources, such as the DSM-5, to develop a diagnosis for constructing an appropriate treatment plan and offer psychotherapy services for the treatment of the mental illness and disorders.

Dissimilarities: Clinical Psychology differs from Psychiatry in many aspects, as made clear in Table 1.1 as follows.

Table 1.1 Distinction between Psychiatry and Clinical Psychology

Psychiatry	Clinical Psychology
1. Psychiatry is the branch of medicine focused on the diagnosis, treatment, and prevention of mental, emotional, and behavioral problems and disorders.	1. Clinical psychology is an applied branch of the subject of psychology focused on the diagnosis, prevention, and treatment of mental, emotional, and behavioral problems and disorders.
2. Psychiatry is known for its specialty in gaining an understanding how the body—especially the brain and nervous system—affects people's behavior.	2. Clinical psychology also to some extent provides training in understanding how the body—especially the brain—affects behavior, but this is not its specialty.
3. Psychiatry provides a unique insight into mental disorders through the provision of studying brain and central nervous system functioning.	3. On the other hand, Clinical Psychology emphasizes gaining insight into mental disorders through the study of mental processes of the affected people in the context of their behavioral functioning.
4. Psychiatry is known for its specialty in understanding the use of medicines for the treatment of mental illness and disorders and thus enabling professionals to prescribe medicines to patients.	4. Clinical Psychology has no such specialty in its study and training and thereby clinical psychologists in general are not authorized to prescribe medicines for the treatment of mental illness and disorders.
5. In the study of Psychiatry the main emphasis is on knowing and understanding the human body system in terms of its structure and functioning much like the understanding of a machine or hardware in terms of its construction and functioning.	5. In the study of clinical psychology, on the other hand, the emphasis is on understanding individuals in terms of their general behavioral functioning, much like understanding the role of software in terms of input, processing, and output in the human machinery.
6. Psychiatry emphasizes making use of biological and medical lenses and means for the diagnosis and treatment of mental illness and disorders.	6. On the other hand, Clinical psychology emphasizes using psychological lens and means for the diagnosis and treatment of mental illness and disorders.
7. In general, the study and practice in psychiatry does not emphasize psychological testing for assessment of the mental, emotional, and behavioral problems and disorders of their patients.	7. The study and training of clinical psychology is well known for equipping its professionals well in the use of psychological testing for the assessment and diagnosis of mental, emotional, and behavioral problems and disorders of their clients.
8. In general, psychiatry as a medical discipline restricts the use of its theory and practice for providing medical diagnosis and treatment of mental illness and disorders of patients in a hospital and clinical setting.	8. The scope of the theory and practice of clinical Psychology is quite wide. In addition to providing diagnosis and treatment of mental disorders, it prepares professionals for working in a diverse array of settings such as community centers, individual and group counseling services, and generally for people's physical, mental, emotional, and social well-being.
9. The study and training carried out in Psychiatry enables one to provide therapy without a therapy license.	9. The study and training provided in Clinical Psychology cannot by itself equip one for providing therapy. He or she needs to obtain a therapy license before practicing therapy with clients.

Clinical Psychology and Counseling Psychology

Similarities: Clinical Psychology and counseling psychology share a number of common features, as follows.

1. Both represent applied branches of the larger discipline psychology.
2. They make use of similar methods and approaches for conducting research, studying the behavior of individuals, and providing therapies and treatment.
3. Both are aimed to help individuals, families, and communities for resolving the psychology-related problems of their day-to-day life by making use of the theory and practice of psychology.
4. In dealing with the problems of their clients both try to see these problems through psychological and sociological perspectives instead of making use of the medical lenses as happens in the case of Psychiatry.
5. Both try to look after the overall physical, mental, and social well-being of individuals instead of limiting themselves to the task of providing treatment for mental illness and disorders.
6. Study of both disciplines enables the professional to acquire a license for being termed a "licensed psychologist," and as such, to work independently as health care providers.

Dissimilarities: Clinical psychology and Counseling psychology differ in the ways as shown in Table 1.2.

Table 1.2 Distinction between Counseling Psychology and Clinical Psychology

Counseling Psychology	Clinical Psychology
1. True to its name, it is more concerned with helping individuals in the form of counseling them as necessary for the resolution of their problems.	1. Its services are more extensive and not limited to providing advice and suggestions, but rather toward providing a workable clinical solution to their problems.
2. In general, it focuses on helping individuals who have less severe psychological problems —normal people who are experiencing daily life issues in marriage, career choice, studies, work, relations, health and so on.	2. In general, it pertains to resolving the more severe psychological issues of individuals concerning mental, emotional, and behavioral problems and disorders.
3. In terms of carrying out assessment and diagnosis, it is more concerned and focuses on vocational and career assessment of healthy individuals instead of patients suffering from mental illness or disorders.	3. It mainly focuses on the assessment and diagnosis of patients/clients suffering from mental illness and disorders and for this purpose provides proper knowledge and understanding of the different testing and diagnostic devices, including projective techniques.
4. Assessment and diagnosis carried out in counseling psychology does not lead to description of the characteristics of people suffering from mental illness or disorders, and thus not does not help in the development of a classification systems such as the DSM and ICD.	4. Assessment and diagnosis work carried out in clinical psychology has helped much in describing the characteristics of people suffering from mental illness or disorder leading to the development of the classification systems such as the DSM and ICD.

(Continued)

Table 1.2 (Continued)

Counseling Psychology	Clinical Psychology
5. In relation to making use of therapies for dealing with psychological problems, counseling psychology does not equip one with a varied and diversified theoretical orientation and practical training. It usually remains confined to ascribe to humanistic and person-centered theoretical orientations meant for counseling clients.	5. In contrast, clinical psychology tries to equip one for gaining knowledge and practical training in the use of a number of various therapies including psychoanalytic, behavioral, cognitive, humanistic, family and group therapies in a well-balanced and integrated way for treating mild as well as serious types of mental ailments and disorders.
6. Counseling psychology may be seen to rely and lean toward the developmental perspective to focus on the strengths and adaptive strategies of an individual across the life span.	6. Clinical psychology seeks to understand the underlying causes and nature of the mental, emotional, and behavioral problems of individuals for their proper treatment.
7. Counseling psychology equips one to provide his or her services to clients in the form of counseling in various settings, including private practice, but it is usually confined to provide counseling services for the solution of their day-to-day problems instead of providing treatment of mental illness and disorders.	7. Clinical Psychology equips one to provide his or her services to society in a variety of diversified settings, and engage in private practice for providing help, including the meaningful diagnosis and treatment of mental ailments and disorders.

Clinical Psychology and School Psychology

Similarities: Clinical Psychology and School Psychology exhibit similarities in a number of ways, as follows.

1. Clinical and school psychology both represent specialized branches of the broader discipline of Psychology.
2. Both apply the theory and practice of psychology for studying the behavior of individuals in specified environments.
3. Both make use of scientific ways and methods for their study and research work.
4. Both are known to help their clients in overcoming their mental, emotional. and behavioral problems.
5. The knowledge and skills acquired in both disciplines help professionals to assess, diagnose, and build and implement treatment plans for helping clients overcome their problems.
6. The study and skills acquired in both disciplines make their professionals eligible for earning licenses to practice.

Dissimilarities: Clinical psychology, while having a lot of similarities with School Psychology, is found to be dissimilar in a number of ways as discussed in Table 1.3.

Clinical Psychology and Social Work

Many of us choose the discipline known as social work for our study (by earning degrees like master of social work—MSW) toward a career in social services. It bears a number of similarities and dissimilarities with clinical psychology, as demonstrated next.

Table 1.3 Distinction between School Psychology and Clinical Psychology

School Psychology	*Clinical Psychology*
1. In school psychology we study the behavior of individuals in relation to the school situation or environment.	1. In clinical psychology we study the behavior of individuals in relation to the clinical setup or environment.
2. School psychology represents a specialty or applied branch of the discipline of psychology enabling professionals to combine their knowledge of education and psychology principles to deal with school-related issues relating to children, families, parents, school organizations, and teachers.	2. Clinical psychology represents a specialty or applied branch of the discipline of psychology enabling professionals to apply the theory and practice of psychology for dealing with a variety of mental, emotional, and behavioral problems and disorders of a wide range of individuals, groups, families, and communities.
3. The study and training provided in the discipline of school psychology is limited in its dealing with the problems of school-aged children and school-related issues, and does not concern itself much with long term therapy and psychopathology as done by clinical psychology. Its main focus is to enable professional to address behavioral and learning concerns of children in school.	3. The study and training provided in the discipline of clinical psychology equips one to assess, diagnose, and treat a wide range of mental, emotional, and behavioral problems and disorders of individuals of all ages aiming toward their overall well-being. In this way, the scope and field of operation of clinical psychology is quite diversified.
4. The study and training in school psychology includes the topics related to the streams of education, school organization, special education, instructional methods, and classroom management helpful in dealing with school-aged children and school-related issues.	4. The study and training in clinical psychology may vary depending on the provision of specialty earned, but it rarely includes topics related to the streams of education, school organization, special education, instructional methods, and classroom management.
5. The use and application of school psychology, true to its name, is very much confined to take care of the mental health and well-being of school-aged children.	5. The study and training in clinical psychology may equip professionals to address a broad range of mental, emotional and behavioral problems and disorders for patients of all ages.
6. Like clinical psychology, the study and training in school psychology also enables professionals to develop treatment plans for helping clients in getting rid of their problems; however, limited to their learning and school-related issues.	6. The study and training of clinical psychologists equips its professionals to develop treatment plans that include assessment, diagnosis, and treatments for a wide range of problems and disorders.
7. The study and training provided in school psychology may enable one to work as a licensed psychologist after getting a postgraduate degree in psychology or in the specialization of school psychology within the discipline of clinical psychology. Contrary to clinical psychologists, however, they are not authorized to prescribe medications to their clients.	7. The study and training in clinical psychology requires prospective professionals to earn a doctoral degree in a relevant field of clinical psychology for working as a licensed psychologist. At some places, they are authorized to prescribe medications to their clients.

Similarities

1. Social work and Clinical psychology are both designated and termed as Behavioral Sciences.
2. Both provide us the necessary knowledge and skills needed to help people deal with problems that interfere with their day-to-day life activities.
3. The minimum degree of prescribed qualification is required by professionals of both disciplines for doing their jobs.

Dissimilarities: Clinical psychology may be seen do differ with the discipline of Social Work in the manner as discussed in Table 1.4.

Table 1.4 Distinction between Social Work and Clinical Psychology

Social Work	Clinical Psychology
1. The study and training provided in the discipline of social work may enable the social worker to help people with direct services and assist clients in solving problems interfering with their day-to-day life such as legal issues, human rights or poverty and their mental, behavioral or emotional malfunctioning.	1. The study and training provided in clinical psychology does not aim to equip its professionals to provide their services in dealing with such daily life problems of clients. It is limited to the diagnosis and treatment of mental illness and disorders.
2. The study and training in social work enables professionals to help individuals, families, communities, and society as a whole in overcoming their daily social problems and improving their quality of life.	2. The study and training in clinical psychology may also equip professionals to work with individuals experiencing difficulties in their lives, but typically in doing so they work one-on-one with individuals rather than families or other community groups.
3. The study and training in social work equips social workers to be employed or provide their services in a wide and diversified settings such as community centers, public health services, schools, business centers, industrial establishments, rehabilitation centers, nursing homes, prisons, and government agencies.	3. The study and training in clinical psychology aims to equip professionals to practice and offer their services limited to work in the clinical setting for dealing with the mental, emotional, and behavioral problems and disorders of the clients/patients.
4. Social workers are found to be easily approachable and accessible to the community people in dealing with their day-to-day problems including their mental health, illness, and disorders. They assist problem-ridden people by referring them to clinical psychologists and working with clinical psychologists and family members for the proper diagnosis, assessment, prevention, and treatment of mental illness and disorders.	4. Clinical Psychologists are not so much mixed with and accessible to the community as happens in the case of social workers. It is a relatively costly and more effortful affair in comparison to interaction and consultation with social workers. Clinical psychologists are approached by people for overcoming problems typically related to their mental illness and disorders for the needed diagnosis and treatment.
5. The individuals who wish to study and join courses related to the discipline of social work for adopting the profession as a social worker must earn a degree of Master of Social Work (MSW) to be eligible.	5. The path to get a practicing license to work as a clinical psychologist is arduous in comparison to becoming a social worker. Here in India, one must earn an M Phil degree in clinical psychology after doing postgraduate work in psychology/clinical psychology accompanied with rigorous practical experience and training to earn the desired license.

To Sum Up

Regarding the relationship existing between clinical psychology and some other disciplines like psychiatry, counseling psychology, school psychology, and social work, it may be seen that all of them bear resemblance with clinical psychology in respect to their serving clinical purposes. However, in doing so, they differ a lot from clinical psychology in their nature and functioning in a variety of ways, such as:

Psychiatry (a branch of medicine) differs from clinical psychology (an applied branch of the subject psychology) in respect to using biological and medical lenses for the diagnosis and treatment of mental disorders instead of psychological means and methods utilized in clinical psychology.

The task of counseling psychology is confined to providing counseling services to the needy for the solution of their daily life issues including less severe psychological problems. It does not equip one to have specialization in the diagnosis and treatment of severe psychological problems.

The task of school psychology is confined to providing solutions to problems related to teaching-learning and school education, including care of the mental health of the concerned persons. It does not equip one with the skills for the diagnosis and treatment of mental disorders.

The discipline of social work has a wide social responsibility in comparison to clinical psychology in terms of equipping social workers to provide their services directly to the community in assisting people with their day-to-day life problems and working as an easily accessible caretaker for seeking ease of their mental health issues with clinical psychologists.

The Scope of Clinical Psychology

The scope of a subject, in general, may be stated and described by pointing out (i) What is studied or what type of topics and contents are included in the study of that subject, and (ii) What is its field of operation and application, or for what use its study can be put to clients? Let us try to analyze and discuss the scope of clinical psychology from these angles one by one.

What is Included in the Study of Clinical Psychology?

Clinical psychology, in all its ways and means, forms and shapes, purposes and objectives, stands for studying and explaining the behavior of individuals in the context of clinical situations for helping them in overcoming their mental, emotional, and behavioral problems and disorders with a broad objective of working toward their overall well-being.

As a result, its study must include the topics helpful in dealing with its nature and the what, how, when, where and why of the things needed for improving mental health as well as the overall well-being of individuals, including care for their physical, emotional, personal, social, and professional well-being. Consequently, the following topics and study material are generally included in the study of the discipline of clinical psychology:

• Discussion and clarity about the meaning and concept of clinical psychology as an applied branch of the broader discipline psychology.

- The nature of clinical psychology as a scientific discipline and its relationship with the other related branches of applied psychology as well as other disciplines and related fields such as psychiatry, counseling psychology, school psychology, and social work.
- Preparations of professionals in clinical psychology regarding performing various duties and providing various types of services in their world of work, their jobs, the nature of their duties, the types of training provided, and the competencies expected from them for working as a licensed clinical psychologist.
- Developments in the field of clinical psychology, especially with respect to new research findings, methods of study, and clinical practices.
- The methods used for conducting studies and research work in clinical psychology addressing various issues related to the development of its theory and practice such as the experimental method, correlation method, field study and survey method, naturalistic observation method, case study method, and so on.
- The concepts of mental health and hygiene and the distinction between what is termed good and poor mental health.
- Knowledge of the concepts of normality and abnormality of human behavior and different criteria for its description.
- Knowledge of the concepts of mental illness and mental disorders, including their etiology or inherent causes for their occurrence.
- Discussion of classification systems available in the form of the DSM and ICD developed by the American Psychiatric Association (APA) and the World Health Organization (WHO).
- Discussion of the major disorders with respect to their meaning and concept, types, etiology (causes of their occurrence), diagnosis, prevention, and treatment, with special reference to psycho-physical disorders, psychoneurotic disorders (neurosis), Psychotic disorders (psychoses), Neurodevelopmental disorders, Disruptive, Impulsive control and Conduct disorders, Substance-related and Addictive disorders, Sexual deviations and disorders, Elimination and Eating disorders, Sleep disorders, Old age or degenerative disorders, and so on.
- Discussion about Clinical assessment—the ways and means of conducting assessment and diagnosis of the prevalence of specific mental illness or disorder among clients/patients with special reference to the use of psychological tests such as intelligence tests and personality assessment tests as well as techniques including the standardized personality inventories and projective techniques, anxiety and depressive scales, clinical interviews, neurological testing, and so on.
- Discussion about the treatment and cure of mental illness and disorders in the form of preparing and implementing treatment plans with the use of various psychotherapies based on suitable therapeutic approaches such as psychodynamic therapies, behavior therapies, cognitive or cognitive-behavioral therapies, humanistic therapies, family and group therapies, and so on.
- Discussion about the clinical rehabilitation of patients by adopting suitable measures such as at-home care and clinical advice, environmental modification by enlisting the cooperation of family and community members, seeking proper social, vocational, and professional rehabilitation, and so on.

Specializations Available for Students in Clinical Psychology

Besides gaining expertise on topics and contents related to the subject of clinical psychology, students may also get opportunity to opt to study specializations such as the following:

Forensic Psychology

Defined by the American Psychological association (APA), Forensic psychology as a specialization in clinical psychology stands for "the application of clinical specialties to the legal arena." Here, attempts are made to make use of psychological knowledge and methods for answering legal questions arising in civil or criminal proceedings. The knowledge and skills gained through its study equips students to become a forensic psychologist professional for working as practicing witnesses in court cases involving criminal insanity pleas, child custody, and discrimination issues.

Clinical Child Psychology

Clinical child psychology represents a specialty in clinical psychology that provides knowledge and skills related to the assessment, diagnosis, and treatment of the mental health issues of infants, toddlers, children, and adolescents. Its subject matter is based on a sound understanding of the principles of developmental psychology and the biological, psychological, and social problems faced by the younger generations.

Health Psychology

Health psychology as a specialty in the field of clinical psychology focuses on promoting people's health as well as the prevention and treatment of their disease and illness—physical as well as mental. It considers one's mental health and physical health to be highly related and thereby lays due emphasis on adopting a healthier and more positive lifestyle for overall well-being. For this purpose, it tries to apply the knowledge and principles of psychology for bringing needed modification in ways of thinking, feeling, and behaving. The knowledge and understanding acquired on the part of the health psychologist professionals help them in better understanding health and illness, studying the psychological factors that impact the health of the people, and contributing to the healthcare system and health policy of the state/country.

Clinical Neuropsychology

Clinical neuropsychology represents a specialty of Clinical Psychology that is based on the relationship between the brain and behavior. The knowledge and skills gained in the field of Clinical neuropsychology help the professionals understand the relationships between brain and behavior, particularly in reference to the application of these relationships to the diagnosis of brain disorders, assessment of cognitive and behavioral functioning, and the design of effective treatment plans for the affected individuals. Since the malfunctioning of one's neurological organs, particularly the brain, is found to cause a number of neurological disorders and dysfunction of the cognitive functioning of the affected individuals, the clinical neuropsychologist professionals may be found most often to assist clients with traumatic brain injuries, tumors, dementia and other problems hindering their normal cognitive functioning.

Clinical Geropsychology

Clinical Geropsychology is a specialty of Clinical Psychology, the knowledge and understanding of which helps professionals gain competency in knowing and understanding the needs and problems of older persons, and help them in dealing with these problems and consequential ailments and disorders. In essence, it caters to the needed task of assisting elders and their families to cope with their age-related ailments and disorders, end-of-life decisions, loss of independence, and self-care with the purpose of helping them in achieving their maximum potential for overall well-being.

The Use and Applications of Clinical Psychology

Another way to describe the scope of the subject of clinical psychology centers around the discussion and description of its field of operation and applications; the uses for which its study can be put. Let us analyze and discuss the scope of clinical psychology from this very angle. In this concern, we may find that the knowledge and skills acquired and attitudes formed through the study of clinical psychology may be applied to serve various causes, as discussed next.

1. Applications in the Field of Mental Health and Illness

Clinical psychology is well known for serving a great purpose in the field of mental health and illness. Its main contributions in this concern may be outlined as follows:

- Helping in the study of the behavior of individuals in a clinical setting or environment in a scientific way by availing the necessary means, methods, and tools on this account.
- Acquainting us with the concepts of normality and abnormality of human behavior.
- Building knowledge and understanding of the etiology of human abnormal behavior, maladjustment, and mental health problems.
- Acquainting us with the concept of mental health and hygiene and their significance in our lives.
- Providing continuous help in the development of standardized classification systems such as DSMs and ICDs; describing their unique characteristics, features, and symptoms for the purpose of their proper identification and diagnosis at the hands of clinical practitioners.
- Helping clinical psychologists and other practitioners in their job of diagnosing and treating people affected by mental illness and disorders by equipping them with the abilities and skills needed for

  ◦ Performing various types of assessment tasks related to their intellectual and achievement potential, personality traits and make-up, state/scale of their anxiety, stress and frustration, the status of their adjustment to self and environment, and so on.
  ◦ Holding Diagnostic interviews and seeking case history of the problems affecting the patient, their family members, and friends.
  ◦ Making diagnosis and drawing a picture of the problems and disorders faced by the patient/client.
  ◦ Considering therapies/psychological treatments for helping the patient/client in overcoming their affliction.
  ◦ Chalking out a treatment plan and working toward its implementation by skillfully applying therapeutic techniques and seeking cooperation of the patient and family members.
  ◦ Evaluating the outcomes of treatment efforts and making decisions regarding its continuance or modification as needed in the situation.

2. Applications in Terms of Performing the Task of Overall Well-Being

The scope of clinical psychology in terms of its utilization is widened when we see that it not only concerns mental health and illness, but goes much beyond that by caring for people's overall happiness and well-being, involving the physical, emotional, social, and aspects of their living. Let us explore how this happens.

- There exists an inseparable relationship between one's body and mind—the physiological and mental aspects of one's well-being. Therefore, the looking after of mental aspects by clinical psychology, thus keeping one mentally healthy, contributes toward one's physical wellness. Clinical psychology, thus, may well stand for providing the needed mental strength for the physical well-being of individuals.
- There is also a close link between one's emotional and mental health. The development of emotions as well as their appropriate expression is governed by one's cognitive health, and cared for through the knowledge, skills, and attitudes acquired through the study and practice of clinical psychology.
- What happens in our personal, social, and professional life in terms of our adjustment and maladjustment is also governed by the state of our mental health and well-being, and there is no denying of the fact that services of clinical psychology are well availed for to support one's proper adjustment and well-being.

3. Applications in the Field of Community and Social Services

There are multiple avenues available in communities and societies for looking after well-being, such as community centers, welfare societies, NGOs and social workers. In addition to helping people with their problems, the persons belonging to the field of clinical psychology also do a great service in the prevention of maladjustment, mental illness, and disorders among the community due to reasons including the effects of natural calamities, accidents, violence, terrorism, and war by collaborating with the efforts of government, social workers, and volunteers.

4. Applications in the Field of Guidance and Counseling

There are occasions where help is sought by people in seeking guidance and counseling from others capable of steering them toward well-being. The work for this purpose is conducted by guidance and counseling personnel, professional counselors, family and marriage counselors, and counseling psychologists. In doing their job, they may more often need the services of the clinical psychology personnel, especially in connection with mental illness and disorders, and often refer these cases for the necessary consultation with professional clinical psychologists. Additionally, they may seek collaboration and assistance from practitioners of clinical psychology for understanding the underlying problems of their clients for counseling them properly. There is no denying the fact that clinical personnel are well equipped with the training of studying and practicing clinical psychology to provide such counseling assistance.

5. Applications in the Field of Business and Industries

The field of industry also benefits immensely through the services provided by clinical psychology personnel, and this is why businesses are increasingly enlisting such personnel as consultants for supporting the mental health and professional adjustment of their managerial and working staff. We may know very well that like other fields of life, the business and industrial world is also very much engulfed with tensions, conflicts, mutual rivalries, unhealthy competitions, frustrations, stresses, and turmoil, giving rise to mental illness or issues in the workforce. Unless resolved satisfactorily, these may prove quite costly—not only to individual victims, but also to the overall functioning and future of the whole establishment. The understanding and applications of the theory and practice of clinical psychology can well serve the purpose in this situation.

6. Applications in the Field of School Education and University Teaching

Clinical psychology also shows its usefulness in the field of school education and university teaching. Let us first consider school education. For managing the psychological concerns of school organization and management, including the welfare of students and staff, it is not unusual on the part of school authorities to enlist the services of school psychologists. When school psychologists are faced with issues concerning complex mental health issues, they seek collaboration or assistance from the clinical psychology personnel equipped with the knowledge and skills of the discipline.

Another area in which the services of personnel equipped with the knowledge, skills, and practice of clinical psychology is very much needed is in working as faculty members for the teaching and training of students at the graduate and postgraduate departments of colleges and universities. Such training of prospective candidates is essential for serving the cause of the discipline in terms of its existence, development, and transmission. The scope of clinical psychology is thus extended to providing its services in the teaching and training of future clinical psychologists.

7. Applications in the Field of Research and Innovations

Study and training in clinical psychology equips students, trainees, and practicing clinical psychology personnel with the methods, tools, and techniques for conducting useful research in the field of clinical psychology for the development of its theory and practice related to the assessment, diagnosis, prevention, and treatment of the mental, emotional, and behavioral issues affecting mental health and causing mental and behavioral disorders among individuals.

8. Applications in the Field of Crime and Legality

The field of clinical psychology involves forensic psychology as one of its specializations, the knowledge and understanding of which has an immense utility for providing testimony in a court of law in cases involving criminal insanity pleas, child custody, and discrimination issues. In pleas of criminality insanity, the convicted take a plea that they have not committed the criminal act with their full consciousness; they are mentally disturbed persons. The court in such cases requires a proper testimony of their mental state from a certified and licensed clinical psychologist. In this way, the knowledge and understanding reached through the study of clinical psychology may prove its worth in various unique ways in the field of crime and legality.

9. Applications in the Field and Areas of Rehabilitation

Upon getting treatment for their problem, clients/patients require proper rehabilitation—adjusting and going back to their normal life. Clinical psychology also plays a substantial role here, as follows:

- Clinical psychology personnel may provide their services outside the clinic by visiting community rehabilitation centers for clients recovering from addiction, and centers supporting people with intellectual disabilities, ADHD, autism, conduct and impulsive disorders, sexual perversion, and neurobiological impairments.

- They can provide their services to discharged patients at homes/residences for providing needed aftercare, guiding family members and caretakers, and instructing them about the precautions necessary to prevent incidences known to trigger their mental, emotional, or behavioral problems.
- They collaborate with counselors, social workers, and NGOs for support in the patient's occupational/vocational rehabilitation, personal, social, and community life, and adjustment and adaptation to normal living.

In this way, it may be seen that the scope of clinical psychology in terms of its breadth of material as well as its uses and applications is quite wide and extensive. It does not limit itself to the task of assessing, diagnosing, preventing, and treating mental illness and disorders, but goes quite beyond that, encircling all aspects of our functioning—physical, mental, emotional, social, and moral—supporting overall happiness and well-being across the life span in varying cultures and at all socioeconomic levels.

To Sum Up

We can discuss the scope of the subject of clinical psychology in two ways: by pointing out what is studied here in terms of the topics and contents (including the specializations available in the field of clinical psychology), and by stating its uses and applications in our day-to-day life. Such a discussion demonstrates that the scope of clinical psychology is quite wide. It studies and explains all that is needed for supporting mental health and preventing and treating mental illness and disorders.

Review Questions

1. What is clinical psychology? Discuss its meaning and nature.
2. Define the term clinical psychology and throw light on its nature.
3. To what extent may we term the nature of clinical psychology scientific? Discuss.
4. What do you understand about the scope of the subject of clinical psychology?
5. Generally, what must be included in terms of contents and subject matter in the study of clinical psychology?
6. Name and discuss some of the important specializations available to students in the discipline of clinical psychology.
7. Discuss its scope in relation to its uses and applications in day-to-day life.

References

American Psychological Association (2012), About clinical psychology, retrieved from http://www.apa.org/div12/aboutcp.html

Korchin, S. J. (1986), *Modern clinical psychology: Principles of intervention in the clinic and community*, New Delhi: CBS Publishers & Distributors.

McFall, R. M. (1991), Manifesto for a science of clinical psychology, *Clinical Psychologist*, 44: 75–88.

Myers, D. G. (2013), *Psychology* (10th ed.), New York, NY: Worth.

Sexton, V. S., & Hogan, J. D. (Eds.), (1992), *International psychology: Views from around the world*, Lincoln, NE: University of Nebraska Press.

Truax, P. (2002), Behavioral case conceptualization for adults, In M. Hersen (Ed.), *Clinical behavior therapy: Adults and children* (pp. 3–36), New York, NY: John Wiley & Sons Inc.

References (On line)

1. Collins Dictionary, Definition of clinical psychology, retrieved from www.collinsdictionary.com/dictionary/english/clinical-psychology

2. *Merriam-Webster.com Dictionary*, Merriam-Webster, definition of clinical psychology, retrieved from www.merriam-webster.com/dictionary/clinical%20psychology

3. Encyclopedia, Britannica, Definition of clinical psychology, retrieved from www.britannica.com/science/clinical-psychology

4. N., Sam M. S., Definition of clinical psychology, retrieved from https://psychologydictionary.org/clinical-psychology/

5. Canadian Psychological Association, Definition of clinical psychology, retrieved from https://cpa.ca/docs/File/Sections/Clinical%20section/What%20is%20Clinical%20Psychology.pd

6. American Psychological Association, Definition of clinical psychology, retrieved from www.apa.org/ed/graduate/specialize/clinical

Chapter 2

Clinical Psychologists—Functions and Training

Learning Objectives

After going through this chapter, you will be able to:
- Define the term clinical psychologist.
- Discuss where clinical psychologists work.
- Discuss in what aspects clinical psychologists differ from other mental health professionals.
- Distinguish and differentiate clinical psychologists from psychiatrists, counseling psychologists, school psychologists, and social workers.
- Name some activities done and functions performed by clinical psychologists.
- Throw light on the procedure involved in the education and training of clinical psychologist professionals in our country.
- Discuss the education and training of prospective clinical psychologists in the United States and United Kingdom.
- State how to become a licensed clinical psychologist in India.

Who are Clinical Psychologists?

In its simple meaning, we may think of clinical psychologists as professionals who make use of the theory and practice of clinical psychology in conducting their professional activities. Let us learn more about the term clinical psychologist with the help of its meaning in the dictionary.

According to the Merriam Webster Dictionary (Online), the term Clinical psychologist is used for "a licensed psychologist with an advanced degree who assesses, diagnoses, and treats mental, emotional, and behavioral Issues."[1]

According to another popular English Dictionary, The American Heritage Dictionary (2016), a clinical psychologist is "a person who is trained and licensed to diagnose and treat people with mental disorders."

These definitions highlight the following characteristic features of clinical psychology professionals:

- To become a clinical psychology professional, one must (i) obtain a required degree by going through a course comprising theory and practice of clinical psychology, and (ii) get the license by fulfilling the requirements of a license providing authority.
- As a professional, a clinical psychologist's task is to assess, diagnose, and treat the mental, emotional, and behavioral issues or disorders of their clients/patients.

DOI: 10.4324/9781003398325-2

However, the tasks performed and services provided by clinical psychologist professionals cannot be limited to such a narrow extent as diagnosing and treating the mental, emotional, and behavioral problems or disorders. We have seen in the previous chapter that the scope of clinical psychology in terms of its uses and applications is quite extensive and wide. Its study and

> **Clinical Psychologists**
>
> Properly qualified and licensed health professionals possessing the required competency for the assessment, diagnosis, and psychological treatment of mental illness and disorders with a broader view of assisting clients/patients to improve overall well-being in their lives.

training equip individuals to play a diversified role in terms of executing many functions and providing various services to people of all ages and cultures in helping them improve their well-being in all aspects of life and work, by taking due care of mental health, illness, and disorders.

Consequently, we may term clinical psychologists as *the properly qualified and licensed health professionals who are equipped with sufficient knowledge of the theory and practice of clinical psychology for the assessment, diagnosis, and psychological treatment of mental, behavioral, and emotional issues or disorders of clients/patients with a broader view supporting their overall adjustment, happiness and well-being in their personal, social, and professional lives.*

Where Do Clinical Psychologists Work?

The knowledge and understanding reached, skills acquired, and attitudes formed in the study and training of clinical psychology make clinical psychologist professionals capable of providing their services in a wide variety of settings. In our country, their services are of use in the settings listed as follows:

- Medical hospitals and institutes, both General and psychiatric, run by Governments—local, state and central—including the military, railway hospitals, and so on.
- Medical hospitals and clinics, both General and psychiatric, run by private individuals and organizations.
- As teaching and research faculty in Colleges, Universities and other institutions of higher learning running departments of clinical psychology.
- Community mental health centers run by the NGOs and community welfare agencies.
- Diverse mental health settings such as Substance abuse centers, Prisons, Juvenile remand homes, or working with mentally or physically disabled and geriatric patients.
- Engaging in private practice in their own clinics or providing at-home services.
- Providing consultancy services to various government and private businesses and organizations.
- Collaborating and assisting other mental health professionals, such as psychiatrists, counseling psychologists, marriage and family counselors, school psychologists, sports psychologists, and social workers.
- Serving the courts in assessing defendants and potential parolees.
- Serving volunteer agencies and organizations supporting the victims of natural and manmade disasters and violence.

To Sum Up

Clinical psychologists have job opportunities in a wide variety of settings such as medical hospitals, institutes and clinics, teaching and research faculties of colleges and universities, prisons and juvenile remand homes, serving in community centers and the projects run by voluntary agencies, private practice in their own clinics, providing home-care to the mentally ill and disabled, assisting psychiatrists and other mental health professionals, working as consultants, and serving the courts as witnesses of mentally ill convicts.

Aspects in which Clinical Psychologists Differ from Other Mental Health Professionals

There are other mental health professionals like psychiatrists, counseling psychologists, school psychologists, and social workers whose work and status overlap with those of clinical psychologist professionals. Specifically in this regard, we may notice that each of these professionals contribute toward the preservation and promotion of mental health and well-being. For avoiding the underlying confusion, it therefore becomes important on our part to know in what aspects clinical psychologists differ from other mental health professionals. Let us proceed in this direction.

Distinguishing Clinical Psychologists from Psychiatrists

Clinical psychologists differ from Psychiatrists in the manner shown in Table 2.1.

Table 2.1 Distinction between Psychiatrists and Clinical Psychologists

Psychiatrists	Clinical Psychologists
1. Psychiatrists are medical doctors who complete studies in medical colleges. As well as their specialization in psychiatry, they are primarily trained as Physicians. They are licensed as physicians and are well authorized to prescribe medication to their patients.	1. Clinical psychologists are not medical doctors; they are psychologists/counselors and study in colleges and universities. They are licensed as clinical psychologists for dealing with the mental health problems of their clients and in general are not authorized to prescribe medication to their clients.
2. Psychiatry training emphasizes biology to such an extent that they tend to view mild to severe abnormalities and mental disorders as the outcome of physiological abnormalities of the brain. Psychiatrists tend to prescribe medication, or use measures such as electroconvulsive therapy or brain surgery. This does not mean that psychiatrists do not first use other means of treatment. They certainly respect and resort to other means of treatment, such as psychotherapy and counseling, but they favor and generally prefer to make use of biological and medical lenses and means for the diagnosis and treatment of mental illness and disorders.	2. Clinical psychology training also certainly appreciates the biological aspects of their clients' problems, but it does not orient them to view and address them through physiological correction. Instead, it lays stress on viewing their mental health problems as behavioral, cognitive, emotional, and employs the psychological lens and means for the diagnosis and treatment of mental illness and disorders. Accordingly, the practicing clinical psychologist are very much required to gain proficiency in making use of various types of psychological testing, assessment and diagnostic devices as well as psychotherapies.

Distinguishing Clinical Psychologists from Counseling Psychologists

Clinical Psychologists differ from counseling psychologists in the manner discussed in Table 2.2.

Distinguishing Clinical Psychologists from School Psychologists

Clinical psychologists differ from School psychologists in the ways discussed in Table 2.3.

Distinguishing Clinical Psychologists from Social Workers

Clinical psychologists are found to differ from social workers in the manner as discussed in Table 2.4.

Table 2.2 Distinction between Counseling Psychologists and Clinical Psychologists

Counseling Psychologists	Clinical Psychologists
1. The main task and function of counseling psychologists is to counsel individuals as needed to help them in the resolution of their problems.	1. The main task and function of the clinical psychologists is to provide suitable therapy for treating mental illness or problems.
2. Counseling psychologists are more likely to work with or counsel less pathological clients.	2. Clinical psychologists are more likely to work with seriously disturbed individuals.
3. On account of their working with less seriously disturbed individuals, counseling psychologists tend to work and complete internships in university counseling centers and working in the community.	3. On account of their working with more seriously disturbed individuals, clinical psychologists tend to work and complete internships more often in settings such as hospitals and inpatient psychiatric units.
4. In dealing with their clients, counseling psychologists tend to endorse soft approaches (humanistic and client-centered) more than do clinical psychologists.	4. Clinical psychologists tend to endorse behaviorism more strongly than do counseling psychologists.
5. Counseling psychologists are equipped to provide their services to clients in the form of counseling at various settings, but they are usually confined to provide counseling services for the solution of their day-to-day problems instead of providing treatment of mental illness and disorders.	5. Clinical psychology equips one to provide his or her services to society in various diversified settings as well as private practice for providing help to clients/patients, including the meaningful diagnosis and treatment of mental ailments and disorders.
6. Counseling psychologists tend to be more interested in vocational testing and career counseling.	6. Clinical psychologists tend to be more interested in applications of principles of psychology to medical settings—seeking treatment for mental health problems.

Table 2.3 Distinction between School Psychologists and Clinical Psychologists

School Psychologists	Clinical Psychologists
1. To become a school psychologist one must earn a postgraduate degree in psychology with a specialization in School psychology. In some cases, they must obtain an MPhil or PhD degree to become a licensed school psychologist.	1. To become a licensed clinical psychologist, one must earn an MPhil or PhD degree in Clinical psychology after having completed a postgraduate degree in Psychology or Clinical Psychology, along with internship experience.
2. The task of school psychologists is limited in its dealing with the problems of school-aged children and school-related issues and does not concern itself with long-term therapy and psychopathology, unlike clinical psychologists. Its focus is to address behavioral and learning concerns of children in schools.	2. The task of clinical psychologists encircles a wide and diversified area, including the assessment, diagnosis, and treatment of various mental, emotional, and behavioral problems and disorders of individuals of all ages aiming toward their overall well-being.
3. School psychologists usually work in schools, and in settings such as daycare centers or correctional facilities, with the primary objective of helping students in their needed adjustment, learning, and overall development. Additionally, they provide help to school personnel in the organization and management of school affairs.	3. Clinical psychologists work in a wide variety of settings including hospitals and private clinics, community health centers, business establishments, and other organizations for providing care, counseling, and therapeutic treatments to problems associated with mental health.
4. The primary function of school psychologists is to enhance the intellectual, emotional, social, and developmental lives of students.	4. The primary function of the clinical psychologist is to provide psychological therapy or treatment for helping individuals with their mental health issues.
5. On account of their concern for the learning and developmental needs of the students, school psychologists engage in psychological testing such as conducting intelligence and achievement tests and Administrating specialized tests, scales and inventories to diagnose mental deficiency, learning disorders, emotional disturbances and ADHD among students, and then adopt suitable measures for helping them.	5. Clinical psychologists are not confined to the learning and developmental issues of students. They engage in psychological testing and assessment work for the diagnosis of a wide variety of mental, emotional, and behavioral problems and disorders of people of all ages living and working in diverse social and cultural settings.

Table 2.4 Distinction between Social Workers and Clinical Psychologists

Social Workers	Clinical Psychologists
1. For being eligible to work as a professional social worker, in our country one must earn a postgraduate degree in social work, known as a Master's of Social Work (MSW).	1. For working as a licensed clinical psychologist in our country one must earn an MPhil degree in clinical psychology after doing postgraduate work in psychology/ clinical psychology.

(Continued)

Table 2.4 (Continued)

Social Workers	Clinical Psychologists
2. Social workers have easy access to the people in a community for rendering direct help and assisting them in solving the problems interfering with their day-to-day life such as legal issues, human rights, poverty, and their mental, behavioral, or emotional malfunctioning.	2. Clinical psychologists are not easily accessible as they do not get so much mixed with the community people. They do not help them directly as happens in the case of social workers in their day-to-day life problems and are approached by the people only for getting rid of the problems typically related to their mental illness and disorders.
3. Social workers help their clients by connecting them with social services, such as welfare agencies, disability offices, or job-training sites (Fossum et al., 2016).	3. Clinical psychologists rarely engage in practices such as social services; they are professionals conducting their own practices.
4. Social workers provide their services in a diversified setup such as community centers, public health services, schools, business centers, industrial establishments, rehabilitation centers, nursing homes, prisons, and government agencies.	4. Clinical psychologists limit their services to the clinical setting for helping clients care for their mental, emotional, and behavioral problems and disorders.
5. The education and training of social workers is quite different from that of clinical psychologists. It lays more emphasis on rendering direct help to people through social service or community welfare means, and includes very little on research methods, psychological testing, physiological psychology, and psychotherapies.	5. The education and training of clinical psychologists are specialized and rigorous, enabling them to execute their functions related to the research, assessment, diagnosis, and treatment of mental illness and disorders. It necessarily includes the contents related to research methods, psychological testing, physiotherapy, and physiological psychology.

To Sum Up

The work of professionals such as psychiatrists, counseling psychologists, school psychologists, and social workers overlaps with the work of clinical psychologists in respect to their contribution toward the preservation and promotion of mental health and well-being. However, they differ from clinical psychologists various ways.

Psychiatrists are trained as medical doctors and thus make use of biological and medical lenses and means for the diagnosis and treatment of mental illness and disorders, in comparison to the psychological means and methods preferred by clinical psychologists.

The work done by counseling psychologists in providing mental health services is limited to counseling people in terms of the solution of their day-to-day life problems or mental health issues of a less severe nature. They can only assist clinical psychologists if enlisted to, rather than providing treatment of mental illness and disorders on their own.

The task of school psychologists in providing mental health services is limited in its dealing with the problems of school-related issues affecting the adjustment and mental health of children. Their main function is to address behavioral and learning concerns, instead of providing long term therapy and psychopathology, as done by clinical psychologists.

Social workers, who have easy access to the general public, render direct help to the community as a whole in their mental health issues through social service and community welfare means. However, in doing so their work is limited to that of a mediator between patients and clinical psychologists, or providing necessary support to the mentally ill, rather than providing diagnosis and treatment to the affected individuals, as done on the part of clinical psychologists.

The Functions Performed by Clinical Psychologists

The range of functions performed by clinical psychologists across varied employment and working sites are quite diversified, as demonstrated next.

1. Carrying Out the Task of Assessment and Diagnosis

The main work expected of a clinical psychologist is to support treatment for mental health problems or disorders. The adoption of any treatment measure requires a preliminary assessment and diagnosis toward the following objectives:

- To identify the exact nature and kind of mental health problem or disorder experienced by the client.
- To evaluate the client's potential and capabilities (e.g., intelligence and cognitive functioning, personality, achievement level, interests, attitudes and level of adjustment, anxiety, depression, frustration. etc.) for diagnosing a particular mental health problem or disorder.
- To gather information relevant to planning therapeutic measures.

> **The Functions performed by Clinical psychologists**
>
> - Assessment and diagnosis of mental illness and disorders
> - Treatment of mental illness and disorders
> - Teaching and training
> - Research and writing work
> - Providing consultancy services
> - Assisting and collaborating with other mental health professionals
> - Performing supervisory and administrative duties
> - Participating in clinical conferences.

In gathering necessary information about the client's problem and disorder as well as their potential and capabilities, clinical psychologists engage in activities like those listed subsequently.

(i)   They conduct interviews with the clients, their family members, friends, professional colleagues, and so on.
(ii) They go through naturalistic observation of the behavior of the clients.
(iii) They try to compile a case history of their clients.

(iv) They administer psychological tests (e.g., intelligence tests, academic achievement tests, personality tests, projective techniques, self-administered questionnaires, personality inventories, self-concept tests, adjustment inventories, attitude and interest tests, scales for measuring anxiety, mood, depression, and frustration, and so on).

After collecting this information, clinical psychologists engage in the process of drawing interpretations and conclusions for the purpose of composing a therapy plan.

2. Carrying Out the Task of Providing Treatment

A major activity area of clinical psychologists is concerned with providing intervention and treatment for the mental health problems and disorders of their clients. The tasks and activities performed in this concern begin with their earnest attempts to develop and maintain functional therapeutic relationships with clients. Then, they engage in providing treatment to the client on the basis of the assessment and diagnosis carried out earlier. In this concern, they are found to engage in the task of providing a suitable psychotherapy for the treatment of the client's problem/disorder by opting for a single appropriate psychotherapy or adopting an eclectic approach by drawing on a combination of several therapeutic techniques—behavior therapy, cognitive behavior therapy, client centered therapy, group therapy, family therapy, psychoanalysis, and so on. They conduct occasional evaluations of the impact of the introduced treatment and on this basis, continue or modify their treatment approach, with a clear-cut objective of helping the client improve their welfare.

3. Engaging in the Task of Teaching and Training

A number of clinical psychologist professionals opt for their career the task of teaching and training in colleges, universities, and other medical or behavioral science institutes. In fulfilling their responsibilities in this regard, they teach courses prescribed for graduate, postgraduate, MPhil and PhD degrees in the discipline of clinical psychology, such as Abnormal psychology, Physiological psychology, Psychological testing, Clinical Interview, Personality theories, Advanced psychopathology, Counseling psychology, Clinical intervention and Psychotherapies, Research methodology and Statistical techniques, and so on. In addition to providing theoretical orientation, they also train students in assessing and diagnosing mental health issues and employing therapeutic techniques, as well as supervising them in internships and guiding them in their research pursuits.

4. Conducting Research and Engaging in Writing Work

An important and useful task in which we see a number of clinical psychologist professionals engaged concerns conducting, guiding, and evaluating research, as well as publishing papers in journals and writing books on the theory and practice of clinical psychology. In this area, the clinical psychologist professional can make their most needed and distinctive contributions, as research and publications add to the development of theory and practice of mental health techniques. In general, the research and publication activities of clinical psychology professionals cover four main dimensions of mental health issues: (i) etiology or causes of underlying mental disorders, (ii) diagnosis and assessment of mental health problems and disorders, (iii) the process of performing psychotherapy, and (iv) evaluation of the outcome or suitability of psychotherapy for types of mental disorders.

5. Providing Consultancy Services

Many clinical psychologists work as consultants on a full-time or part-time basis in different settings for serving various purposes. The list of their places of work may include educational institutions, government departments and offices, business organizations and establishments, medical hospitals and clinics run by local, state, and central governments, private health clinics, community health centers, private residential colonies and homes, and so on. The consultancy services provided at these places may cover a wide range of activities for serving specific purposes. The goal of consultancy may be stated as "to help and increase the effectiveness of those who are already working thereby imparting them some degree of expertise for helping others or their own self in the prevention and treatment of the mental, emotional and behavioral issues." In this way, clinical psychologists provide consultancy on issues related to the prevention, diagnosis, and treatment of the mental health problems of individuals or an entire organization, for serving their individual interests as well as the healthy functioning of the organization as a whole.

6. Providing Assistance and Collaborating with Other Mental Health Professionals

Another significant activity area of clinical psychology is concerned with providing assistance and collaborating with other mental health professionals working in different settings, such as psychiatrists, counseling psychologists, marriage and family matter specialists, school psychologists, forensic psychologists, and social workers engaged in seeking health and overall well-being. Let us examine how.

- Clinical psychologists are not qualified to provide medical treatment in the form of shock therapy, drugs, psychosurgery, and handling serious cases of mental illness and disorders. However, in this latter concern they do perform two useful tasks: (i) to refer these cases to practicing psychiatrists along with their own initial observation and treatment report, and (ii) to assist and collaborate with them in determining which approach to use, in evaluating the progress of therapy, and in applying psychotherapy when the patient is amenable to it.
- They work with counseling psychologists, marriage and family matter specialists, and school psychologists in assisting with matters especially related to the diagnosis and psychotherapeutic treatment of mental issues and disorders.
- They assist and collaborate with psychologist colleagues specializing in Forensic psychology for providing expert testimony in the court of law.
- They make themselves available to the community and community health workers for assistance and collaboration in matters related to the prevention, diagnosis, and treatment of mental disorders. They assist in recommending serious cases of mental illness to specialist counselors and psychiatrists, and provide help in the rehabilitation of the patients such as recovered addicts, social and sexual deviants, and patients recovering from mental health problems and disorders. They also work with social workers to promote the health, quality-of-life, and psychological well-being of the community.

7. Doing Necessary Supervision, Performing Administrative Duties, and Participating in Clinical Conferences

Clinical psychology professionals are also engaged in the tasks and activities related to supervision, administrative duties, and contributing to professional seminars and workshops. In this regard, we may find them engaged in the activities such as the following:

- Supervision of (i) trainees doing internships for earning degrees in the discipline of clinical psychology, and (ii) the practice work of degree holders, making them eligible for obtaining practicing licenses, (iii) the work of junior clinical psychologists rendering clinical services to patients.
- Administrating the organizational setup and functioning of a mental health center, clinic or hospital in reference to its infrastructure, instruments, and facilities of conducting assessment, diagnosis, and treatment of mental disorders, assigning and supervising the functions of the working psychologists and other staff, arranging meetings with patients and their family members, and seeking cooperation of the community and other government agencies for day-to-day running of the activities of the mental health center.
- Keeping up-to-date regarding the development of theory and practice in their profession, staying aware of the latest research findings in the area of mental health and disorders, being conscious of the activities of different professional organization in their field, and making themselves available for professional activities such as journal publications, holding conferences, seminars and workshops, and so on.

The Education and Training of Clinical Psychologists

Clinical psychologists occupy an essential place in society as mental health professionals, not only for the well-being of its people but also for its own progress as a whole. To realize this purpose, they work in diversified clinical settings and fulfill varied responsibilities, specifically related to the prevention, diagnosis, and treatment of the mental illness and disorders. To face this challenge, they must be equipped with the necessary knowledge and understanding of the theory and practice of clinical psychology by undergoing courses of study and specialized training appropriately planned and designed for this purpose. This education and training must be examined and certified by an accepted and recognized authority that stands for issuing license to prospective clinical psychologists for enabling them to engage in private clinical practice, seek useful employment for working in the varied clinical settings, and becoming recognized as clinical psychologist professionals. Each country and even states/regions may have their own regulations, minimum academic level in terms of the attainment of particular degrees, regulating and accreditation bodies for developing prescribed courses, and training schedules and license issuing authorities. For example, in the United States, the responsibility of accreditation of courses and training schedules meant for the preparation of clinical psychologist professionals lies on the shoulders of the American Psychology Association (APA), and the task of issuing licenses is done by the respective state governing agencies. In our country, both these tasks are performed by a single authority, the Rehabilitation Council of India (RCI)—a statutory body enacted in 1993 through the RCI Act by the Parliament of India. Remember that there is no direct option for obtaining this license from license-providing authorities. For this purpose, candidates must go through some specific duration of study courses and training schedules, earn specified academic/professional degrees, and fulfill other requirements as fixed by the respective license issuing authorities and country/state governments. Globally, there is now a growing trend to fix the attainment of a doctoral degree in clinical psychology (PhD or PsyD) on the part of candidates as an essential requirement for earning licensing. What are these degrees and prescribed study courses and training schedules? Let us explore them.

Of these two types of programs, known as PhD and PsyD, PhD is a more traditional, research-based professional degree, while the purpose of PsyD is to place a greater focus on preparing the individual for professional practice, with less research training built into the curriculum. The decision to strive for either degree depends on what the aspiring clinical psychologist wishes to do in their professional life. If they choose to adopt a career in academia, (to become a full-time teacher, trainer, or researcher in the discipline clinical psychology), the PhD in clinical psychology would certainly be more advantageous to them because of its research-based emphasis. However, if they are planning for a career centered on applied clinical practice (to run their own private practice or serve in a clinical environment), then certainly, PsyD is the better choice for them, because of its practice-based emphasis. Nowadays, the increasing demand for practicing clinical psychologists, due to the growing prevalence of mental illness and disorders, the global trend among prospective clinical professionals is toward working in a clinical setting helping people and society as a whole in the task of dealing with psychologically based disorders and ailments. Thereby, most clinical psychologists (irrespective of their education and training as PhD or PsyD scholars), prefer to be in the domain of the clinical practice instead of academia and research.

The question arises what type of education and training is provided in institutions for obtaining the degrees PhD and PsyD in clinical psychology, and what are the eligibility and qualifications for getting entry into these programs? And how, then, is one finally licensed as a clinical psychologist? Let us explore one such process abroad through the example of the United States.

The Education and Training of Prospective Clinical Psychologists in the United States

There are two types of doctoral programs (PhD and PsyD) in the United States for the education and training of prospective clinical psychologists. The courses covered, practical work done, and pre-doctoral internship work undertaken in both programs culminating in PhD and PsyD differ in the sense that while in the former places much emphasis on orienting prospective clinical psychologists to work as teacher, trainer, and researcher, the latter aims to orient them more as a practicing clinician. Candidates seek admission in their referred program suiting their academia-related or practice-oriented interests.

To seek admission in clinical psychology doctoral programs (PhD or PsyD), the minimum academic qualification is a bachelor's degree in clinical psychology or a bachelor's degree in psychology with a specialization in clinical psychology. Most candidates trying to seek admission hold such degrees; however, some aspirants may have earned a master's degree from a "terminal" master's program in clinical psychology.

The duration of education and training for those entering such a program with only a bachelor's degree is five years. However, it is shortened by two years for those who already have a master's degree. During the period of five years, the education and training of prospective clinical psychologists is undertaken, as summarized subsequently.

(i) During the first four years, students must complete intensive, full-time coursework helpful in understanding and applying the theory and practice of clinical psychology. In general, it comprises courses on psychotherapy, psychological testing, abnormal psychology, diagnosis and assessment of metal disorders, statistics, research methodology, biological bases of behavior, cognitive-affective bases of behavior, social bases of behavior, individual differences, rehabilitation of treated patients, and specializations such as health psychology and forensic psychology, as well as other subjects. The nature, number, and depth of these courses vary according to their research-based and practice-based requirements of the PhD and PsyD programs.

(ii) In addition to theoretical understanding of these courses, the students are also required to go through practical work during the four years period of completing a master's thesis, doctoral dissertation, and the practicum in which students accumulate supervised experience doing clinical work.

(iii) Once on-campus course responsibilities are complete, students in their fifth and final year move on to the task of pre-doctoral internship, in which they must take on greater clinical responsibilities and obtain supervised experience on a full-time basis in an APA-approved, applied clinical setting (i.e., a psychiatric hospital, a university counseling center, a community mental health center, a medical school, or another agency where clinical psychologists work).

The Task of Getting Licensed as a Professional Clinical Psychologist in the United States

One does not automatically become licensed after obtaining a doctoral degree (PhD or PsyD); after graduation, one must undergo formalities such as the following:

1. In some US states, candidates who have completed their pre-doctoral internship and obtained the doctoral degree, must undergo a postdoctoral internship for licensure as a psychologist. During this internship of one to two years, the candidates take on more responsibilities (under close supervision of senior and experienced clinical psychologist professionals) than they had carried as pre-doctoral interns. Some states are considering abolishing this requirement, as it puts an additional burden on candidates who have spent so much time already on their education and training.

2. After this comes another requirement—passing the following licensure examinations.

   (i) *The Examination for Professional Practice in Psychology (EPPP):* A standardized examination consisting of multiple-choice questions on a broad range of topics studied and practiced during their years of training to become PhD and PsyD. To become eligible for licensure, candidates must earn a minimum score on this examination.

   (ii) *A state-specific examination on laws and ethics:* An examination (written or oral) focused on legal issues relevant to the ethical code of clinical psychology practice in the state.

A similar process is employed, albeit with variation, among other leading progressive democratic countries such as Canada, the United Kingdom, Australia, and New Zealand. Let us see what happens in the United Kingdom.

In the UK, clinical psychologists undertake a Doctor of Clinical Psychology (D. Clin. Psych.) degree, a practitioner-doctorate with both clinical and research components. This is a three-year full-time salaried program sponsored by the National Health Service (NHS) and based in universities as well as the NHS. Entry into these programs is highly competitive and requires at least a three-year undergraduate degree in psychology, plus some form of experience, usually in either the NHS as an Assistant Psychologist or in academia as a Research Assistant. It is not unusual for applicants to apply several times before being accepted into a training course, as only about one-fifth of applicants are accepted each year. These clinical psychology doctoral degrees are accredited by the British Psychological Society and the Health Professions Council (HPC). The HPC is the statutory regulator for practitioner psychologists in the UK. Those who successfully complete clinical psychology doctoral degrees are eligible to apply for registration with the HPC as a clinical psychologist.

In India, we employ a unique process for the education, training, and licensure of prospective clinical psychologists, as discussed next.

How to Become a Licensed Clinical Psychologist in Our Country?

As a student or reader of this text, you will surely be interested to know what needs to be done on one's part in terms of getting education and training for becoming a properly licensed clinical psychologist in our country. Let us discuss it.

We already know well that for doing practice and getting recognized as a clinical psychologist professional, one must obtain a certified license for this purpose from a license-issuing authority. In our country, such authority is vested in the Rehabilitation Council of India (RCI), a statutory body enacted in 1993 through the RCI Act by Parliament of India. There is no direct option to get this license from RCI; the candidate must pursue a prescribed course known as MPhil. in Clinical psychology, or have a doctoral degree in Clinical psychology, such as PhD or PsyD.

The M.Phil. in Clinical Psychology course is a two-year hospital-based post-graduate course conducted by several universities and medical institutes in our country. The list of institutions recognized for running this course, as well as the course's syllabus and eligibility for entry, is available on the RCI website. The main features of this course along with admission requirements are summarized as follows.

1. The minimum educational requirement for admission to this course is a two-year MA/MSc degree in Psychology from a university recognized by the UGC with a minimum of 55% marks in aggregate (50% marks in aggregate for SC/ST category). Candidates fulfilling this minimum educational requirement must appear in an entrance examination (a written test consisting of multiple-choice questions regarding multiple psychological topics). The merit list is drawn on the basis of entrance test scores, thus constituting a criterion for providing admission to aspiring candidates.
2. The courses and training provided during the two-year period aims to provide students the necessary knowledge and skills for performing diversified responsibilities as a qualified professional clinical psychologist. It consists of the following.

    (i) The study of clinical psychology through various course papers such as: Psychosocial Foundation of Behavior and Psychopathology, Statistics and Research Methodology, Psychiatry, Biological Foundations of Behavior, Psychotherapy and Counseling, and Behavioral Medicine.
    (ii) Emphasis on "Practicum" related to the skills of psychological testing, diagnosis, and psychotherapies through experiences gained in clinical work settings under the supervision of faculty members of their institution or clinical psychologists working in the centers.
    (iii) Dissertation work under the guidance of a qualified clinical psychology faculty member.

After obtaining the degree in MPhil Clinical psychology, prospective clinical psychologists are required to approach RCI for their registration as a licensed clinical psychologist.

Their registration in the appearance of their names as clinical psychologist practitioners in the register maintained by RCI, then, makes them legally eligible to provide their services as a practicing clinical psychologist anywhere in India.

The objective of becoming a licensed clinical psychologist may be properly achieved in our country by obtaining the MPhil clinical psychology degree. One can then conduct their own practice as clinical psychologist or provide their services in the diversified mental health service sectors including providing testimony in the courts. However, the MPhil program bears some serious limitations, such as the following.

- It is merely a practice-oriented program aimed to equip trainees with necessary knowledge and skills for working in the mental health sectors as a properly licensed clinical psychologist.
- It does not have a provision of providing enough clinical experience in the form of internship in the clinical setting for dealing with the diagnosis and treatment of mental health problems and disorders.
- It neither prepares them as a scientist enabling them to do needed research in the area of clinical psychology, nor orients them to take up the task of teaching and training at the postgraduate level.
- Moreover, it merely equips them in a generic manner, and does not prepare them for a future career in specialty areas related to clinical psychology.

For overcoming these limitations, individuals who have completed their MPhil degree must obtain an additional degree— the PhD (the traditional doctoral degree earned in the university setting) and/or go through specific skill training for earning the required abilities to become practitioners in a sub-specialization. It costs them much in terms of time, money, and labor.

Questions may arise as to what options, other than doing MPhil Clinical psychology, are available for candidates to become a clinical psychologist professional in our country. Let us make it clear.

- If you intend to become a licensed clinical psychology practitioner in a generic form suitable for the diversified services including private practice in the mental health sector, then MPhil clinical psychology is the best option before you.
- If you intend to make your career in academia (as a researcher, teacher, and trainer in clinical psychology), then doing PhD in Clinical psychology will be a better choice for you.
- If you intend to train yourself as a practitioner (more competent and capable than being trained in MPhil clinical psychology course) cum scientist (capable of performing responsibilities as a researcher, teacher, and trainer) then certainly obtaining a PsyD doctoral degree in clinical psychology will be the most beneficial choice.

Let us explore more about this latter program, which is fully endorsed and recognized as the highest available degree in clinical psychology on the part of the RCI, the authority responsible for maintaining the required standard for education and training of prospective clinical psychologists along with their licensing as practicing-cum academic clinical professionals. The RCI website lists the institutions recognized for running PsyD programs as well as details about the admission requirements, course contents, and work required to complete the programs. However, for the interest of our readers, we provide a summary as follows:

(i) The PsyD program, four years in duration, is conducted in institutions recognized by the RCI. There may be two types of trainees in this program: those who join the course in the third year of the program as a lateral entry after registering with RCI as clinical psychologists following two-year MPhil clinical psychology degree, and those who join the course from its beginning as a direct entry having a MA/MSc degree in Psychology from a university recognized by the UGC with a minimum of 65% marks in aggregate (60% for SC/ST/OBC category).

(ii) Both the lateral and direct entry candidates must appear and seek merit in the entrance test examinations held separately for both categories of candidates for admission in the recognized institutes running PsyD programs.

(iii) During the first two years, course papers studied include: Psychosocial Foundations of Behavior, Biological Foundations of Behavior, Psychopathology, Psychiatry, Psychotherapy and Counseling, Behavioral Medicine, Evidence-Based Practice and Clinical Research Issues, and Statistics and Research Methodology.

The practicum undertaken in these two years is focused on acquiring skills for conducting psychological assessment, diagnosis, and psychotherapy for mental health problems and disorders.

(iv) During the third year, trainees must acquire advanced proficiency in two sub-specialization areas depending on their interest, chosen from a given list of twenty-one options, including Applied Behavior Analysis, Behavior Therapy, Behavioral Medicine, Cardiac Rehabilitation, Clinical Child and Adolescent Psychology, Clinical Neuropsychology, Cognitive-Behavior Therapies, Community Mental Health, Crisis Interventions, Forensic Clinical Psychology, Geriatric Psychology, Human Sexuality and Dysfunctions, Marital and Family therapy, Mental Retardation, Pain Management, Palliative Care, Psychoanalytic Therapies, Psycho-oncology, Rehabilitation of Mentally Ill, School Psychology, and Substance Abuse.

(v) During the fourth and final year, the trainees are required (a) to complete one-year rotation internship assignments supervised by a professional clinical psychologist who may or may not be a faculty member, and (b) submit an empirical research thesis in one of the elective areas the trainee has chosen to acquire advanced proficiency under the guidance of a faculty member holding a PhD/PsyD degree.

As per the updated list issued by the Rehabilitation Council of India (RCI) as of October 4, 2022 (www.rehabcouncil.nic.in/writereaddata/approved_inst.pdf), the following universities/institute/hospitals are recognized to provide MPhil Clinical Psychology and PsyD courses for the academic season of 2022–23. RCI changes their list of approved institutions every year, so further changes in the following list are possible. Therefore, readers are advised to look for these changes in the coming years on the RCI website.

List of RCI-Approved Institutions offering MPhil Clinical Psychology Course

1. Lokopriya Gopinath Bordoli Regional Institute of Mental Health, Tezpur—784001, Dist. Sonitpur, Post Box no. 15, Assam
2. Government Medical College & Hospital, Department of Psychiatry, Level—V, Block—D, Sector—32, Chandigarh—160030
3. Post Graduate Institute of Behavioural & Medical Sciences, Opp. Rajkumar College, Swami, Atmanand Marg, Raipur, Chattisgarh
4. Central India Institute G.E. Road Dewada Chowk, Kopedih Road, Gram Dewada, Dist-Rajnandgaon Chhatisgarh-491441
5. Institute of Human Behaviour & Allied Sciences (IHBAS), P.O. Box no. 9520, Dilshad Garden, Delhi—110095

6. PGIMER, Dr. Ram Manohar Lohia Hospital, Baba Kharag Singh Marg, New Delhi—110001
7. B.M. Institute of Mental Health, Near Nehru Bridge, Ashram Road, District—Ahmedabad, Gujarat—380009 P.D. (CL.Psy)
8. Institute of Behavioural Sciences, Gujarat Forensic Sciences University 18/A, B/H Police Bhawan, Gandhinagar, Gujarat—382007
9. Rashtriya Raksha University At Lavad, Ta. Dahegam, Distt-Gandhinagar, Gujarat-382305
10. Department of Audiology & Speech Language Pathology, Amity University Haryana, Amity Education Valley Distt. Gurgaon (Manesar), Haryana—122413
11. Shree Guru Gobind Singh Tricentenary University, Chandu-Budhera Gurgaon-Badli Road, Gurgaon—122505.
12. Post Graduate Department of Psychiatry, Govt. Medical College Kathi Darwaza, Rainawari Srinagar—190003
13. Ranchi Institute of Neuropsychiatry & Allied Sciences Kanke, Ranchi (RINPAS)—834006
14. Central Institute of Psychiatry (CIP) Post—Kanke, District—Ranchi, Jharkhand—834006
15. Department of Clinical Psychology, School of Allied Health Sciences, Manipal University, Manipal, Karnataka—575 104
16. Dharwad Institute of Mental Health & Neurosciences (D.I.M.H.A.N.S.), District—Dharwad, Karnataka
17. J.S.S. Medical College (Deemed to be University) Sri Shivarathreeshware Nagara, Dist-Mysuru—570015
18. Kateel Ashok Pai Memorial Institute of Allied Health Sciences, Manasa Trust "vinodini Building", Park Extension, Durgigudi, Shivamogga, Karnataka—577201
19. Amrita School of Medicine, Amrita Institute of Medical Sciences & Research Centre AIMS Ponekakara PO, Kochi, Ernakulam District, Kerala—682041
20. Institute of Mental Health & Neurosciences (IMHANS), Govt. Medical College campus Kozhikode—673008.
21. Gwalior Mansik Arogyashala Jail Road, Gwalior, M.P. 474012
22. Amity Institute of Behavioural & Allied Sciences, Amity University Madhya Pradesh, Opposite Airport Maharajpura, P.O.: Gole Ka Mandir Tehsil: Morar Gwalior, Madhya Pradesh
23. Amity Institute of Behavioural and Allied Sciences (AIBAS) Amity University Bhatan, P.O. Somathne Taluka—Panvelo, Mumbai—410206
24. Department of Mental Health Institute of Naval Medicine, (INHS) Asvini Colaba, District—Mumbai, Maharashtra—400005
25. Maharashtra Institute of Mental Health, Sassoon General Hospital Campus, Pune, Maharashtra
26. Regional Institute of Medical Sciences, (RIMS), Lamphelpat, Imphal—795004
27. Mental Health Institute (COE in Mental health) SCB Medical College & Hospital, Cuttack, Odisha—753007
28. Amity Institute of Behavioural & Allied Sciences (AIBAS) Amity University Rajasthan Kant Kalwar, NH—11C, Jaipur-Delhi National Highway Jaipur, Rajasthan—303002
29. Mahatma Gandhi Medical College & Hospital Faculty of Medicine—RIICO Institutional Area, Sitapura, Iaipur, Rajasthan—302022
30. MJRP College of Education, Mahatma Jyoti rao Phoole University SP 2 & 3 Ram Kalwar, RICCO Industrial Area, Lala Mode, Achrol, Jaipur, Rajasthan—303103
31. Sri Ramachandra Institute of Higher Education and Research (Deemed to be University) Dept. of Clinical Psychology, Sri Ramchandra Faculty of Allied Health Sciences, Sri Ramchandra Institute of Higher Education and Research (Deemed University) Porur, Chennai—600 116

32. National Institute for Empowerment of Persons with Multiple Disabilities, East Coast, Muttukadu, Kancheepuram Dist., Kovalam Post, Tamilnadu—603112.
33. SRM Medical College Hospital & Research Centre, SRM Deemed University, SRM Nagar, Potheri, Kattankulathur Post, Kancheepuram Dist., Tamilnadu—603 203
34. Institute Of Mental Health, Medavakkam Tank Road, Kilpauk, Chennai, Tamilnadu—600010.
35. Sweekar Academy of Rehabilitation Sciences, Upkaar Complex, Upkaar Circle, Picket, Secunderabad, Telangana—500 003
36. The Institute of Chartered Financial Analyst of India (ICFAI) University, PO.Kamalghat, Sadar, Mohanpur, Tripura (West)—799210.
37. Amity Institute of Behavioural (Health) & Allied Sciences (AIBHAS), Amity University, Amity Campus, Sector-125, Plot No. 4, Gautam Budh Nagar, Noida
38. Institute of Mental Health and Hospital, Billochpura, Old Mathura Road, Agra, Uttar Pradesh—282002
39. King George's Medical university, Department of Psychiatry, KGMU Chowk, Shahmina Road, Lucknow, Uttar Pradesh—226003
40. Gautam Buddha University, Near Yamuna Expressway, Greater Noida, Dist. Gautam Budh Nagar, Uttar Pradesh—201308
41. Amity University, Malhore, Near Railway Station, Gomti Nagar Extension, Lucknow, Uttar Pradesh—226 028
42. Nai Subah (Institute of Mental Health & Behavioural Sciences) Khanav, near Water Tank, PostBachav, District-Varanasi—221011
43. Department of Psychology, University of Calcutta, University Colleges of Science, Technology and Agriculture, 92, Acharya Prafulla Chandra Road, Kolkata West Bengal—700009
44. Institute of Psychiatry, IPGME&R, 7 D.L. Khan Road, Kolkata, West Bengal—700025,
45. Amity Institute of Behavioural and Allied Sciences (AIBAS) Major Arterial Road, Action Area—II Rajarhat, New Town Kolkata—700135

List of RCI Approved Institutions Running PsyD Clinical Psychology Courses

1. Sweekar Academy of Rehabilitation Sciences, Secunderabad, Telangana
2. Amity Institute of Behavioural (Health) & Allied Sciences (AIBHAS), Noida, Uttar Pradesh

---

To Sum Up

For working as a clinical psychologist professional, one must go through the prescribed courses and training programs, earn a particular degree from a recognized institution, and obtain a license certified by a recognized authority of one's country. Each country for this purpose has its own functioning system, rules, and regulations.

For example, in the United States, the minimum requirement for being eligible to get licensed to work as clinical psychologists is the attainment of a doctoral degree in clinical psychology (PhD, or PsyD). In this concern, the responsibility of accreditation of the courses and training schedules for the PhD or PsyD degree lies on the shoulders of the American Psychology Association (APA), and the task of issuing licenses is done by the respective state government agencies.

Out of these two, PhD is a more traditional, research-based professional degree, while the purpose of the PsyD is to focus on preparing the individual for professional practice. The candidates have the choice of opting for either of these two degrees depending upon their desire to enter into a research-based or practice-oriented profession.

In our country, there are three different programs for the preparation and training of prospective clinical psychologists, providing three types of degrees, namely MPhil, PhD, and PsyD in clinical psychology. Candidates may choose either of these three according to their needs. The PhD in clinical psychology is meant for those who prefer to enter teaching or research work. For those who are less interested in academic pursuit (research or teaching) and intend to become a licensed clinical psychology practitioner, doing MPhil clinical psychology is the best option. The option to earn a PsyD doctoral degree in clinical psychology is meant for those who intend to equip themselves with higher competency in both areas—academic (research and teaching) and practicing as a capable clinical psychologist professional.

While obtaining a postgraduate degree in clinical psychology occurs through universities governed by UGC rules and regulations, the responsibility of accreditation of the courses and training schedules for the MPhil and PsyD in clinical psychology lies on the shoulders of a national agency—the Rehabilitation Council of India (RCI). Additionally, the RCI issues licenses to certified clinical psychology professionals once they have achieved the minimum eligibility degree requirements.

Review Questions

1. Who are clinical psychologists? Where do they work and what activities do they usually perform?
2. Discuss in what aspects clinical psychologists differ from other mental health professionals, such as psychiatrists, counseling psychologists, school psychologists, and social workers.
3. Discuss in detail the procedure involved in becoming a certified licensed clinical psychologist in the United States.
4. Throw light on the education and training of clinical psychologist professionals in India, including the certification and licensing process.
5. Describe in detail what one must do to become a clinical psychologist practitioner in our country.

References

American Heritage Publishing Company (2016), American Heritage Dictionary of the English Language—Fifth Edition, New York, NY: Houghton Mifflin Harcourt Publishing Company.

Fossum, T. A., Logeais, M. E., & Robiner, W. N. (2016), Related mental health professions, In J. C. Norcross, G. R. VandenBos, D. K. Freedheim, & L. F. Campbell (Eds.), *APA handbook of clinical psychology: Education and profession* (pp. 455–468), Washington, DC: American Psychological Association.

Reference (On line)

Merriam-Webster, Merriam-Webster.Com Dictionary, definition of clinical psychologist, retrieved from www.merriam-webster.com/dictionary/clinical%20psychologist

Chapter 3

Clinical Psychology—Historical Perspectives and Present Position

Learning Objectives

After going through this chapter, you will be able to:

- Describe the historical roots of clinical psychology.
- Discuss the birth of clinical psychology and its development in the early half of the 20th century.
- Throw light on developments in clinical psychology from 1951 onward.
- Describe the present position and developmental status of clinical psychology.
- Discuss the historical roots of clinical psychology in India.
- Throw light on the development of clinical psychology in British and Independent India.
- Name some clinical journals published in India and abroad.
- Name some of the clinical psychology associations working in India and abroad.

Introduction

Let us survey the historical development of the subject of clinical from its earlier roots, formal origin, and subsequent development.

A. The Historical Past and Earlier Roots of Clinical Psychology

Clinical psychology as a scientific discipline examines problems related to mental health—specifically the diagnosis and treatment of mental illness and disorders. The existence of problems related to mental health, illness, and disorders is as old as the emergence of the first primitive men and women on earth. Thus, if we try to locate a time period of the first attempts to define, diagnose, and treat such issues, we may find their existence since the beginning of the civilizations in the world. This earliest era in the history of identifying and treating mental health problems, before the emergence of the discipline of psychology and its applied offshoot, clinical psychology, may be distinguished by various in the manner as briefed as follows.

1. *The earliest period—the dominance of superstitions:* The identification and treatment of abnormality, mental illness, and disorders was completely under the cloud of superstitions during the

DOI: 10.4324/9781003398325-3

earliest phases of the ancient eras. It was believed that devils, evil spirits, and other supernatural powers are responsible for mental illness and abnormality in one's behavior. As historical evidence, we find several early writings of the Egyptians, Chinese, Hebrews, Greeks, and Indians locating the cause of mental disorders inherent in the roles of demons and evil spirits. They also provide testimony for the treatment of these disorders at the hands of *priests* and *tantriks* consisting of various techniques to make evil spirits leave the body of the sufferer. Some were treated by prayer, charms, and sacrifice to appease the Gods, as well as other measures such as noise making, flogging, starving, burning, and ingesting wine, dung, and urine, in an attempt to make the body of the sufferer so unholy or unpleasant a place that spirits would be driven out.

2. *Brighter period of the Humane outlook and naturalistic medical treatment:* After the ancient era, there came an enlightenment period in which ancient civilizations like Greek, Roman, and Ancient Indian took a lead in developing a humane outlook and naturalistic medical approach for the diagnosis and treatment of mental health issues. Notable moments include the following:

   - Hippocrates (460–357 BC), the Greek physician lauded as the "father of the modern medicine," along with his followers developed "naturalism." According to this doctrine, demons, spirits, and heavenly bodies had nothing to do with mental disorders; they were now seen as the results of natural causes requiring treatment in the same manner as physical diseases. Hippocrates initiated the pathological or medical approach by explaining abnormalities and mental health problems in terms of diseases of the brain. He also emphasized that hereditary predisposition, environmental, and emotional stress can damage one's body and mind. He classified all mental disorders into three general categories—mania, melancholia, and phrenitis. For the treatment, he advocated a regular clinical observation with proper records. In this way, Hippocrates brought about a revolution in the history of mental health.
   - Among the Roman physicians, Asclepiad (124 BC) was the first to discriminate between acute and chronic mental illness and to distinguish between illusions, delusions, and hallucinations. He was opposed to undesirable measures such as bleeding, purging, and mechanical restraints, and strongly advocated for making patients more comfortable. He favored humanism and recommended the use of music as a therapy.
   - Later, another Roman physician called Aretaeus (second century AD) became known for the insight he gained regarding the importance of emotional factors and the pre-psychotic personality of the patient. He was the first to describe the various phases of mania and melancholia and to consider these two pathological states expressions of the same illness.
   - There was a significant prevalence of a well-organized system of diagnosing and treating mental disorders in ancient India, as described in the earlier treatise Vedas (Atharvaveda and Ayurveda) and Sanhitas (Charak Sanhita) advocating treatment based on rituals, diet, and medicine, and later by Patanjali in practicing yoga as an approach for dealing with mental health problems.

Thus, the enlightenment period of the ancient era contributed much to the diagnosis and treatment of mental disorders, through Hippocrates and other Greek and Roman physicians as well as the ancient systems of medicine and psychological treatment prevailing in India. Many of our modern concepts of mental illness and its treatment bear unique resemblance to the views advocated during this period.

3. *The return of superstition and ill treatment:* After the collapse of the Greek and Roman civilizations in the fifth century AD, and the diminishing of the glory of the Vedic and Upanishad period, the diagnosis and treatment of mental disorders reverted to the practices prevalent in the early ages of superstition and demonology. Notably, the emergence of religious heads and saints as a

dominating force paved the way for utter ignorance and blind superstition across world societies. Some of the so-called religious heads or saints proclaimed to have special powers in ridding evil spirits or demons possessing people. They established sacred shrines where victims went to be cured. Here, the curative measures were varied. In some cases, holy water, ashes, lying on hands (a practice adopted for paying respect to God), sanctified ointments, relics, and visits to holy places were thought to have a magic effect for curing mental illness. At other times, inhumane tortures such as burning, starving, flogging, and painful immersion in hot or cold water were undertaken to rid evil spirits from the body and mind of the mentally disturbed people. During the later part of this period (the fifteenth to seventeenth centuries), beliefs involving religion, evil spirits, and demons took a turn for the worse. The old belief that disturbed people were unwillingly seized by evil spirits as a punishment by God for their sins was replaced by the belief that the individual, willingly, had made a pact or friendship with Satan, the devil. The mentally ill came to be considered as heretics and witches responsible for storms, floods, crop failures, injuries to their enemies, sexual impotence, death, and diseases. Consequently, measures were taken for the detection and punishment of witches and witchcraft. People with mental illness were often accused of witchcraft and subjected to unimagined tortures such as cutting of the tongue, twisting delicate parts of the body, burning alive, beheading, strangling, and mutilation.

4. *Return of the Humane outlook and the Era of Reason*: With a continuous struggle by courageous individuals, even at the risk of their life, against the hollow concepts of witchcraft and demonology, there emerged an era of reason and a humane outlook toward mental illness and disorders. The major contributions in this regard are noted as follows.

   • Paracelsus (1490–1541), a Swiss chemist, was one of the first to point out that the phenomenon of dancing mania was not a creation of good or bad spirits but a form of disease. He also put forth the idea of psychic causes for mental illness and advocated "bodily magnetism," which later developed into hypnotherapy, in his treatment. However, he had to pay dearly for his unconventional views under continuous persecution—ultimately, with his life.

   • In the same period, another voice of reason emerged in the physician and writer Johann Weyer (1515–1588). He published a book on witchcraft and pointed out that a considerable number of those imprisoned, tortured, and burned as witches were sick, mentally, or physically. He was one of the first specialists in mental disorders. For his progressive views on mental illness, he is regarded as the real founder of modern psychiatry. Being ahead of his time, he was met with vehement protest and condemnation, and his works were banned by the Church and remained so until the 20th century.

   • Reginald Scot (1538–1599) is known for his publication *The Discovery of Witchcraft*, in which he argued that mental disorders had no connection with demons or evil spirits, and so-called witches were merely unfortunate women affected by mental illness. His views were also attacked, and King James I of England personally refuted and ordered the burning of his book.

   • Another person who, at the risk of his life, condemned demonology and witch horror was St. Vincent de Paul (1576–1660). He boldly declared that mental diseases were no different from bodily diseases and advocated the medical and humane treatment of people with mental illness.

5. *The establishment of Asylums for people with mental illness:* The voices of reason, raised against the maltreatment of people with mental illness, helped in diminishing the influence of religious heads in dealing with the mentally disturbed. As a result, for the first time in the history, King Henry VIII of England was inspired to convert the monastery of St. Mary of Bethlehem in London into a mental hospital in 1547. Hospitals called asylums were also

established later in other parts of Europe and in the Americas. But the early asylums were run like prisons, and patients were treated more like wild animals than sick human beings. They were placed in dark cells and chained to posts, walls, and beds in such a way that they could eat from bowls of food fit only for animals. Severe measures such as starvation, solitary confinement, cold baths, and other methods of torture were often employed to exercise control over the inmates. These asylums became places where the unfortunate inmates lived and died amidst the most inhuman conditions. Critiquing this state of affairs of these asylums, there emerged several voices and movements in Europe and the United States for bringing reforms to asylums and the treatment of inmates. Let us look into such notable attempts.

- One of the first to raise their voice against these asylums was the French physician Philippe Pinel (1745–1826), who was in charge of the La Bicêtre mental hospital in Paris. He began treating the inmates of this asylum as sick human beings and insisted on their chains being removed. The authorities, who were very reluctant to approve the daring plan, were astonished to see the success of the humanitarian approach.
- What Pinel pioneered in France was similarly done in England by William Tuke (1732–1822), who also sought to reduce the plights of asylum inmates in his country. He took a leading step of establishing a residential treatment center, named York Retreat (by collecting donations from the community people), and devoted his entire life to improving the living conditions and treatment of people with mental illness.
- In the United States, the task of adopting a genuine humanistic approach to treating people with mental illness was carried out by leading physicians and others, summarized as follows:

  (i) Benjamin Rush (1745–1813), known as the father of American psychiatry, paved the way for scientific theories and therapies regarding the treatment of mental illness, which in turn led to the mental hygiene movement for prevention and cure of mental disorders and preservation and promotion of mental health.
  (ii) Eli Todd (1769–1833), a physician in Connecticut who was much influenced by Pinel's efforts in France, established "The Retreat" in Hartford, Connecticut in 1824 for treating people with mental illness in a humane and dignified way.
  (iii) Dorothea Dix (1802–1887), while working in 1891 as a Sunday school teacher in a jail in Boston, noticed that many inmates were there as a result of mental illness and intellectual disability, rather than crime. She devoted the rest of her life to improving the lives and treatment of people with mental illness. Her efforts resulted in the establishment of more than 30 state institutions for the mentally ill throughout the United States (and even more in Europe and Asia), providing more decent, compassionate treatment for the mentally ill than they might have otherwise received (Reisman, 1991).

6. *Emergence of modern thoughts in understanding and treating mental illness:* The age of reasoning leading to a more humane approach in dealing with mental illness then paved the way for the emergence of modern thoughts representing two viewpoints: the organic and the psychological. Let us examine the developments in this regard.

(i) Organic viewpoint: The development with regard to the use of the organic viewpoint in dealing with abnormality and mental disorders may be briefed as follows.

   - The first systematic presentation of the organic viewpoint was made by the German physician Wilhelm Griesinger (1817–1868), who asserted that every mental illness or abnormality could be explained on the basis of brain pathology.

- Griesinger was followed by Emil Kraepelin (1856–1926), who furnished a classification of mental diseases and disorders in terms of an organic basis. He regarded mental diseases and disorders to be characterized by a group of symptoms called a syndrome. He also emphasized that each mental illness was distinct from others, with unique, symptoms, and courses of treatment, in much the same way as of measles, smallpox, and other physical ailments. His assertions that schizophrenia is caused by a chemical imbalance in the body, and manic-depressive psychoses are due to irregularities in the metabolism, are evidence of his organic viewpoint for the explanation of mental disorders.

(ii) Psychological viewpoint: The second viewpoint involving a psychological approach was the result of the failure to reveal a satisfactory organic cause in several cases. This new approach explained that mental illness was caused by psychological rather than organic factors. The developments in this regard are summarized as follows.

- Historically, this viewpoint first came from Anton Mesmer (1734–1815), an Austrian physician practicing "Mesmerism," a form of hypnosis, to cure hysteria. The method that he followed to induce mesmerism was so crude that he was branded a charlatan by his medical colleagues and was forced to flee the country. However, during the latter part of the 19th century, Mesmer's contribution aroused the interest of a number of medical practitioners in hypnosis.
- French physicians such as Ambroise-Auguste Liébeault (1823–1904) and Hippolyte Bernheim (1840–1919) were able to demonstrate the success of hypnosis (suggestion technique). Another personality who became interested in the research on hysteria during this period was Jean Charcot (1825–1893), a French neurologist. He subsequently did much to promote an understanding of the role of psychological factors in various mental disorders. Pierre Janet (1859–1947) was another Frenchman whose findings on hysteria further served to popularize the psychological viewpoint.
- The use of the psychological approach gained further support from Josef Breuer (1842–1925), a physician in Vienna. He introduced a new method, known as catharsis, for curing hysteria. In this method, the patient is made to discharge emotional tension associated with repressed traumatic material by expressing it freely.
- Josef Breuer's approach was soon joined by Sigmund Freud (1856–1939), another Viennese physician in the practice of treating hysteria using catharsis, and the two collaborated in publishing a book called *Studies in Hysteria*, which advocates the doctrine of non-organic interpretation of mental disorders. Going further, Freud put forward the doctrine of psychoanalysis, in which he replaced catharsis with a new technique known as Free Association.
- Freud was followed by his students Alfred Adler (1870–1937) and C.F. Jung (1875–1961). While agreeing with the psychological approach to the understanding of mental illness, they differed with the views of their teacher and ultimately developed their own systematic approaches known as "individual psychology" and "analytical psychology." The viewpoints emphasized by these two eminent doctors, coupled with the unique contribution of Freud, sought to establish sufficient ground for understanding and curing mental illness or abnormality on the basis of psychological causes.
- During the same period, while proceeding along somewhat different lines, the psychologists such as Ivan Pavlov (1849–1936), a Russian, and J.B. Watson and B.F. Skinners, Americans, put forth a view point that normal or abnormal behavior is a learned act, and many mental disorders are the product one's life experiences. These ideas have contributed

significantly to our understanding of mental illness and disorders, establishing the role of psychological or socio-psychological factors in relation to behavioral disorders.

The developments narrated thus far resulted in (i) a phasing out of the false notions and superstitions surrounding mental illness, (ii) the development of humanistic approaches in improving asylums, mental hospitals, and the treatment of mental illness, and (iii) widespread adoption of the psychological approach for the diagnosis and treatment of mental problems and disorders. However, until recently, there was nothing like the subject or discipline of clinical psychology in studying the behavior of individuals in clinical settings through scientific methods. For this purpose later came the efforts of an American psychologist named Lightner Witmer, whom we will describe in our subsequent discussion.

To Sum Up

The existence of problems related to mental health, illness, and disorders is as old as the beginning of the world's civilizations. Therefore, the early roots of clinical psychology may be traced to various practices prevalent during the ancient eras for the identification, classification, and treatment of mental illness. In this connection, *the earliest dark period* was completely dominated by superstitions; mental disorders were attributed to superpowers—good or bad—and were cured through *mantras*, magic, and severely inhumane treatment by some priests and *tantriks*. After this there emerged the *enlightenment period*, bringing a somewhat more humane outlook and naturalistic as well as pathological approach to the understanding and treatment of mental disorders through the notable contributions of Greek and Roman physicians like Hippocrates, Asclepiades, and Aretaeous. It was followed again by another relatively dark period extending from the 5th to the 17th century, in which superstitions fueled the fear of witchcraft, often considering mental illness as a deliberate association with the devil. What followed was a *reappearance of the scientific approach*, pioneered by great men like Paracelsus, Johann Wayer, Reginald Scot, and St. Vincent de Paul, who challenged the concept of witchcraft and demonology and paved the way for the return of naturalistic pathological treatment of mental disorders. This resulted in the establishment of mental hospitals called asylums. The inhumane conditions prevalent in the early asylums were later improved, giving rise to the mental hygiene movement in the 18th century through the attempts made by Pinel (France), Tuke (England), and Rush (United States). As a further departure from the ancient past there emerged in the nineteenth and the earlier part of the 20th century an era of *modern thought* with the application of modern science in the understanding and treatment of mental disorders. In this era, men like Griesinger and Kraepelin advocated for organic or physiological bases of mental disorders; others, such as Mesmer, Charcot, Janet, Breuer, Freud, Adler, Jung, Pavlov, Watson, and Skinner established the role of psychological or socio-psychological factors for the understanding and treatment of mental disorders.

B. *The Birth of Clinical Psychology and Development in the Earlier Half of the 20th Century*

Lightner Witmer (1867–1956), a student of Wilhelm Wundt and a professor at the University of Pennsylvania, is credited for establishing in 1896 the first psychological clinic at the University of Pennsylvania for studying mental health problems by applying the principles of psychology.

In his clinic, Witmer and his associates worked with children whose problems related to their learning and behavior, referred by their schools, parents, physicians, or community authorities (McReynolds, 1997). However, through their experimental work, it was successfully demonstrated that whether the subject is a child or an adult, the examination and treatment may be conducted through scientific psychological methods. Witmer trained many doctoral students in psychology at the University of Pennsylvania in such clinical methods.

In addition to establishing his clinic, Witmer is also known for his memorable contributions such as (i) founding the first scholarly journal in the field, called *The Psychological Clinic* in 1907, (ii) authoring the first article in the first issue of this journal, titled "Clinical Psychology," and (iii) coining the term clinical psychology in that very article, and providing its definition as "the study of individuals, by observation or experimentation, with the intention of promoting change." It was his leadership and inspiration that lead others in establishing their psychological clinics, and soon, by the year 1914—before the beginning of World War I—there were 26 similar clinics in the United States.

However, the work done by Witmer and others in these psychological clinics was limited to helping children with learning disabilities and behavioral problems, and thus at this stage of its evolution, clinical psychology "was a glimmer, a baby just catching its first breath, drawing its life from the new science of psychology" (Reisman, 1991, p. 44).

At this beginning stage of clinical psychology, the task of providing treatment to patients with mental disorders and illness was considered to fall in the domain of psychiatrists and neurologists. However, with the growing influence of psychology in its applied form, clinical psychologists were also making inroads, due to their increasing skill at psychological assessment helpful in the diagnosis and identification of mental, emotional, and behavioral problems and disorders of affected individuals. The eruption of World War I in the year 1914 provided opportunity for them to make use of the available psychological assessment tools in the form of intelligence tests and personality assessment measures for recruiting the personnel for the nation's military. The success story of making use of such assessment tools proved too helpful in raising the reputations of clinical psychologists as assessment experts, and it led the task of assessment to become a core discipline of clinical psychology for the coming years, well up to eruption of World War II.

However, the situation changed when World War II broke out in 1939. Soldiers of the war-embroiled countries were found to be grappling with serious mental disturbances upon returning from combat, such as *posttraumatic stress disorder*. Family members of the soldiers fighting on the front were also found to develop symptoms of mental illness and disorders of various natures. Therefore, there was a great shortage of experts who could provide treatments to such great numbers of soldiers and civilians experiencing serious mental problems. Necessity is the mother of invention; all over the globe, demand rose for well-trained clinical psychologists to meet the requirements of the developing situation. Organized efforts for educating and training clinical psychologists to take charge of the diagnosis, assessment, and psychotherapeutic treatment of patients, were thus advanced during the period of 1946–50.

During this period the other mentionable development in the field of clinical psychology was the establishment of the American Association of Clinical Psychology in 1917. It was later merged in 1945 with the American Psychological Association (APA) in the form of its Division 12. Psychological societies and associations in other English-speaking countries developed similar divisions for clinical psychologist professionals, including Great Britain, Canada, Australia, and New Zealand.

World War I and II necessitated and brought significant changes and developments in the field of clinical psychology, not just in America but globally as well. The notable developments occurring in various aspects related to clinical psychology during the first half of the 20th century, such as classification and causation, diagnosis, assessment, and treatment of mental disorders as well as the professional training of clinical psychologists, are described subsequently.

1. Development of the Ways of Classifying Mental Illnesses and Disorders

The credit for first suggesting an official way of classifying mental illnesses and disorders goes to Emil Kraepelin (1855–1926), considered the "father of descriptive psychiatry" (Reisman, 1991, p. 30). He regarded mental diseases and disorders to be characterized by a group of symptoms called a syndrome. He also emphasized that each mental illness was distinct from others, with unique causes, symptoms, courses of treatment, and outcomes, in much the same way as of measles, smallpox, and similar physical ailments. He proposed a two-category system for the classification of mental illness and disorders—exogenous disorders (caused by external factors) and endogenous disorders (caused by internal factors)—and suggested that exogenous disorders were the far more treatable type than the endogenous disorders. Kraepelin also provided the nomenclature to the specific examples of disorders in the broad exogenous or endogenous categories such as *paranoia, manic depressive psychosis, involutional melancholia, cyclothymic personality*, and *autistic personality*, and thus set a precedent for the creation of diagnostic terms that eventually led to the evolution of the DSMs and ICDs in the coming years.

2. Developments in the Field of Assessment and Diagnosis

The task of clinical psychology during this period was facilitated by the development of assessment devices in the form of intelligence tests and personality assessment measures, as we shall now describe.

INTELLIGENCE TESTING

In 1905, Alfred Binet, along with Theodore Simon, created the Binet-Simon scale for testing intelligence. This test significantly distinguished children with intellectual disabilities from their typically developing peers. Later, in 1916, Lewis M. Terman revised and standardized Binet's test and published norms for it using sizable groups of children of different ages. Terman's revision was called the Stanford-Binet Intelligence Scales. For meeting the demand of testing the intelligence of adults, David Wechsler in 1939 developed an intelligence test named the Wechsler Adult Intelligence Scale (WAIS). In 1949, Wechsler released a children's version of his intelligence test named the Wechsler Intelligence Scale for Children (WISC). It included verbal as well non-verbal scales; not only could it assess one's overall IQ, but it could also provide subtest scores.

PERSONALITY ASSESSMENT

The task of assessing personality characteristics with the use of objective and projective techniques holds a unique significance in the diagnosis and assessment of mental illness and disorders. In this regard, the significant development taking place before the end of the first half of the 20th century may be described as follows.

- In 1921, Hermann Rorschach, a Swiss psychiatrist, published a test popularly known as the *Rorschach Inkblot test*, containing a set of ten inkblots. This test was based on the projective technique of assessing the personality.

- In 1935, Christiana Morgan and Henry Murray launched another projective technique-based personality assessment test known as Thematic Apperception Test (TAT), consisting of a number of cards depicting people in scenes or situations that could be interpreted in a wide variety of ways. Clients were asked to build stories on the basis of their own interpretation of the scene depicted in the cards for psychological assessment.s
- In 1949, Leopold Bellak and Sonya Sorel Bellak developed a projective test known as the Children Apperception Test (CAT) for assessing the personality characteristics of the children aged three to ten.
- Besides the aforementioned projective tests, there were several other projective technique-based tests that came into existence during the first half of the 20th century. The notable among them were the following.

   (i)   Goodenough's "draw-a-man" test developed by Florence Goodenough in the year 1926.
   (ii) Menninger Word Association Test developed by Raport, Gill, and Schafer in 1946.
   (iii) Machover "draw-a-person" test developed by Karen Machover in 1949.
   (iv) Rotter Incomplete Sentence Blank Test developed by Rotter and Rafferty in 1950.

- Along with the emergence of projective technique-based tests, objective personality tests also appeared on the scene during this period for carrying out the objective assessment of the personality characteristics of the clients in the form of well-standardized questionnaires and inventories. Among the most mentionable clinical assessment tools of this sort developed during the first half of the 20th century was the Minnesota Multiphasic Personality Inventory (MMPI). It was developed by Starke Hathaway and J. C. McKinley in 1943 and consists of 550 true/false statements (in its first version) for response on the part of the subjects.

3. Development in the Field of Psychotherapeutic Treatment

In the early development of the field of clinical psychology, the main focus of the work done by clinical psychologists was diagnosis and assessment, while the task of curing and treating people with mental illness was left entirely to medical professionals, physicians, and psychiatrists. Moreover, during this early period clinical psychologists were mostly working as academicians—engaging in teaching and research rather than as practitioners in the field of clinical psychology. It was not until the fallout of World War II that the need for enlisting the help of clinical psychologists in the task of curing and treating mental illness was aroused. The war-torn countries all over the globe were forced to take the services of the clinical psychologists for meeting the increased demand for mental health professionals, and for this purpose during the period of World War II and afterwards in the years of the mid-20th century, the use of psychotherapy rose to a more prominent place in the history of clinical psychology. The kind of psychotherapy that was first developed and employed by clinical psychologists was none other than the psychodynamic or psychoanalytic therapy created and popularized through the efforts of the famous psychoanalyst Sigmund Freud. The other psychotherapeutic approach available in the 1940s for the use of clinical psychologists was the client-centered or person-centered approach to psychotherapy developed and popularized by the humanitarian psychologist Carl R. Rogers.

4. Professional Development of the Field and Preparation of Clinical Psychologists

After its birth in the first half of the 20th century, the field of clinical psychology exhibited development in the field of professional development and preparation of clinical psychologist professionals in the manner as discussed next.

PROFESSIONAL DEVELOPMENT OF CLINICAL PSYCHOLOGY

In terms of the establishment of a professional body or organization in the field of clinical psychology, initiative on this account was taken in 1917 with the foundation of the American Association of Clinical Psychologists (AACP), with the purpose of establishing professional standards, in particular regarding the assessment and diagnostic activities on the part of clinical psychologists. It was later merged in 1945 with the American Psychological Association (APA) in the form of its Division 12. Psychological societies and associations in other English-speaking countries developed similar divisions for clinical psychologist professionals, including Great Britain, Canada, Australia, and New Zealand.

PREPARATION OF CLINICAL PSYCHOLOGIST PROFESSIONALS

In terms of organizing training and certification for clinical psychologist professionals there was a practice prevailing during the 1920s in some US universities to require a one-year, full-time internship as a necessary part of training for clinical psychologists who wished to provide services to the public. However, most university psychology departments were following the tradition of training clinical psychologists primarily for research rather than service activities. The situation changed after World War II with the initiation of a well-organized move to standardize training in clinical psychology, not only in the United States but also in other parts of the globe. In the United States, the American Psychological Association took responsibility of setting up a formal system for accrediting training in clinical psychology. The recommendations for such training put forward by the APA were formally ratified by a national conference held in Boulder, Colorado in 1949, resulting in the emergence of the "Boulder" or scientist-practitioner model of clinical training. In this way by the end of the first half of the 20th century, there became availability in the United States as well in elsewhere across the globe two types of models for the training and preparation of prospective clinical psychologist professionals, known as the PhD Clinical Science model (heavily focused on research), and the PhD science-practitioner model (integrating scientific research and practice). The adoption of these two models of clinical psychologist training helped in preparing students for entering careers involving both research and service, and thus enabling them to work either in universities teaching, in research departments, or in clinics as clinical practitioners.

To Sum Up

The credit for giving birth to clinical psychology goes to Lightner Witmer, who established the first clinical psychology clinic at the University of Pennsylvania in 1896. Besides this, Witmer is also known as the founder of the first scholarly journal in the field, *The Psychological Clinic* in 1907, as well as for authoring the discipline's first article, titled "Clinical Psychology," in which he established the term clinical psychology along with its definition. With his inspiration and leadership many more clinical psychology clinics were established soon in different parts of the United States. However, the work done in these clinics was very much limited to helping those with intellectual disabilities and children with behavioral problems. The task of providing treatment for cases of mental disorders and illness was considered to fall in the domain of psychiatrists and neurologists. The eruption of World War I and II in the year 1914 and 1949 created a great demand for experts who could make use of psychological tools such as intelligence and personality tests for recruiting military personnel, as well as providing treatments to vast numbers of soldiers and civilians suffering from serious mental problems. All over the globe, thus, the services of well-trained clinical psychologists grew to increasing demand. Adoption of necessary measures for their education and training, and efforts done in the field of experimentation and research in the first half of the 20th century, thus resulted in the following notable developments:

- Emil Kraepelin (1855–1926) for the first time ventured to provide a two-category system for the classification of mental illness and disorders in the name of exogenous disorders (caused by external factors) and endogenous disorders (caused by internal factors).
- Development in the field of clinical assessment devices in the form of intelligence tests, such as the Binet-Simon scale in 1905 (followed by its revision by Terman in 1916), the Wechsler Adult Intelligence Scale in 1939 (followed by its child version, WISC, in 1949). In the field of personality assessment, the mentionable developments were the Rorschach Inkblot test in 1921, TAT in 1935, MPPI in 1943, and CAT in 1949.
- The use of psychotherapy occupied a prominent place in the treatment of mental disorders, particularly in the form of psychoanalytic therapy popularized by Sigmund Freud, and the client-centered approach developed by the Carl R. Rogers.
- The formation of the American Association of Clinical Psychologists (AACP) in 1917 and its merger in 1945 with the American Psychological Association (APA) in the form of its Division 12. Besides this, the task of the preparation of clinical psychologist professionals in an organized way, picked up its momentum in the first half of the 20th century and consequently by the century's end, there became available in the United States as well in other parts of the globe two types of models for the training and preparation of clinical psychologists in the names of PhD Clinical Science model, and PhD science-practitioner model.

C. Development in Clinical Psychology from 1951 Onwards

The notable developments occurring in various aspects related to clinical psychology (such as classification and causation, diagnosis, assessment, and treatment of mental disorders, as well as the professional preparation of clinical psychologists for carrying out these tasks) from 1951 onwards may be outlined as follows.

1. Development in the Systems of Classifying Mental Illnesses and Disorders

The fall outs of the two world wars resulted in a tremendous increase of cases of mental illness and disorders, and the subsequent expansion of psychiatric services all over the world created an urgent need for a standardized system for the classification of mental illnesses and disorders for facilitating the treatment of these disorders and diseases with their proper symptom-based diagnosis. With the initiative taken in this regard by the American Psychiatric Association

(APA) and World Health Organization (WHO), two types of classification systems known as the DSM (Diagnostic and Statistical Manual of Mental Disorders) and the ICD (International Classification of Diseases), and their subsequent revisions, came into existence during the years after 1951, as follows.

- The first official publication of the Diagnostic and Statistical Manual of Mental Disorders in the name of DSM-1 was released by the APA in 1952. It contained the classification and diagnosis for 128 mental disorders and diseases. Since, then a number of revisions have been brought out by APA for meeting the increased demand of including the classification of newly discovered mental illnesses and disorders in the names of (i) DSM-II in 1968, (ii) DSM-III in 1980, (iii) DSM-III-R in 1987, (iv) DSM-IV in 1994, (v) DSM-TR in 2000, and (vi) the latest one, DSM-V in 2013, which contains the classification and diagnosis for 541 mental disorders and diseases.
- In 1865 the World Health Organization (WHO) published a classification system known as the International Classification of Diseases (ICD-8) containing Section V on mental disorders. It has been followed by a number of revisions in subsequent years for meeting increased demands of the description and classification of newly discovered ailments and diseases, such as (i) ICD-9 in 1977, (ii) ICD-10 in 2010, and (iii) the recent version, ICD-11 in 2019.

2. Development in the Field of Assessment and Diagnosis

The field of assessment and diagnosis in terms of the development and utilization of psychological tests in assessing intelligence and personality characteristics has also been enriched from 1951 onward, as described next.

INTELLIGENCE TESTING

In reference to intelligence testing the sequence of developments taking place since 1951 may be briefed as follows.

- During this period there appeared numerous revisions and re-standardizations of intelligence tests previously developed by Wechsler for adults, including the WAIS in 1955, the WAIS-R in 1981, the WAIS-III in 1997, and the WAIS-IV in 2008. Similarly, Wechsler's intelligence scale for children (WAIS) reappeared as the WISC-R in 1974, the WISC-III in 1991, the WISC-IV in 2003, and the WISC-V in 2014. Moreover, as a new development, in 1967, Wechsler developed an intelligence test for very young children named the Wechsler Preschool and Primary Scale of Intelligence (WPPSI). It was later revised in the years 1989, 2002, and 2012, respectively.
- In the year 2003, there occurred the most recent revision of the previously developed Stanford-Binet intelligence test in the name of the Stanford-Binet Intelligence Scales—Fifth Edition (SB5).
- Many more intelligence tests, verbal, nonverbal, and performance-based, were developed during this period. The most mentionable one, developed in the year 2015, is the Universal Nonverbal Intelligence Test-2 (UNIT-2). However, usage of such tests has remained uncommon in the field of clinical psychology. The Stanford-Binet and Wechsler tests are the only ones that have been in widespread use in their original and translated forms worldwide.

PERSONALITY ASSESSMENT

Regarding the development of testing devices for the assessment of personality characteristics of clients helpful in the diagnosis of their mental health problems, the developmental activities taking place from 1951 onward may be outlined as follows.

- Projective Tests: In the field of projective technique-based testing, the notable tests include (i) Michigan Picture Test, developed by G. Andrew and Associates in 1953, (ii) Kinetic Family Drawing Test (KFD) developed by R.C. Burns and S.H. Kaufman in the year 1970, (iii) Senior Apperception Technique (SAT) developed by L. Bellak. And S.S. Bellak in 1973, (iv) Rosenzweig Picture Frustration Study developed by S. Rosenzweig in 1978, and (v) Children's Apperception Story-Telling Test developed by M.F. Schneider in 1989.
- Objectivity Tests: Regarding the development of standardized objective tests progress entailed the following.

(1) Personality Inventories: The main clinical devices developed are outlined as follows.

   (i) In the continuity of its earlier publication, the second version of the Minnesota Multiphasic Personality Inventory was released in 1989 in the name of MMPI-2. It was followed in 1992 by its adolescent version, the Minnesota Multiphasic Personality Inventory-Adolescent (MMPI-A).
   (ii) Another personality assessment measure in the name of the NEO Personality Inventory (NEO-PI) was developed by P.T. Costa Jr. and R.R. McCrae in 1985. Its revised versions in the names of NEO-PI-R and NEO-PI-3 were brought out in 1992 and 2005, respectively.

(2) Use of specific measures: A number of instruments for the measurement of specific mental states and personality traits of clients have also been developed during this era, such as the Beck Depression Inventory developed by A.T. Beck and R.A. Steer in 1993, and the Beck Anxiety Inventory developed by A.T. Beck, R.A. Steer, and G.K. Brown in 1996.

3. Development in the Field of Psychotherapeutic Treatment

As described earlier, the early period of clinical psychology up to the first half of the 20th century saw two main types of psychotherapies—psychodynamic and client-centered humanistic therapies. On account of the reaction mounted against them for not being grounded on empiricism, and the emergence of behaviorism as the dominating force in the field of psychology, behavioral therapies (based on the principles of classical and operant conditioning) appeared with great force on the platform of clinical psychology during the periods of the 1950s and 1960s, and have occupied a significant place since then. In sequence, another significant approach and method of psychological treatment emerged in the 1970s in the name of modeling as a therapeutic technique. It was based on the principles of observational learning propagated in the year 1973 by the famous psychologist Albert Bandura. In the 1950s and 1960s, the dominance of psychodynamic and behavioral perspectives in the psychological treatment of mental disorders was challenged by cognitive psychology and its principles, paving the way for the emergence of cognitive and cognitive-behavioral therapies that began to flourish by the 1980s. Among the popular cognitive therapies being developed during this period, we may name Rational Emotive

Behavior Therapy (REBT), developed by Albert Ellis, and Cognitive Therapy, developed by Aaron Beck. Along with the use of these therapies applied to individuals on a person-to-person basis, there emerged other useful therapies at the beginning of the 21st century that could be applied to groups of individuals, on a collective and group-interaction basis. Mentionable among them were the emergence of Group Therapy and Family Therapy. We will be discussing the nature and use of such therapies in Chapter 19 of this text.

4. Professional Development of the Field and Preparation of Clinical Psychologists

Professional Development of Clinical Psychology

The professional organizations of clinical psychology organized as divisions of their respective psychological associations and societies during the 1940s in the United States. Since 1951, other countries of the world have embarked upon the realization of objectives set in the interest of the development of the clinical profession. In this mission, for the reputation and professional competency of clinical psychologists, the American Psychological Association published the first edition of its ethical code in 1953, in which it provided a significant discussion of clinical activities, reflecting a new level of professional establishment for clinical psychology (McFall, 2006). Another important activity undertaken on the part of such professional organizations is the publication of their official journal; notably, *The Journal of Abnormal Psychology*, a peer-reviewed scholarly journal in clinical psychology. It was started by Morton Prince in 1906 and later given by him to the American Psychological Association. The APA published another valuable peer-reviewed journal in clinical psychology, *The Journal of Consulting and Clinical Psychology*. Similar journals helpful in the professional development of clinical psychology are published by their respective professional organizations, such as the publication of *The British Journal of Clinical Psychology* by the British Psychological Society.

Preparation of Clinical Psychologist Professionals

Before the second half of the 20th century, in general, there were two types of models for the training and preparation of prospective clinical psychologists—the PhD Clinical Science model (focused heavily on research), and the PhD science-practitioner model (integrating scientific research and practice). Since then, the demand for clinical practitioners was increasing day by day, and a large number of prospective clinical professionals wanted to have a mode of training and preparation in which they might get more scope for building competency in clinical practice; the concept of a practice-oriented degree was thus on the rise and was debated in the 1960s on a large scale. Eventually, in the United States, a national conference at Vail, Colorado in 1973 endorsed this "practitioner" training model referred to as the PsyD practitioner-scholar model (focusing on clinical theory and practice), in which education and training programs, while including skills and a scientific understanding of psychology, would focus mainly on producing highly trained professionals, similar to programs in medicine and law. Similar training models leaning heavily on clinical practice were adopted soon in other parts of the world. For example, in the United Kingdom this trend yielded into a process of offering professional training and awarding Doctor of Clinical Psychology (DClin Psych.) to trainees for making them eligible to work as clinical professional practitioners.

To Sum Up

Development in clinical psychology from 1951 onwards in its various aspects

- This period saw the development of two types of classification systems, known as the DSM (developed by APA) and the ICD (developed by WHO), with their revised versions coming out from time to time. In 2019 the APA published the most recent edition, the DSM-5, and in 2019 the WHO published its recent revision in the name of the ICD-11.
- Regarding the developments taking place during this period in terms of intelligence and personality tests, we may find that in addition to the occasional revision of the previously developed measures, several new measures also came into existence. Among them, the notable ones were the Universal Nonverbal Intelligence Test-2, developed in 2015, and the NEO Personality Inventory (NEO-PI), which was first published in 1985, and its revised versions were brought out in 1992 and 2005. Additionally, measures like the Beck Depression Inventory and the Beck Anxiety Inventory were developed in 1993 and 1996 for the measurement of specific mental states and personality traits.
- During this period, several new approaches and treatment techniques were added to the previous options for methods of treatment. such as behavioral therapies, modeling techniques, and cognitive and cognitive-behavioral therapies in the 1960s, 1970s, and 1980s, respectively. The beginning of the 21st century witnessed the emergence of other useful therapies such as group therapy and family therapy for treating several individuals in a group.
- Regarding the professional development of the field during this period the noteworthy developments may be named as the publication of the APA's first edition of its ethical code in 1953, and the publication of *The Journal of Abnormal Psychology* (a peer-reviewed scholarly journal in clinical psychology) by Morton Prince in 1906, followed by the publication of *The Journal of Consulting and Clinical Psychology* on the part of the APA. Similar journals in clinical psychology such as *The British Journal of Clinical Psychology* were also published in other parts of the globe.
- Regarding the development in the field of preparation and training of clinical psychologists during this period, the most mentionable development may be named as the addition of a third model in 1993 in the name of the PsyD practitioner-scholar model, focusing on clinical theory and practice for producing highly trained clinical psychology professionals.

The Present Position and Developmental Status of Clinical Psychology

With its subsequential development, progress, and expansion, Clinical psychology at present is showing all-around progress and development in the various aspects and dimensions of its study and applications summarized in the manner as follows.

- It has risen to the full-fledged status of being an independent discipline in the realm of applied psychology.

- There has been quite a rise in terms of opportunities available for education and training in the discipline of clinical psychology at the graduate, postgraduate, and doctorate levels in universities and other institutions in the academic and clinical setup.
- Several useful streams or specializations have emerged, such as forensic psychology, child psychology, adolescent psychology, and health psychology.
- With the availability of the latest classification systems, research performed, and experiences gained in clinical psychology practice on the part of clinical psychology professionals and psychiatrists, there has been significant progress in the diagnosis and prognosis of mental illness and disorders.
- Improvement in the assessment methods and devices for carrying out diagnosis and estimation of the nature of a client's disorder, with the employment of sophisticated technological and digital means.
- Efficiency gained in the use of previously known psychotherapies by the clinical psychologists according to the need of the situation as well as their own preference and expertise.
- A growing trend on the part of clinical psychologists all over the globe for the use of psychotherapies in combination (either in eclectic or integrative ways), with full cognition of the nature of the client's disorder as well as his cultural belongingness.
- The running of three types of programs for the education and training of the prospective clinical psychology professional, namely (i) the traditional research-oriented PhD Clinical Science model (heavily focused on research), (ii) PhD science-practitioner model (integrating scientific research and practice), and (iii) PsyD practitioner-scholar model (heavily focused on clinical practice).
- The growing support for clinical psychologists to be authorized to write prescriptions for their clients, as do medical doctors/psychiatrists.
- The increasing use of sophisticated technological and digital means for the education and training of clinical psychologists as well as for the diagnosis, prognosis, prevention, and treatment of mental health problems.

To Sum Up

Regarding the present position and developmental status of clinical psychology we may find that with the increasing demand for clinical psychologists, there is a great expansion in terms of opportunities for their education and training worldwide, the acceptance of clinical psychology as a full-fledged discipline, and adoption of all three types of models (PhD Clinical Science model, PhD science-practitioner model, and PsyD practitioner-scholar model) available for this purpose. There has been all-around progress in the methods and techniques employed for the diagnosis and treatment of mental disorders in terms of the latest classification systems, assessment instruments, and psychotherapeutic measures. The trend is to employ an eclectic approach suiting the nature of the disorders of the clients, and make use of the latest research findings and technological means for dealing with their problems. Professionally, there has also been much rise in the status of clinical psychologists with the growing support of allowing them to write prescriptions to their clients much like medical doctors and psychiatrists.

Important Historical Events in the Creation and Development of Clinical Psychology

- Opening of the first psychological clinic at the University of Pennsylvania by Lightner Witmer in 1896.
- Publishing of Binet-Simon intelligence test in France in 1905.
- Launch of the first professional journal of clinical psychology, *The Psychological Clinic*, and coinage of the term clinical psychology in the first article of this journal by Lightner Witmer in 1907.
- Publishing of Stanford-Binet Intelligence Test (as translated by Terman) in the United States in 1916.
- Founding of American Association of Clinical Psychologists in 1917.
- Publishing of Rorschach inkblot technique in 1921.
- Publishing of Thematic Apperception Test in 1935.
- Publishing of Wechsler-Bellevue Intelligence Test for adults in 1939.
- Publishing of Minnesota Multiphasic Personality Inventory (MMPI) in 1943.
- Emergence of scientist-practitioner training model in Boulder conference held in 1949.
- Publishing of Children Apperception Test (CAT) by Leopold Bellak and Sonya Sorel Bellak in the year 1949.
- Prevalence of psychodynamic and client-centered humanistic therapies up to the first half of the 20th century.
- Emergence of behavioral therapies in the 1950s and 1960s.
- Publishing of Diagnostic and Statistical Manual of Mental Disorders (DSM) in 1952.
- Publishing of the first edition of its ethical code by American Psychological Association in 1953.
- Publishing of Wechsler Adult Intelligence Scale (WAIS) in 1955.
- Publishing of International Classification of Diseases (ICD-8) containing Section V on mental disorders by the WHO in 1965.
- Publishing of the DSM-II in 1968.
- Emergence of PsyD and practitioner-scholar training model in Vail conference held in 1973.
- Emergence of modeling as a therapeutic technique based on observational learning in 1973.
- Emergence and flourishing of cognitive and cognitive-behavioral therapies in the 1980s.
- Publishing of ICD-9 in the year 1977.
- Publishing of NEO Personality Inventory (NEO-PI) in 1985.
- Publishing of DSM-III in 1987, DSM-IV in 1994, and DSM-IV-R in 2000.
- Publishing of MMPI-2 in 1989 and MMPI-A in 1992.
- Emergence of Group Therapy and Family Therapy in the beginning of the 21st century.
- Publishing of WISC-IV in 2003 and WAIS-IV in 2008.
- Development of ICD-10 in the year 2010.
- Publishing of DSM-5 in 2013.
- Development of ICD-11 in the year 2019.

Development of Clinical Psychology in India—Historical Perspective

The Past and the Roots of Clinical Psychology in India

In its historical past, clinical psychology has passed through both bright and dark phases of its development in our country before its birth as a discipline and subject of study. In this concern, the Vedic and Upanishad periods of ancient India may be termed the brighter period in terms of the roots and historical past of clinical psychology's development. In the writings of the Rig Veda, the Upanishads, Ayurveda, Charak Sanhita, and other ancient religious scriptures, there are indications that there existed a sound system of caring for the mental health of people in our ancient past. It was based on the adoption of a holistic approach to the diagnosis and treatment of mental illness by taking care of the internal and external aspects of human beings, incorporating their mind, body, and soul. The main ideas and practices prevailing in this system may be summarized as follows:

1. In the Rig Veda we find description of surgical procedures. It also contains an important section about prayer as a method of promoting mental happiness, empowering the mind, and building intelligence to aid in the healing and quickness of the mind (Murthy, 2010).
2. In the Upanishads, we find a glimpse of modern ideas related to the science of mental health in the form of theories of consciousness, memory, thought, and perception. There is also description of the concept of personality (called "Prakriti") and the various mental states like dreaming state, waking state, deep sleep state, and Samadhi (Murthy, 2010; Avasthi et al., 2013).
3. According to Ayurveda (the ancient system of Indian medicine) a host of biological, physiological, and social factors may lend to the causation of mental illnesses and disorders. In this perspective, various forces in one's environment are said to interact with the individual, affecting their mind, body, and spirit in a complex way; therefore, the diagnosis, assessment, and treatment of mental health problems were holistic and complex, involving all the possible causative factors in a balanced way. To this end, Ayurveda advises maintaining balance between the five *bhutas* or elements constituting the human body—earth, fire, air, sky, and water—and the three *doshas* or humors— including wind (*vata*), bile (*pitta*), and phlegm (*kaph*)—by supporting the holistic functioning of the body, mind, and soul in a state of tranquility (Wig, 1989).
4. Rishi Charak, the well-known medical expert of ancient India, provided a useful account of this system in his writing Charak Sanhita. Let us look into it in reference to the causation, classification, and treatment of mental illnesses and disorders.

   (i) *Causation*: According to Charak, the factors responsible for the causation of mental illnesses and disorders may be stated as:

   - One's improper dietary intake (e.g., incompatible, vitiated, and unclean food substances)
   - One's improper conduct (e.g., disrespect to Gods, elders, and teachers)
   - Mental jerk or shock due to emotions such as excessive fear and joy
   - Faulty body activity.

   (ii) *Classification*: According to Charak, mental illness and disorders may be classified as:

   - Purely psychological and emotional disorders (e.g., inflicted with jealousy, fear, sense of inferiority, grief, etc.)

- Unspecified/exogenous disorders (mental illness or diseases caused by negative occurrences on account of the anger of Gods)
- Psychosomatic disorders such as compulsive-obsessive disorders, hysteria, epilepsy, and so on.

(iii) *Treatment:* Charak tried to propose the following types of treatment for these aforementioned disorders:

- For the treatment of psychological and emotional disorders he recommended the use of psychological means helpful in dealing with their psychological and emotional problems.
- For dealing with the unspecified/exogenous disorders, he recommended the use of a combination of ritual, religious, and spiritual practices such as chanting mantras, bearing precious stones, observing fasting, engaging in auspicious rites, providing offerings, worshiping Gods, and going on pilgrimages.
- For the treatment of psychosomatic disorders, he recommended the use of methods and processes such as cleansing of the body, using appropriate drugs, and adjuvant psychological strategies.

5. The Yoga Shastra, the treatise written by Maharishi Patanjali, provided an authentic and useful means and measure for the prevention and cure of mental health problems by adopting a comprehensive holistic approach focusing on their overall well-being. The eight-stage approach mentioned in this text for this emphasized practicing and absorbing oneself in the activities called Yam (observance of certain principles of conduct), Niyam (Disciplining the mind), Asans (practicing some postures), Pranayam (doing deep breathing exercises), Pratyahara (withdrawal from excessive sensual pleasures), Dharna (concentrating), Dhyan (meditation), and Samadhi (Seeking enlightenment) (Pandurangi et al., 2017).
6. In addition to this, evidence is also available that the system of diagnosing and curing the mentally ill through Indigenous approaches such as herbal or Ayurvedic medicines, yoga, and music prevailed for thousands of years after the ancient Vedic age (Prasadarao and Sudhir, 2001).

In this way, we may see that several useful things were emphasized and practiced in our ancient past for acquainting us with the causation, prevention, diagnosis, and treatment of mental health problems. Many of them are still quite relevant, practical, and fruitful in their usage, not only in the task of preventing and curing mental disorders but also in achieving the goal of overall happiness and well-being for practitioners.

However, in later eras, with the diminishing influence of the preaching and practices prevailing in the ancient Vedic period, and the dominance of religious institutions and ruling classes (known for their ulterior motive of subjugating and befooling the masses), there emerged an extended period of superstitions and misbelief regarding the identification and treatment of abnormality, mental illness, and disorders in the manner as prevalent in the other civilizations of the world. Accordingly, there happened instances in Indian history where we blamed devils, evil spirits, and other supernatural powers as responsible for mental illness and abnormality in one's behavior. It was thus quite customary during this period to involve *priests* and *tantriks* for employing their own invented techniques to make the body of the sufferer so unholy or unpleasant a place that spirits would be driven out. The dark period of such superstition and misbelief continued to dominate the field of causation, diagnosis, and treatment of people with mental illness, right up to the arrival of the scientific era, the emergence of the humane outlook, and the spread of education which brought clinical psychology to the entire world.

To Sum Up

Regarding the historical past of clinical psychology in our country, it may be inferred from the writings of the RigVeda, Upanishads, Ayurveda, Charak Sanhita, Yoga Shastra, and other ancient religious scriptures that there existed a sound system of caring for the mental health of people in our ancient past. It was based on a holistic approach regarding the causation, prevention, diagnosis, and treatment of mental illness by taking care of the internal and external aspects of human beings, incorporating their mind, body, and soul. The things suggested and practiced at that time are still quite relevant and fruitful in their use, not only in the task of preventing and curing mental disorders but also in achieving the target of overall happiness and well-being. However, at a later stage, the ways of caring for mental health passed through dark periods, much like the practices prevalent in other civilizations of the world. Accordingly, there occurred instances in Indian history where we in India were found to believe in devils, evil spirits, and other supernatural powers responsible for mental illness and abnormality in one's behavior, and thereby involved *priests* and *tantriks* for dealing with mental disorders by employing their own strange means and techniques. The dark period of such superstition and misbelief continued to dominate the field right up to the emergence of the scientific era, and the arrival of the modern wave of education in which clinical psychology emerged on the world stage.

The Development of Clinical Psychology in British and Independent India

Upon its creation through the efforts of Lightner Witmer, clinical psychology was getting well on the path of development in the early decades of the 20th century in the United States and Great Britain, while our country was reeling under the subjugation of the British rulers. Therefore, what was transferred to us in terms of the study and practice of psychology and its offshoot of clinical psychology was nothing but the reflection and continuation of what was available to our scholars and students through opportunities to study in Great Britain and the United States. With the advantage and influence of such opportunities, it was the University of Calcutta that took a lead in establishing psychology as an academic discipline in the year 1915 by having the first Department of Psychology under the leadership of Dr. N.N. Sengupta, who had worked under Professor Hugo Munsterberg, a former student of William Wundt (the Founder of the first psychology laboratory in the world). The establishment of psychology as an independent discipline of study rather than being a part of the department of philosophy actually opened the gates of study and research into many of its applied offshoots, including clinical psychology. The progress in this direction was continued under the leadership of Dr. Girindra Shekhar Bose, who succeeded Dr. N.N. Sengupta at Calcutta University. A medical practitioner in the field of clinical psychology, he tried to establish himself as the first clinical psychologist in India by initiating the practice of western psychotherapy in the country. Because of his professional background as a psychoanalyst and his close contact with Sigmund Freud, Mr. Bose became a pioneer in the field of psychoanalysis. He started a postgraduate course in psychoanalysis at Calcutta University, and in 1922 founded the Indian Psychoanalytical Society, affiliated with the International Psychoanalytic Association. As a further boost for the development of the study and research in psychology, it began to be considered as a separate section in the Indian Science

Congress in 1923. Another big development in the field of psychology in India was the founding of the Indian Psychological association in 1924, as well as *The Indian Journal of Psychology* a year later. In subsequent developments during this period of British rule, more psychology departments were established in other Indian universities such as Mysore University, Madras University, and Patna University in the years 1924, 1943, and 1946, respectively, providing opportunities for study and research in clinical psychology for those interested.

After gaining independence in 1947, the study and research in psychology and its applied branches, including clinical psychology, caught momentum with the establishment of departments of psychology in several Indian Universities, an encouraging increase to 32 departments by 1960. At present, it has increased significantly, as most Indian universities, including private ones, now have departments of psychology with an optional paper in the name of clinical psychology. The other notable developments in the field of clinical psychology and mental health may be accounted as follows.

1. The government of India established the All India Institute of Mental Health at Bangalore, currently known as the National Institute of Mental Health and Allied Neuro-Sciences (NIM-HANS). In the year 1955, advanced training programs in the field of clinical psychology were introduced to this institution. Since its inception, this institution has played a major role in training prospective clinical psychologists and providing psychotherapeutic services to patients in need.

2. Another national-level institute known as the Central Institute of Psychiatry, Ranchi (renamed as such on April 1, 1977 from its previous name Hospital for Mental diseases, Ranchi) has also played a significant role in promoting the cause of clinical psychology development in India since its inception and working as a mental hospital for the mentally ill. Before independence, it was operating under the name of the European Mental Hospital and serving the cause of European and Anglo-Indian Patients. After independence, the name European Mental Hospital was changed to Inter-Provincial Mental Hospital in 1948, and the hospital was opened to all Indians. It was subsequently renamed the Hospital for Mental Diseases in 1952, and in 1954 its administration was taken over by the Government of India. At present the institute is functioning under the administrative control of the Directorate General of Health Services, Ministry of Health and Family Welfare, New Delhi, with the objectives of patient care, manpower development, and research in the field of mental health. With regard to the training of prospective clinical psychologists, it is running postgraduate training courses (which started in 1962) with a Diploma in Psychological Medicine (DPM) and Diploma in Medical and Social Psychology. As a further development, the Diploma in Psychiatric Social Work (DPSW) was started in 1970 followed by MD (Psychiatry) in 1971, PhD in Clinical Psychology in 1973, and Diploma in Psychiatric Nursing (DPN) in 1983.

3. The development of psychology and its applied branches including clinical psychology took a big leap in the year 1969 with the establishment and functioning of the Indian Council of Social Science Research (ICSSR). It began supporting research, training, and publications in the social sciences including psychology. Academic and research work in psychology was, thus, now open to receiving assistance from this national-level organization, including descriptions and reviews in publications such as *The Periodical Survey of Psychological Research* and the journal *Indian Psychological Abstracts and Reviews*.

4. Besides this, another contribution regarding the progress and development in the field of psychology emerged on the scene in the form of the beginning of MPhil and Doctoral Programs with coursework in the discipline among the Indian universities from the 1970s onwards.

It helped much in training future leaders and providing opportunities to scholars for doing research work in the field of psychology and its applied branches, including clinical psychology.

5. In addition, the establishment of psychological associations and the publication of journals in the field of psychology in our country must also be credited for the development of clinical psychology in India. The important events in this concern include (i) the establishment of the Indian Psychological Association (IPA) in 1925 and the commencement of their publication of *The Indian Journal of Psychology (IJP)* in 1926, (ii) the establishment of the Madras Psychology Society in 1944 their publication of *The Journal of Psychological Researches* in 1957 as well as *The Indian Journal of Applied Psychology* beginning in 1964, (iii) the establishment of the Indian Association of Clinical Psychologists (IACP) in the year 1968, (iv) the launch of the journal named *The Journal of Indian Psychology* in the mid-1970s, (v) the formation of the Association of Professional Psychologists in the year 1985, (vi) the establishment of an important psychological organization in the name of the National Academy of Psychology (NAOP) in 1989, (vii) the formation of the National Association of Psychological Science (NAPS) in 2010, and (viii) the establishment of the Association of Indian Psychologists in 2013.

6. After independence there have been major attempts to frame legislative measures for the proper living, treatment, and rehabilitation of persons experiencing mental health problems, illnesses, and disorders. Mentionable in this connection is the enactment of the Indian Lunacy Act of 1912, the Mental Health Act of 1987, and the Mental Health Care Act of 2017.

7. Until the mid-1980s in our country, the public viewed psychology primarily as a remedy for abnormal behavior. Therefore, in the early days, psychology in its applied form was mainly used in clinical settings, and courses focused on training clinical psychologists. In this concern, a mentionable event is the provision made by NIMHANS, Bangalore to teach a postgraduate diploma in medical psychology as a full-time course with supervised internship training in clinical psychology during the 1960s, and the MPhil in clinical psychology as a full-time training course in clinical psychology since 2000. Another national-level institute, the Ranchi Institute of Neuro-Psychiatry and Allied Sciences, is also known for providing such courses and training provisions for clinical psychologists. The provision of training programs and academic learning facilities for clinical psychologists has picked up speed with the establishment of the Rehabilitation Council of India (RCI), a statutory body enacted in 1993 through the RCI Act by the Parliament of India. RCI has been authorized to issue a certified license for doing practice and getting recognized as a clinical psychologist professional in the country to the intended candidates. To become eligible for such a license one is required to earn a degree in the name of MPhil in Clinical psychology or a doctoral degree in Clinical psychology (PsyD). RCI is responsible for drafting the prescribed courses and training programs for these degrees, and also issues sanctions to academic institutions for running these courses. With the establishment and functioning of the RCI with such objectives of standardized training programs and preparation of clinical psychologists, there has been a tremendous increase in the number of academic institutions eligible for running MPhil and doctoral degrees in clinical psychology in government as well as private setups (recognized by the Rehabilitation Council of India, New Delhi, and affiliated Indian universities recognized by the University Grant Commission). The departments of psychology working in various universities all over the country are also running specialized courses in clinical psychology in their MA, MPhil, and PhD courses with the provision of providing students opportunities for doing research and gaining experiences in clinical settings. As a result, there has been a substantial increase in the number of professionals working as clinical psychologists in our country, with a considerable increase in research and practice in the area of clinical psychology.

To Sum Up

Regarding the development of clinical psychology in British India, the initiation occurred with the establishment of the first Department of Psychology (with the acceptance of psychology as an independent discipline) at Calcutta University in 1915, under the leadership of Dr. N.N. Sengupta. Later, his successor, Dr. GirindraShekar Bose, established himself as the first clinical psychologist in India by initiating the practice of western psychotherapy in the country. He started a course in psychoanalysis for postgraduate study in psychology at Calcutta University, and in 1922 he founded the Indian Psychoanalytical Society with its affiliation with the International Psychoanalytic Association. As a matter of another big development in the field of psychology in India, the Indian Psychological association was founded in 1924, and *The Indian Journal of Psychology* appeared a year later. Subsequent developments during this period of British rule saw more departments of psychology established in other Indian universities, such as Mysore University, Madras University, and Patna University in the years 1924, 1943, and 1946, respectively, providing those interested with opportunities for study and research in clinical psychology.

After gaining independence in 1947, study and research in psychology and its applied branches including clinical psychology caught momentum with the establishment of departments of psychology in several Indian Universities with an optional paper in the name of clinical psychology in postgraduate studies. Other mentionable developments in the field of clinical psychology and mental health may be accounted as (i) the starting of advanced training programs in the field of clinical psychology by the National Institute of Mental Health and Allied Neuro-Sciences (NIMHANS) in 1955, (ii) the establishment of the Indian Association of Clinical Psychologists (IACP) in 1968 (iii), the establishment and functioning of Indian Council of Social Science Research (ICSSR) since 1969 with the purpose of supporting research, training, and publications in the social sciences including psychology, (iv) the beginning of MPhil and Doctoral Programs with coursework in the discipline among Indian universities from 1970s onwards, (v) the functioning of an important national-level institute known as the Central Institute of Psychiatry, Ranchi since 1971, with the objectives of patient care, manpower development, and research in the field of mental health, (vi) the enactment of the Indian Lunacy Act of 1912, Mental Health Act of 1987, and Mental Health Care Act of 2017 for the proper living, treatment, and rehabilitation of persons suffering from mental health problems, (vii) starting of the journal named *The Journal of Indian Psychology* in the mid 1970s, (viii) the establishment of the Association of Indian Psychologists in the year 2013, and (ix) the establishment of RCI as the national authority to issue a certified license for doing practice and getting recognized as a clinical psychologist professional in the country after earning a degree, in the name of MPhil. in clinical psychology or a doctoral degree in clinical psychology (PsyD), from the institutes recognized by RCI and affiliated to Indian universities recognized by the University Grant Commission.

Important Events in the Development of Clinical Psychology in India

- The establishment of a separate department of psychology in Calcutta University in 1916, headed by Professor N.N. Sengupta.

- Foundation of the Indian Psychological Association in the year 1924.
- Publication of the first psychology journal in India, *The Indian Journal of Psychology* in 1926.
- Establishment of Departments of Psychology in Mysore University, Madras University, and Patna University in the years 1924, 1943, and 1946.
- Introduction of a certificate course in Applied and Abnormal Psychology in Calcutta University in 1945.
- Introduction of a one-year program in clinical psychology in BHU in 1951.
- Starting of the first postgraduate course in clinical psychology in AIIMH (now NIMHANS) in 1955.
- Establishment of the National Institute of Mental Health and Neuroscience (NIMHANS) at Bangalore in 1955.
- Establishment of the Hospital for Mental Diseases in Ranchi in the year 1962.
- Replication of the program for clinical psychology in the Central Institute of Psychiatry, Ranchi in 1962.
- Establishment of the Association of Clinical Psychologists in 1968.
- Establishment and functioning of the Indian Council of Social Science Research (ICSSR) in 1969 in the form of support giving agency for research, training, and publications in the field of Social Sciences, including psychology.
- Starting of MPhil and Doctoral Programs with coursework in the discipline among Indian universities and higher institutions (including IITs) from the 1970s onwards.
- Enforcement of legislative measures in the name of the Mental Health Act of 1987.
- Establishment of the National Academy of Psychology (NAOP) in 1989.
- Establishment of the National Association of Psychological Science (NAPS) in 2010.
- Establishment of the Association of Indian Psychologists (AIP) in 2013.
- Enactment of the Mental Health Care Act of 2017 by the Indian Parliament.

However, what has occurred in the field of clinical psychology after gaining independence in the country so far is in no way said to be a satisfactory affair. It needs to be pushed and revolutionized in tune with the present-day situations and needs of our country in the manner as briefed next.

- With the sudden arrival of dreadful viral diseases such as Covid-19 and its numerous variants, conflicts, and clashes among groups and countries, terrorism and religious fanaticism, unhealthy and competition-based improper lifestyle, there has been a rise in cases related to mental health problems, illness, and disorders. We need more mental health and specialized clinical psychology professionals for taking care of these rising cases. A special initiative therefore should be launched for creating more opportunities and places for the education and training of clinical psychologists and mental health professionals. There should be a sizable increase in the establishment of clinical psychology departments in universities (private and public sectors) and other apex national institutes with increased opportunities of earning MPhil and doctoral degrees in clinical psychology. However, with such expansion, it should also be remembered that the quality of the training should not get sacrificed; it should essentially match the expertise needed for taking care of the complexity of mental health cases.

- There is a significant need for preparing clinical psychology professionals for working among various client populations of the country. We have significant cultural diversity among the client population as well as variations in the etiology of mental health cases, requiring much sensitivity in providing the needed psychotherapeutic treatment to clients. We may need Indigenous ways of treating them, as many of the westernized ways and methods may not be applied to all clients in their typical mode.
- We are in need of revolutionizing the types of research carried out at present in the field of clinical psychology in our country. The blind imitation of work done abroad should be discouraged and stopped. We should create through our research endeavors what we truly need for the diagnosis, assessment, prevention, and treatment of mental health problems of the Indian people in the best and most economic way possible. For providing required boosts to research programs, there should be substantial increase in research-promoting agencies in both public and private sectors, including more professional organizations, associations, and reputed research journals. Besides this we here in India essentially need the functioning of a responsible professional organization much like American Psychiatric Association.
- There is a need to take stock of the competency of clinical psychology practitioners in a more objective and sincere way, such as enforcing immediate bans on self-styled practitioners by regulating and framing a legal code of conduct and creating a more conducive and functioning national licensing board. For this purpose, there is a need to establish an autonomous body involving the collaborative efforts of government machinery (e.g., the Medical council), the Indian Psychological Association, and the Indian Association of Clinical Psychologists. Besides this, In India, there is a need for a professional body (much like the American Psychological Association or British Psychological Society) to become involved in guiding research and formulating training, certifying and improving the continuous professional development of clinical psychologists.
- Much attention must be paid to technological advancement and digital technology in the theory and practice of clinical psychology. The education and training of clinical psychology professionals, as well as research and clinical practice work (involving diagnosis, prognosis, prevention, and treatment of mental health problems), should be guided by technological advancement and digital technology available for this purpose.

To Sum Up

What we have at present in the field of clinical psychology needs to be pushed further in tune with the present-day situations and needs of our country in the manner such as:

(i) Making sincere attempts to create more opportunities and places for the education and training of clinical psychologists and mental health professionals, (ii) Researching and adopting Indigenous ways of dealing with and treating the culturally diversified population of our country, (iii) Bringing improvement to the type and methodology of clinical psychology research, in tune with the needs and applicability of Indian clients, (iv) Adopting more appropriate and valid measures for competency certifications to work as clinical psychology practitioners by framing laws and codes of conduct, and creating a more conducive and functioning national licensing board, and (v) Laying more emphasis on the use of technological advancement and digital means in the theory and practice of clinical psychology.

Table 3.1 Clinical Psychology Journals (Published in India and Abroad)

Name of the Journal	Year of First Publication– Status at Present	Frequency of Publication	The Present Publisher/Sponsor or Collaborator
1. Journal of Consulting and Clinical Psychology	1937–Present	Monthly	American Psychological Association, USA
2. Journal of Clinical Psychology	1945–Present	Monthly	John Wiley &Sons
3. Indian Journal of Clinical Psychology	1974–Present	Biannually	Indian Association of Clinical Psychologists
4. Indian Journal of Psychological Medicine	1978–Present	Bimonthly	Sage Publishers on behalf of Indian Psychiatric Society
5. British Journal of Clinical Psychology (formerly called British Journal of Social and Clinical Psychology)	1981–Present	Quarterly	Wiley-Blackwell on behalf of the British Psychological Society, UK
6. Clinical Psychology Review	1981–Present	Monthly	Elsevier, Amsterdam, Netherlands
7. Journal of Social and Clinical Psychology	1983–Present	Bimonthly	Guilford Publications Inc. New York
8. Clinical Psychology & Psychotherapy	1993–Present	Bimonthly	John Wiley &Sons
9. Clinical Psychologist	1993–Present	Quarterly	Australian Psychological Society's College of Clinical psychologists
10. Journal of New Zealand College of Clinical Psychologists	1993–Present	Half Yearly	Clinical Psychology Association, New Zealand
11. Clinical Psychology— Science and Practice	1994–Present	Quarterly	Wiley-Blackwell, New York
12. Journal of Clinical Psychology in Medical Settings	1994–Present	Quarterly	Springer, New York
13. Clinical Child and Family Psychology	1998–Present	Quarterly	Springer, Berlin, New York
14. Clinical Psychological Science	2013–Present	Bimonthly	Sage Publications on behalf of the Association for Psychological Science, USA

Clinical Psychology Associations (Working in India and Abroad)

1. **The American Psychological Association (APA):** This is the largest scientific and professional organization of psychologists, including clinical psychologists, in the United States. It was founded in 1982 and has its headquarters in Washington, D.C. It serves the interests of the profession of Clinical Psychology with the special provision of establishing specialized professional organizations, such as the following:

   (i) The **Society of Clinical Child and Adolescent Psychology** (SCCAP) first appeared in the American Psychological Association under the division of clinical psychology (Division 12) in 1962. However, for meeting the increased need for encouraging the development and advancement of clinical child and adolescent psychology, it later was listed separately in Division 53 of the American Psychology Association.

(ii) **The Society of Clinical Psychology** Division 12 of the APA includes APA members who are active in practice, research, teaching, administration, and/or study in the field of clinical psychology. Membership includes a subscription to the journal, *Clinical Psychology: Science and Practice*, and the quarterly publication *The Clinical Psychologist*.

2. **Association for Psychological Science (previously called The American Psychological Society):** This is a professional organization of American psychologists including clinical psychologists. It was founded in 1988 and its headquarters are located in Washington, D.C. A mentionable contribution of this organization is the running of the National Institute of Mental Health Centers for Behavioral Science Research, helping to translate basic behavioral science into its applications.

3. **American Mental Health Counselors Association (AMHCA):** This is a professional organization of clinical mental health professionals, particularly licensed mental health counselors, in the United States. Besides publishing a popular journal called *The Journal of Mental Health Counseling*, it also enforces standards of education, licensing, and ethics for American mental health counselors. It was founded in 1976. Its headquarters are located in Alexandria, Virginia.

4. **British Psychological Society (BPS):** This is a representative body and the main professional organization for psychologists including clinical psychologists working in the United Kingdom. It was founded in 1901. Its headquarters are located at St Andrews House, 48 Princess Road, East Leicester, United Kingdom. **The Division of Clinical Psychology** is the largest division within the BPS. It is subdivided into thirteen faculties serving the objective of promoting mental health and welfare in every aspect.

5. **Australian Psychological Society (APS):** This is the largest representative body and professional organization for psychologists including clinical psychologists in Australia. It was founded in 1966 and presently has its headquarters located at Level 11, 257 Collins Street, Melbourne, Australia. Three important journals are published by APS, namely *The Australian Journal of Psychology*, *Australian Psychologist*, and *Clinical Psychologist*.

6. **Indian Psychoanalytical Society:** This is a professional organization of clinical psychologists in India. It was founded in 1922 by Dr. Girindrashekhar Bose. Its headquarters are located at ParsiBagan Ln Machuabazar, Kolkata, West Bengal. It is affiliated with the International Psychoanalytical Association and is devoted to serving the cause of mental healthcare and treatment of mental disorders. It provides affiliation with a six-month certificate course on the basic theories of psychoanalysis, conducted by the Department of Psychology at West Bengal State University, Barasat.

7. **Indian Association of Clinical Psychologists (IACP):** This is a well-reputed national organization of clinical psychologists belonging to India with the objective of promoting mental health. It was founded in 1968. It is well known for its flagship publication, a journal entitled *The Indian Journal of Clinical Psychology* (IJCP).

Review Questions

1. Provide a detailed description of the historical development, before the birth of clinical psychology as a discipline, regarding the diagnosis and treatment of mental illness and disorders.
2. Discuss the birth of clinical psychology at the hands of Lightner Witmer and throw light on the subsequent development occurring in the field of clinical psychology in the earlier half of the 20th century.

3. Provide a detailed description of the development occurring in the various aspects of clinical psychology during the period of 1951 onwards.
4. Discuss the present position and developmental status of clinical psychology.
5. "We in India, have a glorious past in dealing with the mental health of the people"—justify this statement by describing what was happening in our glorious past.
6. Discuss the roots of clinical psychology and its past in our country.
7. Throw light on the development of clinical psychology in British India and describe in detail what happened after gaining independence.
8. Give an account of the clinical journals published as well as clinical psychology associations working in India and abroad.

References

Avasthi, A., Grover, S., & Kate, N. (2013), Indianization of psychiatry utilizing Indian mental concepts, *Indian Journal of Psychiatry*, 55: 136–144.

McFall, R. M. (2006), Doctoral training in clinical psychology, *Annual Review of Clinical Psychology*, 2: 21–49.

McReynolds, P. (1997), *Lightner Witmer: His life and times*, Washington, DC: American Psychological Association.

Murthy, S. (2010), From local to global contributions of Indian Psychiatry to International Psychiatry, *Indian Journal of Psychiatry*, 52: 30–37.

Pandurangi, A., Keshavan, M., Ganapathy, V., & Gangadhar, B. (2017), Yoga: Past and present, *American Journal of Psychiatry*, 174: 16–17.

Prasadarao, P. S. D. V., & Sudhir, P. M. (2001), Clinical psychology in India, *Journal of Clinical Psychology in Medical Settings*, 8(1): 31–38.

Reisman, J. M. (1991), *A history of clinical psychology* (2nd ed.), New York, NY: Hemisphere.

Wig, N. (1989), Indian concepts of mental health and their impact on care of the mentally ill, *International Journal of Mental Health*, 18: 71–80.

Chapter 4

Research and Methods of Investigation in Clinical Psychology

Learning Objectives

After going through this chapter, you will be able to:

- Define research or investigation.
- Name the goals of clinical psychology research or investigation.
- Name the different types or kinds of research conducted in clinical psychology.
- Name and discuss the different methods used in clinical psychology research or investigation.
- Discuss the nature and use of the experimental method in the studies of clinical psychology.
- Throw light on the nature and use of the systematic or naturalistic observation method in clinical psychology studies.
- Explain how the survey method can be used as a method of investigation in clinical psychology.
- Elucidate the use of the correlation method in clinical psychology research studies.
- State the nature and application of the case study method in clinical psychology research studies.
- Describe the meta-analysis method used in clinical psychological research.
- Reflect on the ethical issues in clinical psychology research.

What is Research or Investigation?

The word research in its simple meaning stands for inquiring about or learning something new about a thing, person, phenomenon, or event. The generalized day-to-day meaning of the word research may emerge through examples of people finding answers to their queries, in the situations like the following:

1. A housewife may try to know what combinations of sugar, salt, or food contents make a dish tasty and presentable.
2. A coach may try to find out the best possible way to provide coaching to his hockey team.
3. A worker may try to find out the technique of getting better output from the machine.

DOI: 10.4324/9781003398325-4

4. A traveler may try to find out the shortest way of his journey.
5. A clinical psychologist may try to find the best possible mode of psychotherapy used for the treatment of their client.
6. A teacher may try to find out the best method of teaching their students.

> **Research or scientific investigation**
>
> A well-thought out scientific process involving definite steps for arriving at something new or adding modifications to the existing stock of knowledge helpful in solving the confronted problems.

All the above individuals are trying to find solutions to their problems. In other words, it may be said that all are engaged in the task of inquiry or research in their own way. However, as far as the real meaning of the concept of inquiry or research is concerned, it is quite possible that none of the above persons are carrying out research in its true sense. They may seek a solution to their problems or answer to their queries from experts in their respective fields or may acquire the desired knowledge from reading literature or get it through mere chance and trial.

Let us now consider some dictionary definitions and the writings of well-known authors for understanding the meaning of the term research or scientific investigation in a proper way.

The Advanced Learner's Dictionary (1952:1089): Research is "careful investigation or inquiry especially through search for new facts in any branch of knowledge."

Merriam Webster Seventh New Collegiate Dictionary (1966:730): Research is a "careful or diligent search" or "studious inquiry or examination; especially investigation or experimentation aimed at the discovery and interpretation of facts, revision of accepted theories or laws in the light of new facts, or practical application of such new or revised theories or laws."

Young (1966:15): Research is "the systematic method of discovering new facts or verifying the old facts, their sequence, interrelationships, causal explanations and the natural laws which govern them."

Kothari (1990:20): "The term research refers to the systematic method consisting of enunciating the problem, formulating a hypothesis, collecting the facts or data, analysing the facts and reaching certain conclusions either in the form of solution(s) toward the problem concerned or in certain generalizations for some hypothetical formulations."

Best and Kahn (2006:25): "Research may be defined as the systematic and objective analysis and recording of controlled observations that may lead to the development of generalizations, principles, or theories, resulting in prediction and possibly ultimate control of events."

A close analysis of the definitions provided above may reveal the following things about the meaning and nature of the term research or scientific inquiry.

- Research is always conducted with a definite purpose or objective in view. It is aimed to serve purposes such as (i) to provide the answer to the question raised and problems felt, (ii) to seek reliable information or acquire new knowledge of a subject or its utilization for the needed practical applications.

- Research is not conducted in a haphazard way. It represents systematized efforts, studious inquiry or examination, and scientific or critical investigation involving well-planned and definite steps of a scientific method or approach for realizing its set goals or objectives.
- Research is a process and not a product. It can be employed as a tool, means, or method of manipulating the things, concepts, and available data for arriving at reliable and valid conclusions for serving the goals or objectives of the research.

After getting, acquainted with what research is, it becomes essential for us to examine some of the pertinent questions regarding the conduct of research work in clinical psychology in the form of:

1. What are the purposes or goals of research studies in clinical psychology?
2. What types or kinds of research are undertaken in clinical psychology?
3. What methods and techniques are used in collecting information or data in clinical psychology research?
4. What is Meta-Analysis as a method used by researchers in clinical psychology for the reliability and validity of research findings?
5. What type of ethical principles or codes of conduct need to be observed on the part of researchers in clinical psychology?

Let us try to seek answers to these questions one by one.

Goals of Clinical Psychology Research or Investigation

As said earlier in defining the term, research is a purposeful activity undertaken for serving concrete objectives and goals. Now the question arises, what purposes or goals are aimed for, in general, on the part of clinical psychologist researchers? The research work carried out in this concern must help clinical psychologists in their professional preparation and effective exercising of their functions as professional clinical psychologists, such as knowing and understanding the various types of psychological disorders, their prevalence, characteristic symptoms and syndromes, causes of their occurrence, methods of their assessment and diagnosis, and the ways and approaches utilized for their treatment. In light of these different functions associated with research work in clinical psychology, the goals and objectives served through clinical psychology research may be summed up as follows.

1. To gain knowledge and understanding about the existence and prevalence of various types of mental disorders
2. To study the prevalence of one or the other type of mental disorders in a particular segment of the society or population.
3. To gain knowledge and understanding about the symptoms and syndromes related to mental disorders.
4. To gain knowledge and understanding about the causation and development of mental disorders.
5. To help in building systems of classifying mental disorders and investigate the appropriateness of the existing systems of classification.
6. To help in developing methods or devices for the clinical assessment and diagnosis of mental disorders including judging the effectiveness of the available methods.

7. To help in devising necessary measures for the prevention of one or the other types of mental disorders.

8. To help in developing methods or devices for the treatment of mental disorders including judging the relative effectiveness of the available psychotherapies.

9. To assess the appropriateness of the available modes of educating and training clinical psychologists and help in building more suitable ones.

10. To investigate and explore issues related to the professional organization of clinical psychologists and the ethical standards maintained in their clinical practice.

The Types or Kinds of Research Undertaken in Clinical Psychology

The types or kinds of research undertaken in clinical psychology may be broadly classified as experimental research and non-experimental research. Experimental research may be further categorized as experimental and quasi-experimental research, and in the category of non-experimental research we may put the researches like (i) Epidemiological research, (ii) Descriptive or normative survey research, (iii) Developmental research (Longitudinal and Cross-sectional), (iv) Correlational research, and (v) Case study research.

Let us discuss these types of clinical research.

Experimental Research: This type of research in clinical psychology is undertaken to establish the existence and demonstration of a cause-and-effect relationship between two variables of the research study, referred to as independent and dependent variables. One must manipulate the independent variable while observing or measuring the subsequent changes in the dependent variable to know whether or not the changes in the independent variable are accompanied by the changes in the dependent variable. For having valid observations (change in the independent variable causing or not causing change in the dependent variable),

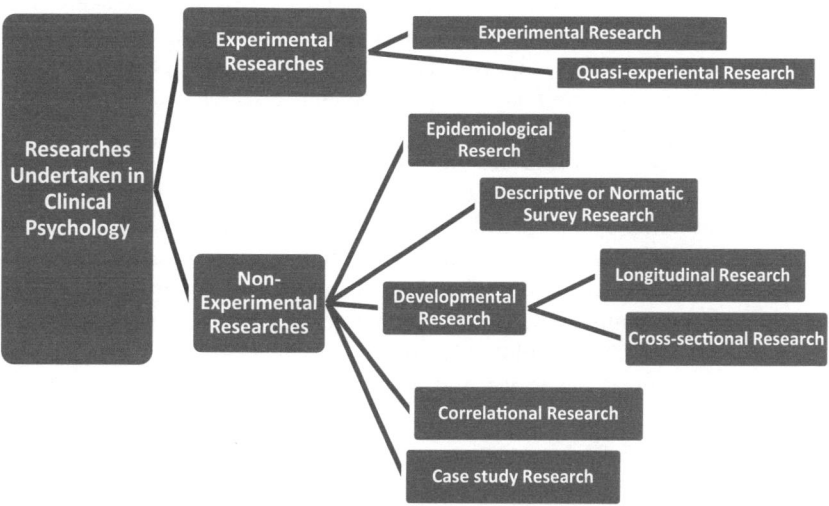

Figure 4.1 Types or Kinds of Research Undertaken in Clinical Psychology

all other extraneous variables (that may influence the results of the study) must be controlled to ensure they do not influence the two variables being examined.

Epidemiological Research: This type of research in clinical psychology is undertaken for studying the incidence, prevalence, and distribution of mental illness or disease in a given population. By the term incidence, we mean the rate of new cases of illness developing within a given period of time. It gives us an idea of whether or not new cases of an illness or disorder are on the increase. The term prevalence, on the other hand, refers to the overall rate of cases (old and new) prevailing within a given period of time in a given population. It helps in finding out the current estimate of the percentage of the population affected by a particular illness or disorder.

As examples of epidemiological research conducted in clinical psychology we may name clinical research such as (i) the rising cases of mental disorders due to the sudden arrival of a dreaded disease or war, (ii) the relationship between the mental disorders of newborns and the alcohol consumption of the pregnant mothers, and (iii) the relationship between schizophrenia and socioeconomic factors/caste/religion, and so on.

In conducting all types of epidemiological research, researchers conduct survey studies through the use of questionnaires and interviews as instruments for data collection.

Descriptive or Normative Survey Research: In this type of clinical research, researchers seek answers to questions related to the current state of affairs. The purpose of descriptive research is to describe variables; in other words, to measure a variable or set of variables as they exist naturally at the time of study. Since this type of research is usually carried out through a normative survey mode it is also designated as normative survey research. As examples of this type of research conducted in clinical psychology, we may name research aimed (i) to know or conform about the symptoms or syndromes associated with one or the other mental illness/disorder, and (ii) the percentage of senior citizens affected with one or the other types of memory disorders in a particular state or region, and so on.

Developmental Research: In tune with its name, developmental research is a particular type of non-experimental research that can be used to study changes in behavior (of individuals) that relate to changes in terms of age, time, or efforts made for such change (Gravetter and Forzano, 2003:23). In this way, the purpose of developmental research is to study and describe the characteristics of a developing individual, particularly as a function of time, and age; for instance, how does the memory ability of individuals undergo change with increasing age?

In answering such questions related to developmental research, the researchers usually try to make use of one of the following two research designs.

Cross-sectional design: With this design, a researcher makes use of different groups of individuals, each group representing a different age. They can also go to match these different groups in terms of the variables acting as confounding variables to influence the memory ability of the participants. In this way, for answering research questions related to the relationship between memory and aging, they may, for example, select from a given population a sample of four different age groups (such as 50 years old, 60 years old, 70 years old, and 80 years old). For carrying out the study, they can then plan for the measurement of the mean memory scores for each group (consisting of 100 people in each group) separately and then draw the necessary conclusions about the effect of aging on the potential of one's memory.

Longitudinal design: In making use of this design, the researcher tries to use only one group of participants (matched in terms of the possible intervening or influencing variables) for carrying out his study, and tries to measure the corresponding changes in the particular behavioral or personality characteristics of the participants (such as memory ability in the present case) over an extended period of time for months or several years. For example, to study the effect of aging on memory while adopting a longitudinal design for the study, the researcher here may be seen to measure memory by a memory test on a group of 50-year-olds, and then measure the same participants of this group again at the ages of 60, 70, and 80 years. In this way, where the adoption of cross-sectional design tends to be easier and more efficient, longitudinal designs, on the other hand, require much longer periods of time. However, while consuming more time, longitudinal studies provide an important view of changes that take place or evolve over time.

Correlational Research: In this type of non-experimental research, the researcher first tries to measure the scores of two or more relevant variables of the study, and then uses these scores for assessing relationships between or among the variables. Typically, these variables are measured as they exist naturally, with no attempt to manipulate or control them. In fact, the purpose of correlational research is to bring into light the variables that show a systematic relationship with each other; for instance, a lack of adjustment to one's environment and poor mental health, the relationship between increasing age and deterioration in memory, and so on. However, the major weakness of correlation research lies in their inability to establish cause-and-effect relationships between variables of the study, despite confirming the presence of a close bond of relationship as well as dependency between them.

Case study Research: This type of research in clinical psychology typically involves an in-depth study and a detailed description of a single individual or a very small group of clients in their real-life context. A case study is also characterized by follow-up work of the introduction or administration of some intervention or treatment to the studied client. When a case study does not include any treatment or intervention, it is often called a case history. The information or data in case study research may be obtained in a variety of ways, such as administering questionnaires, holding interviews with the client or their close relatives, observation of the client in various relevant situations, conducting surveys, and searching archival data. As examples of case study research in clinical psychology, we may name the studies such as (i) the study of a client suffering from a particular type of mental illness or disorder, (ii) the study of individuals or a group engaged in a mass suicide attempt, and (iii) the study of the clients of a particular clinic given a particular therapy for the treatment of a particular mental disorder.

Methods Used in Clinical Psychology Research or Investigation

We have seen that clinical psychologists must engage in various types of research work for serving a number of purposes. Thus, answering a basic question like "why do clinical psychologists get engaged in some or the other research work?" The next pertinent question in this sequence may arise: How do clinical psychologists perform such research work and what methods do they generally employ for conducting research work? Let us know about the nature and use of these various methods.

For this purpose, let us, at present, start with the discussion of the experimental method—the highly used method employed by clinical psychologists and scholars in clinical psychology for their research work.

Experimental Method

The experimental method, in accordance with its name, lays emphasis on performing experiments. In the sciences, while conducting experiments in the laboratory or field we may want to learn, for example, the effect of friction on motion, the effect of sunlight on the growth of plants, and so on. In clinical psychology, we also perform experiments in the laboratory or outside the laboratory in the clinical setting to study cause-effect relationships, for example, the effect of anxiety, drugs or stresses on human behavior, the effect of a treatment measure or therapy in the treatment of mental disorders. In

---

Experimentation Method

This research method aims to establish possible cause-and-effect relationships between the independent and dependent variables of the study through systematic and well-planned observations carried out under controlled conditions.

---

performing such experiments, we try to establish certain cause-and-effect relationships through objective observations of the actions performed and the subsequent changes produced under pre-arranged or rigidly controlled conditions. From these observations, certain conclusions are drawn and theories or principles are formulated.

It is a widely used and favored method of investigation employed by clinical psychologists all over the globe for carrying out the needed research work in clinical psychology. Their choice has merit, as the experimental method may be said to comply with all the requirements needed for a method being called a scientific method, as follows:

- It provides the opportunity to carry out experimental work for researchers to make the *most careful systematic observations of the behavior of clients in controlled conditions* otherwise unavailable through the use of other methods of investigation.
- It provides scope for the *prediction of the behavior* of clients by establishing *cause-and-effect relationships* between two variables (the things and phenomena that stand to vary and change in the social environment) related to clinical behavior.

Understood in this way, the experimentation method, in the shape of a formal definition, may be termed a *type of research method aimed at establishing the possible cause-and-effect relationship between variables under study through systematic and well-planned observations carried out under controlled conditions.*

In this definition, we have mentioned a few terms such as variables and control of experimental conditions for the employment of the experimental method on the part of investigators. Let us know about them.

1. **Variables:** A variable in an experimental study stands for any characteristic or condition (of the clients and the social environment) that is liable to be varied and thus can be attributed with different values. A researcher may encounter a number of variables that need to be manipulated, controlled, or observed as per the requirement of their research study. These variables are known and classified as independent, dependent, and extraneous or intervening variables.

   Independent variable: In an experimental study, the term independent variable stands for the type of variable controlled by the experimenter. The researcher deliberately manipulates and varies it for observing its effects on the dependent variable.

   Dependent variable: In an experimental study, the term dependent variable stands for the type of variable (i.e., aspect of one's clinical behavior) that is supposed to get affected or changed in tune with the introduction and manipulation of the independent variable.

Extraneous or intervening variables: In an experimental study, the concept of extraneous or intervening variables regards all those variables (factors or conditions) that are of no interest to the experimenter. These may influence and interfere with the results and thus must be controlled and neutralized (held constant) by the experimenter to clearly establish the cause-effect relationship between the independent and dependent variables of his study.

2. *Exercising control over conditions:* In an experimental method, it is essential to exercise control over conditions or variables. By this control we can eliminate irrelevant conditions or variables, isolate the relevant ones, and thus become able to observe the causal relationship between the independent and dependent variables by keeping all the extraneous or intervening variables/conditions neutralized or constant. For the purpose of exercising such needed control, an experimenter must make the needed provisions such as the following.

(i) Random assignments of participants to experimental conditions.

To nullify the influence of intervening variables, the experimenter must assign the subjects/participants to varying conditions of the independent variable in a random fashion. Randomization is regarded as the most convenient but powerful tool for controlling a host of extraneous variables (known or unknown) affecting the results of a study. By doing this, the experimenter is capable of providing them equal chance of being exposed to each level of the independent variable, thus ensuring the ruling out of any extraneous effects arising on account of the factors related to participants. The task of randomization may be carried out by using a lottery system, tossing a coin, or making use of a random number table.

Let us try to illustrate the task of exercising control over experimental conditions by adopting the technique of randomization in one of the experimental studies conducted for testing the outcome of a particular therapy given for the treatment of a diagnosed mental disorder. For this purpose, a clinical psychologist may proceed as follows:

- Making attempts to recruit and select a group of volunteer participants who meet the criteria for the diagnosis of the mental disorder in study.

Independent variable: The type of variable or factor in an experimental study that is deliberately manipulated and systematically varied for observing its effects on the dependent variable.

Dependent variable: The type of variable or factor in an experimental study that is expected to change in relation to the introduction and manipulation of the independent variable.

Extraneous or intervening variables: Those variables (factors or conditions) in an experimental study that need to be controlled or nullified on account of their supposed interference with the results of the study.

Random assignments of participants to experimental conditions

A provision made in an experimental study to see that all participants included in the study have an equal chance of being exposed to each level of the independent variable and thus ensuring the ruling out of any extraneous effects arising on account of the factors related to participants.

- Assigning each participant randomly to the experimental group (the group receiving therapy) and the control group (the group not receiving therapy).
- Providing therapeutic treatment to the participants of the experimental group and depriving the control group of such treatment by adopting the measures like placing them on a waitlist, keeping them on a placebo nonspecific treatment, or giving them a "routine" type of therapy.
- Assessing the extent or degree to which the given therapeutic treatment has been successful. For this purpose, in both groups, attempts may be made to assess the target variables (objective measurement of the typical symptoms associated with the diagnosed disorder) at the outset as a baseline and at the end of the study for observing the effect of the actual treatment and placebo nonspecific treatment.

(ii) Holding all other factors other than the independent variable as constant. The employment of this provision demands from the experimenter to hold constant all factors other than the independent variable that may be suspected to influence the participants' behavior. For this purpose, the experimenter may need to carefully consider suitable experimental designs for the conduct of their study. Let us look into these experimental designs.

Experimental Designs Used in Clinical Studies

There are several experimental designs available to clinical psychologists for making use of the experimental method in their research studies. We may broadly classify them as (i) single-group or within-subject designs, (ii) true-experimental or between-subject designs, (iii) designs involving rotation, and (iii) quasi-experimental designs. Let us consider them in detail one by one.

Single-Group or Within-Subjects Design

In such designs, there is no need for two different groups of subjects for the experiment. Here a single group of individuals can work as the subject for the experiment. The researcher here tries to obtain two sets of scores from the same sample of participants (instead of dividing them into experimental and control groups) for the necessary comparison to draw inferences regarding the causal relationships existing between variables. In other words, all the participants included in the study are here first subjected to a particular type of treatment, observed objectively under normal conditions, and then provided another treatment and observed under the changed conditions. The conclusions are then drawn by comparing the differences. Suppose we wish to study the effect of fear stimuli. The psychological laboratory makes available all necessary instruments and materials necessary for the study of fear responses, including changes in respiration, pulse, blood pressure, functioning of the digestive and other internal systems, facial expression, and so on. The initial readings regarding all these functions under normal conditions (when there are no fear stimuli present) are taken by such instruments. Then, all the subjects included in the sample of the study are exposed to sudden fear stimuli such as a snake, loud noise, or darkness, and then the changes in the readings as a result of the intensity of fear responses are recorded by the various instruments. The difference in the second and initial readings will then indicate the different degrees of fear intensity that were aroused on account of the different types of fear stimuli in the participants included in the sample of the study.

True Experimental or Between-Subjects Design

The method of Single-group or Within-Subjects design possesses a serious drawback known as the practice effect. If the subjects or group are subjected to a certain treatment, then it will automatically carry its effect or influence at the time of introduction of some other treatment at the latter stage. Moreover, these designs have no provision for fulfilling the requirements of an experimental study, particularly in terms of exercising proper control over the confounding variables. All such limitations can be properly overcome through the adoption of true experimental or between-subjects designs.

These experimental designs are referred to as true experimental designs due to the fact that they are characterized by the presence of all the essentials to conduct true experiments in clinical studies capable of measuring underlying cause-effect relationships.

The basic procedure in making use of these designs involves activities such as (i) dividing the participants into two equivalent groups, control and experimental, based on randomization or matching, (ii) subjecting them to different treatment conditions and thus getting two sets of scores separately from each group of the participants, (iii) comparing the performances of the experimental and control groups in terms of these two sets of scores, and (iv) drawing conclusions about the relative effectiveness of the introduced treatments.

In a nutshell, a researcher tries to obtain two sets of scores from the two equivalent groups of participants (by dividing them into experimental and control groups) for comparison to draw inferences regarding the causal relationship between variables. For example, in a clinical research study, the researcher examining the appropriateness of a particular psychotherapy may provide this therapy to the participants of the experimental group (diagnosed with anxiety and depression-related mental disorders) by assessing them on a measure of anxiety and depression before and after the treatment. At the same time, the control group is given a placebo nonspecific treatment and tested on the same anxiety and depression measures before and after their treatment. Then the differences in the anxiety and depression scores of the groups are calculated. In cases with significant differences, the results are attributed to the effect of the prescribed psychotherapy.

True experimental designs are also referred to as between-subjects designs because comparison occurs between the subjects/participants of the two separate groups rather than between participants of the same group.

Design Involving Rotation

This design consists in presenting two or more stimulating situations to experimental subjects in as many sequences as necessary to control the serial effects of fatigue or practice. For example, if we want to determine the relative influence of two specified conditions, A and B (say pleasant and unpleasant happenings on one's mood), on a group of subjects, we will not measure all the subjects under condition A and then under condition B. Condition A might cause fatigue, and as such, condition B would not be independent of the fatigue. Here are two alternatives that can be adopted:

(i)   We may obtain half the measures for condition A, all the measures for condition B, and then the other half of the measures for condition A. This technique is sometimes called the A B B A order.

(ii) Another alternative is to separate the subjects into two equal groups, one of which receives treatment A and then B, whereas the other group receives treatment B and then A. Both sets of A results and both sets of B results may then be combined and the difference between them calculated.

Quasi-Experimental Design

There may arise a number of situations in clinical psychology studies in terms of ethical, practical, and other constraints of the variables used in the study where it is not feasible to have true experimental conditions (i.e., pre-selection and randomization of the groups and control over the confounding variables) for arriving at the decision concerning the effectiveness of a particular clinical assessment or treatment method or providing a causal explanation for a clinical phenomenon. Moreover, research work in clinical psychology may often involve the study of things and phenomena as they occur or exist naturally in their physical and social environment. It is not possible for the researchers here to exercise the needed control in terms of manipulating the independent variable at their will for measuring its effect on the dependent variable. In such a situation the researchers are compelled or have no option other than to seek a compromise in the form of employing a quasi-experimental design for their experimental studies.

   For example, let us consider the example of clinical research aimed to study the outcome of a particular psychotherapy for the treatment of a specific anxiety-related depression. To conduct a true experimental study for this purpose, a clinical researcher would need to arrange for the true experimental conditions in the form of taking identical participants, inducing in them identical anxiety states, and then assigning them to different treatment conditions (the prescribed psychotherapy or some alternate psychotherapy) to measure the effectiveness of the prescribed psychotherapy. You may yourself judge the inappropriateness and implausibility of the needed measures ensuring the true experimental conditions for said research. Here the researcher has to face a lot of difficulty including the ethical issues for securing the needed experimental condition for the research study. In case, if he or she somehow tries to seek the formation of two comparison groups by matching them as much as possible, the study will never be as internally valid as a true experimental study. In such a situation, the only appropriate alternative available to the researcher is to opt for a quasi-experimental design for their study. For this purpose, they may enroll participants of the study sample from the roll of the patients coming in for treatment of their anxiety-ridden depressions in various clinics of a region or state, with an acceptance that the participants included in the two comparison groups may be different in the nature and intensity of the anxiety associated with their depression, and also will differ in respect to many other things, such as age, personality characteristics, sociocultural background, and so on.

To Sum Up

Experimental Designs used in clinical studies may be broadly classified as Single-group or Within-subjects designs; True-experimental or Between-subjects designs; Designs involving Rotation; and Quasi-experimental designs.

   In making use of a *single-group or within-subjects design*, the researcher tries to obtain two sets of scores from the same sample of participants (instead of dividing them into experimental and control groups) for the necessary comparison to draw inferences regarding the causal relationships between variables. In making use of a *true experimental or between-subjects design*, the participants are first divided into two equivalent groups–control and experimental–and are then subjected to different treatment conditions for yielding two sets of scores for the necessary comparison to draw inferences regarding the causal relationships between variables. In making use of a *design involving rotation*, the researcher tries to present before the experimental subjects two or more stimulating situations in as many sequences as necessary to control the serial effects of fatigue or practice. The adoption of a *quasi-experimental design* on the part of a researcher is necessitated in a situation when the observance of the requirements for performing a true experimental study seem implausible or unethical.

The Suitability of the Employment of Experimental Method

Regarding the validity of the experimental method used for conducting clinical research, it has been found that employment of this method (along with the adoption of true experimental design) may yield quite favorable

Internal Validity

The term internal validity of the findings of an experimental research stands for making sure that the independent variable, and only the independent variable, influences the dependent variable.

results in terms of its internal validity. By the term internal validity of the findings of experimental research, we mean certainty that the independent variable, and only the independent variable, influences the dependent variable (Campbell and Stanley, 1963).

However, difficulty regarding the maintenance of external validity may still pose a serious question about its usefulness.

By the term external validity in reference to the findings of an experimental study (laboratory or field), we mean the extent to which the results of the study are applied to a similar situation outside the experimental setup. In this connection, here we may find that the findings of the experimental studies are likely to suffer in terms of their lack of external validity. This is often simply because we must make use of small samples of participants, and try to derive conclusions by conducting a particular type of experiment under rigidly controlled conditions. Thus, it is natural to be suspicious about the applicability of research findings of experimental studies to real-life situations.

For this reason, researchers in clinical psychology must carefully consider various methods of investigation that may be helpful in overcoming the problem of external validity with the research findings of their studies. Let us look into the nature and applicability of these methods one by one.

To Sum Up

Regarding the suitability of the experimental method in terms of validity (accuracy and truthfulness of the research findings of an experimental study), we may say that it can be termed to possess the required internal validity to the extent of the proper identification and control of all the possible intervening variables. However, in regard to the external validity of experimental studies—the application of the study's results to a similar situation outside the experimental setup–we may find that results of experimental studies are likely to suffer in terms of their lack of external validity.

Systematic or Naturalistic Observation Method

As the name suggests, in the use of the systematic observation method for studying clinical aspects of behavior, attempts are made to observe the target aspect of the behavior in a systematic way, along with its careful recording for deriving the needed conclusion in view of the objectives of the research study. The nature of such observation thus differs a lot from our routine observation in daily life. It is quite sys-

> **Systematic or Naturalistic Observation Method**
>
> The research method in which the investigator tries to observe and record the occurrence of people's behavior in its natural setting in a systematic way for deriving the needed conclusion in view of the objectives of the research study.

tematic as well as objective in its processing and outcomes. Because it entails the observation and recording of the clinical aspects of one's behavior in its natural setting, it is termed the naturalistic observation method.

In its use and application, this observation method is regarded as one of the most convenient and appropriate methods for investigation employed in clinical psychology. We can get valuable quantitative as well as qualitative information about aspects of peoples' clinical behavior by the systematic and careful observation of their behavioral activities going on in their natural, day-to-day living. A clinical psychologist or researcher may collect valuable data or information regarding the causation, symptoms and syndromes, characteristic features, assessment and diagnosis, and the effectiveness of preventive and treatment measures related to mental illness and disorders of individuals in various physical and social situations of real-life contexts.

Styles and Ways of Carrying Out Observation

The task of observation carried out in the use of the systematic or naturalistic observation method for investigation in clinical psychology may usually take one of the forms and styles known as participant and non-participant observation. Let us examine them.

Participant Observation: In this type of observation, the observer tries to observe the behavior of the individual client or a small group of affected individuals by joining them as an associate or participant in their social activities. For example, the observer may join the individual child or group of children in their play activities, mix with them at their home, school, and other social places with their family/friends/relatives, or accompany them on excursion activities to closely observe them for investigation into aspects of their clinical behavior/mental health problem or disorder. This may provide a good opportunity for the observation of the behavior of the target individuals in a proper way. However, it suffers from a serious limitation, as the presence of an observer may obstruct the natural and spontaneous flow of the behavioral activities of the participants under study.

Non-participant observation: This type of observation tries to do away with the aforementioned defect or limitation of participant observation. Here, the observer observes behavior in such a way that the observed may have no idea that their behavior is in any way being observed. For this purpose, the observer may take their position in such a place and in such a way that while the individuals under observation may not see them, they can clearly watch and hear, if possible, all the behavior in action. There may be a screen or a curtain that hides the observer's presence. The use of modern equipment such as secret cameras, video recording, and audio recording may also serve such a purpose. While sitting at a far distance, the observer may also use a telescope for clear but discreet observation. Whatever means and methods may be employed by the observer, their motive in such an observation is always to come in contact with the natural and spontaneous behavior of the subjects without making them aware of their presence.

After performing the task of appropriate observation and recording of information and data regarding the target clinical or problematic behavior of the client, the researcher needs to get engaged in the subsequent task of analyzing and interpreting the available observed data to derive the necessary interpretation/conclusion about the nature and characteristics of that aspect of one's target behavior. For example, regarding the disruptive behavior of the child client, they may conclude the characteristic features, frequency and intensity, the factors causing the child to react in such a way, and the after-effects of each episode of such behavior on themselves or others, the effectiveness of measures taken for controlling disruptive behavior episodes, and so on.

To Sum UP

In the use of the systematic or naturalistic observation method for investigation in clinical psychology, the investigator tries to observe and record the occurrence of the target problematic or clinical behavior in its natural setting in a systematic way for deriving the needed conclusion in view of the objectives of the research study. The observation for the required purposes may be carried out in ways like participant observation (participation of the observer in the events of observation), and non-participant observation (observing without letting the subjects know). The success of the observation method lies in the proper planning and preparation of the observation task and then carefully observing and recording the events of the observed behavior.

Survey Method

The *Survey method* is also often utilized for investigation in clinical psychology, mainly to collect information about *what exists* by studying and analyzing important aspects of a pattern of a particular clinical aspect of the behavior of individuals with mental illness and disorders. Clinical psychologists and researchers may study and collect information regarding the nature, types, symptoms, and syndromes related to mental illness and disorders existing at present in different populations. They can study the etiology, rate of prevalence, inherent causes, and effectiveness of treatments associated with one or the other mental disorders. The quality of education and training provided to prospective clinical psychologists, and measures to develop them professionally, as well as formalizing their practice according to an accepted ethical

> ### Survey Method
>
> The method of investigation in which the investigator tries to collect information about *what exists* by involving all the members of a population's representative sample to derive the desired specific information about one or the other clinical aspects of people's behavior.

mode, may also be the subjects of survey studies in clinical psychology. Additionally, the opinions, attitudes, and behavioral actions of various segments of the population toward individuals with intellectual disabilities, cognitive malfunctioning, emotional difficulties, memory loss, and severe psychological problems may be properly studied through the use of the survey method.

For this purpose, the needed contact with a wide variety of people of a particular group or region to arrive at a proper conclusion concerning with the objectives of a clinical psychology study can only be possible through survey method. Here instead of a single individual or group, a large population of people as a whole or its representative sample is made a subject of careful and systematic observational study. As a result, we can consider and define survey method *as a method of extensive study for the investigation in clinical psychology involving all the members of a population or its representative sample to derive the desired specific information about one or the other clinical aspects of people's behavior.*

How to Make Use of the Survey Method

The main activities regarding the employment of the survey method in clinical psychology research may be named as follows:

(i)   The selection of a representative sample,

(ii) Making use of survey tools such as questionnaires and interviews for collecting the required data from the representative sample, and

(iii) Analyzing the collected data for drawing necessary inferences to address the research question.

In the application of the survey method, sampling and administration of the survey tools are, thus in fact, the main hubs and centers of a survey study. While making use of the survey method, researchers should take necessary pains in selecting an unbiased and truly representative sample of the targeted population. Regarding the administration of the survey tools (questionnaire/interview schedule) to the chosen sample, keep in mind that these should be administered in such a way as to provide reliable and valid data for addressing the research questions of the study. The modes discussed as follows are popular for the administration of a questionnaire and interview schedule on a representative sample:

Mail surveys: In mail surveys, researchers hand out self-administered questionnaires. In practice, an appropriate questionnaire well developed by the researcher themself (or otherwise available as a standardized tool for conducting the desired survey) is sent by post to the persons belonging to the representative sample with a forwarding letter stating the significance of the survey study and request for returning the questionnaire after responding to it properly. A self-addressed stamped envelope is also enclosed for receiving the response from the respondents.

Group Administered Surveys: In this type of survey, a sample of respondents is brought together and asked to respond to a structural sequence of questions. This type of administration of a survey tool carries several advantages. Here, the researcher may give the questionnaire to those who are present and thus are fairly sure that there would be a high response rate. If the respondents are unclear about the meaning of a particular question, they can ask for clarification. Luckily enough, the researchers for this purpose may often get the already organized setting in the form of sections or classes of schools, assemblies of clubs, and gatherings at religious places.

Door-to-Door Surveys: A less familiar type of survey made with the help of questionnaires is the Door-to-Door survey. In this approach, a researcher goes to the respondent's house or workplace and hands over the instrument to the respondent. In some cases, the respondent is asked to mail it back or the researcher returns to pick it up. This approach attempts to blend the advantages of the mail survey and the group survey and also provides an opportunity for asking follow-up questions by engaging with the respondent in confidence.

Phone surveys: In this type of survey, researchers communicate with respondents in their study sample through available phone services—both landline and smartphone. The services available on smartphones are now at present considered more convenient and suitable for making contact with and receiving responses from survey respondents. One may send messages and make use of audio-video call services available on smartphones for obtaining needed information/data for the research study from the sampled respondents in a convenient, quick, and appropriate way.

Surveys involving Personal or Face-to-Face Interviews: In this type of survey, researchers are required to collect the needed information or data directly from the respondents of their research study sample by seeking personal interviews with them as a member of a certain group or on an individual basis at a mutually agreed upon place and time. These can prove more advantageous and superior to other modes of surveys mainly on the ground that they allow more flexibility to the researcher to bring modification and alteration to the mode of questioning the respondents for bringing more completeness, reliability, and validity to the task of data collection on the spot through face-to-face dialogue.

Online Surveys: In this type of survey, researchers make use of the internet and web-based services provided by modern computer technology for collecting the desired information/data for a research study. Typically, there are three types of internet and web-based surveys (Simsek and Veiga, 2001):

1. An e-mail message with the survey embedded in the e-mail text can be sent to respondents. The respondents simply reply to the e-mail with the answers.
2. An e-mail can be sent with an attachment that the respondents must open, answer, and then send back as an attachment.
3. Researchers can use a URL-embedded message in the text of the e-mail, so the respondent simply clicks on the hypertext link, which then evokes the web browser to present the respondent with the web-based survey.

Whatever the form and shape of its presentation, an internet and web-based survey may prove a handy tool for collecting a pool of desired information or data from a vast population in little time and at negligible cost. The information collected through this mode of survey is systematic, organized, and can be easily subjected to computerized analysis for deriving valid conclusions in a research study. With its multiple benefits, simplicity, and ease of use on the part of researchers and respondents, this kind of surveying mode is becoming quite popular day by day.

To Sum Up

The Survey method is employed mainly to collect information about what exists by studying and analyzing important aspects of a particular behavior or characteristic related to a population of individuals with mental health problems, or from the general population regarding their opinion and attitude toward people with intellectual disabilities and mental illness. Here the desired information is collected from the total population or its representative sample with the help of devices like questionnaires and interviews. In general, methods of administration of the questionnaire and interview schedule to a given population or its representative sample may include survey modes like mail surveys, group-administered surveys, door-to-door surveys, phone surveys, surveys involving personal or face-to-face interviews, and online surveys involving the use of the internet and web-based services.

Correlational Method

It is quite common on the part of researchers in clinical psychology to make use of the method of correlation in answering their research questions pertaining to aspects of clinical behavior associated with mental illness or disorders. The term correlation in the field of investigation and research describes the type of relationship or association between two variables of a research study, and consequently, correlation research and methods in clinical psychology are employed to examine the relationship between two variables of a research study. In this concern, as pointed out by Cohen et al. (2000:193),

---

Correlational Method

The method of research that helps a researcher to determine whether and to what extent variables of the research study are related to each other, thus coming into a position to predict one from the other.

---

the use of the method of correlation in a research study is intended to answer three questions about two variables or two sets of data, first, "Is there a relationship between the two variables (or sets of data)?" If yes, then two other questions follow: "What is the direction of the relationship?" and "What is the magnitude?"

How to Make Use of the Correlational Method

The goal of the use of the correlation method is to determine whether and to what extent the variables of the research study are related to each other. In cases of finding a satisfactory amount of correlation between two variables of the study, it can help us in predicting that if one variable exists in a social situation, the other likely accompanies it. For an illustration of the procedure employed for making use of the correlation method, let us consider a research study aimed to answer a basic question of to what extent the maladjustment of children at home and school is associated with their disruptive or oppositional defiant behavior in social situations. The steps described next may be followed for the use of the correlation method for conducting a research study in this concern.

1. First, the variables of the study are properly identified. In this study, these variables are (i) maladjustment at school and home on the part of children, and (ii) disruptive or oppositional defiant behavior demonstrated by them in social situations.
2. Then, attempts are made to properly measure these variables by making use of appropriate techniques and thus arriving at two sets of measurement. In this study, a researcher may make use of a standardized adjustment inventory for determining the maladjustment scores of the subjects included in the research sample. For getting scores on aggressiveness and violent behavior of the subjects, they may compile the rating scores of the different research assistants employed for taking stock of disruptive or oppositional defiant behavior demonstrated by the subjects at different social encounters in school, at home, playground, school canteen, and so on.
3. Then futher, attempts may be made to compute a coefficient of correlation between these two sets of scores by making use of the appropriate statistical technique. This computed measure will then tell us about the nature and type of association/relationship existing between the two variables, including their ability to predict one on the basis of the other.
4. Note here that the conclusions drawn through a correlation study depend solely on the value of the computed coefficient of correlation, both in terms of its direction–being positive/negative–and its magnitude–the size of its numerical value. Statistically, the computed value of a correlation coefficient can range from -1 to + 1. In the present case, the numerical value (including the positive or negative sign) of the computed correlation coefficient between two sets of scores regarding maladjustment and disruptive/oppositional defiant behavior will be telling about the nature of the correlation/association between these two variables. If it turns sufficiently positive (possessing a positive numerical value such as 0.7 and more), then it will be concluded that maladjustment and disruptive/oppositional defiant behavior travel together. The children who are maladjusted in school and at home are bound to show the symptoms of disruptive/oppositional defiant behavior in social encounters, and vice versa.

In this way, the method of correlation used for carrying out research in social psychology may make a researcher capable of establishing or denying a satisfactory relationship/association existing between the variables of that study. It also carries an appreciable predictive value. The researcher can then predict the presence/absence of one variable on the basis of the presence/absence of the other. For example, if a researcher in their correlation study finds that there exists a positive satisfactory correlation between the variables of their study–for instance, watching pornographic videos and sexual deviations or disorders–the results of the study can be used for predicting the increase in cases of sexual disorders on account of the increasing trend of watching pornographic videos. But here it should also be remembered that it does not mean that watching pornographic videos essentially causes the viewer to have sexual deviations or disorders, clearly portraying the former as the cause and the latter as the effect. In fact, such a cause-effect relationship between two variables of a study cannot be definitively established through the use of the correlation method and for this purpose, the researchers must make use of the experimental method discussed earlier in this chapter.

To Sum Up

Correlational research and methods in clinical psychology are used by researchers to examine the nature, direction, and magnitude of the relationship existing between two variables of a research study for enabling them to predict one from the other. For conducting correlation research, researchers follow steps such as:

- The identification of the variables of the study in a proper way
- To make proper measurements of the two variables by making use of appropriate techniques and thus arriving at two sets of measurement
- To compute a coefficient of correlation between these two sets of scores by making use of the appropriate statistical technique, and
- To make use of the computed correlation coefficient for concluding about the nature and type of association/relationship existing between the variables of the study, including their ability to predict one on the basis of the other.

Case Study or Case History Method

There are numerous special situations that researchers in clinical psychology must face when they conduct a type of study that may help them in describing the characteristics of an individual with an emotional, mental or behavioral problem, illness, or disorder. In these cases, they must make use of a specialized method of investigation, known as the *case study or case history* method.

As a matter of its formal definition, we can term the case study method a method of investigation employed for carrying out descriptive or explanatory research (capable of being generalized to similar cases studied under similar conditions) that may prove helpful as a detailed and in-depth study of a case in its real-life context, directed toward introducing necessary intervention and measures (if needed) in the interest of the case in question or others.

Case Study Method

A method of research adopted for carrying out a detailed and in-depth study of a case (an individual, a small group, event, or phenomenon) in its real-life context, directed toward introducing necessary interventions and measures (if needed) in the interest of the case studied or others.

In light of our formal definition of the case study method, we may list the characteristic features of this method in the following manner:

1. The case study method involves an in-depth, holistic, detailed, and longitudinal (running over a long time period) study of a case (an individual, a small group, a contemporary phenomenon, or a clinical event).
2. Carried out in its natural setting and real-life context, the case study method provides a systematic way of looking at events, collecting data, analyzing information, and reporting results in a descriptive and explanatory way.

3. The case study method helps researchers in gaining a sharpened understanding of why the particular instance/typical behavior pattern happened as it did, and what might be important to look at more extensively in the future.

4. The case study method is helpful in carrying out both descriptive and explanatory types of research work in clinical psychology. In its descriptive form, it may provide a detailed account of the cases studied in reference to the past, present, and future prospectus. In its explanatory form, it can help in establishing a cause-effect relationship for the things observed and investigated in the explanation of problematic behavior of people with a particular mental illness or disorder.

5. The information or data collected in a case study research can be obtained in a variety of ways, by making use of multiple sources of evidence, such as administering questionnaires, holding interviews with the clients (cases under study), and/or their close relatives, conducting surveys, and analysis of archival data.

6. As emphasized by Hitchcock and Hughes (1995:317), the case study method possesses several unique hallmarks such as:

   • It is concerned with a rich and vivid description of events relevant to the case.
   • It provides a chronological narrative of events relevant to the case.
   • It blends a description of events with an analysis of them.
   • It focuses on individual actors or groups, and seeks to understand their perception of events.
   • It highlights specific events that are relevant to the case.
   • The researcher is integrally involved in the case.
   • An attempt is made to portray the richness of the case in writing up the report.

In a nutshell, we may say that when a researcher needs to obtain a straightforward description of a single unit (individual, group, or phenomenon) in-depth and in detail, it is the case study method that may help them in serving this purpose. For this reason, the use of this method is considered quite meritorious as well as interesting to clinical psychologists for revealing unique things about the clinical aspects and behaviors of problem-afflicted individuals. Thus, you may see descriptions of case study work conducted on subjects experiencing mental health problems and disorders across the texts and research literature belonging to the field of clinical psychology. In the present text, we have narrated a number of case studies during the discussion of one or the other mental disorders or behavioral problems, such as case studies of individuals with obsessive-compulsive disorders, phobias, autism, ADHD, eating and sleeping disorders, and neurotic and psychotic disorders. The descriptions given under these case studies may help well in revealing truths about psychological and adjustment problems faced by individuals, the characteristics and symptoms associated with a particular disorder, the underlying causes and factors responsible for the creation and perpetuation of the problem, the effectiveness of the methods employed for its diagnosis, prevention, and treatment, and so on.

To Sum Up

A method of research known as the case study method is used by researchers in clinical psychology in a situation when one must conduct a study that may help in describing the characteristics of an existing individual unit (i.e., an individual, or small group, or a phenomenon) designated as a case through its in-depth and intensive study.

Such case studies are often undertaken by clinical psychology researchers and practitioners for understanding the nature of the problems experienced by their clients in terms of their peculiar symptoms, causation, and the effectiveness of the treatment given to them.

The data collected in case study research can be obtained from a variety of sources by making use of multiple means, such as administering questionnaires, holding interviews with the cases under study including their close relatives, conducting surveys, and analysis of archival data. The case study method in its application proves quite useful in getting a detailed account of the cases studied in reference to their past, present, and future prospectus. It can help also help in establishing cause-effect relationships for the things observed and investigated in the composition of the case studied.

The Use of Meta-Analysis in Clinical Psychology Research

There arise a number of situations in our day-to-day life where we feel it necessary to seek others' reviews or comments about the suitability of a movie to watch, a hotel to stay at, a travel agency for booking a tour, a product to purchase, and so on. The reading of a good or bad review leaves a sizable impression on us. We make a choice for a thing depending on the type of impression left on us through the reading of a review/comment. This effect is more intensified when it comes from different sources (different reviewers say the same thing about the appropriateness or inappropriateness of a thing) or when a professional reviewer or critic presents it by comparing the different available choices.

Reading about conclusions drawn by a researcher in clinical psychology for answering a research question (e.g., is cognitive behavioral therapy suitable for the treatment of obsessive-compulsive disorder?) is much like reading the opinion expressed by a reviewer about the appropriateness of inappropriateness of a thing. Just as it helps to read several independent reviews from different sources, or a composite and comprehensive review of different available choices from an expert reviewer for accepting or rejecting an offer, we as clinical psychology researchers must (i) consider the many findings of independent research studies focused on the workability of cognitive behavioral therapy for the treatment of obsessive-compulsive disorder, and (ii) look to a composite conclusion drawn by an expert through an objective analysis of the findings of several relevant studies focused on the suitability of cognitive behavioral therapy for the treatment of obsessive-compulsive disorder.

It is the latter mode of working that is adopted in applying the technique of Meta-Analysis for evaluating the reliability and validity of particular research findings regarding a particular research question; in this example, the effectiveness of a particular psychotherapy for the treatment of a mental disorder. Although it is certainly informative to read the results of a single study on, say, the benefits of a particular psychotherapy for the treatment of a mental disorder, it can be far more enlightening to read a meta-analysis on the topic that encompasses many comparable studies (Wampold et al., 1997).

What is Meta-Analysis?

In its technical sense and applicability, meta-analysis refers to a specialized statistical method or tool used by researchers, including clinical psychology researchers, to combine results of separate research studies (each focusing on the same research question) for providing a single result or conclusion characterized with more statistical power and thus making it more reliable and valid for its further use in research and clinical practice. In this way, meta-analysis may be termed the study of studies, providing a methodological objective statistical analysis of what is conveyed by several relevant

> **Meta-analysis**
>
> Meta-analysis is the study of studies, in which a researcher tries to make use of a specialized statistical method or tool to combine results of separate research studies for providing a single result or conclusion for answering a specific research question.

independent studies in terms of answering a particular research question related to a particular clinical aspect. Examples of such aspects include: how far are genetic anomalies responsible for causing this mental disorder?; What is the best possible psychotherapy for the treatment of this mental disorder?; To what extent is cognitive behavioral therapy suitable for the treatment of obsessive-compulsive disorders?

Characteristic Features of Meta-Analysis

To expand on the meaning and nature of the method of meta-analysis, let us look into its characteristic features, summarized as follows.

- Meta-analysis is a sophisticated statistical technique employed for summarizing the results of several independent studies focused on the same research question. It helps in systematically synthesizing or merging the findings of several single, independent studies.
- By combining information from all relevant studies, meta-analysis can provide more precise conclusions about the focused research question than those derived from individual studies included within a review.
- A meta-analysis goes beyond critique and integration and conducts secondary statistical analysis on the outcomes of similar studies. It is a systematic review that uses statistical methods to compute an overall or absolute effect for synthesizing and summarizing the results of similar independent studies.
- The findings of meta-analysis can be used for establishing statistical significance with studies that have conflicting results.
- The main goal of a meta-analysis performed on the findings of so many independent studies is to generate the best possible quantitative estimate of the studied phenomena, such as "the effectiveness of a particular diagnosis or intervention program."
- The process of meta-analysis is characterized by a unique ability to remain objective in evaluating several research findings focused on a common aspect. Accordingly, while carrying out meta-analysis—the study of studies—one must remain sure that the method of analysis employed is scientifically sound (Field, 2013).

How to Make Use of Meta-Analysis in Clinical Psychology Research

The process of meta-analysis requires the use of a statistical method of combining results of separate studies (translated into effect sizes) to create a summation (or, statistically, an overall effect size) of the findings (Hedges and Citkowicz, 2015).

For realizing its mission properly, Durlak (2003) recommends the use of the following five systematic steps for its execution on the part of clinical psychology researchers.

Step 1: The research question—Formulate the research question, including reasonable, important, testable hypotheses.

Step 2: Study sample—Obtain a representative study sample. Determine and explain the criteria by which individual studies will be included or excluded. Consider unpublished reports as well as those that have been published.

Step 3: Collection of information or data—Extract summary data or outcomes/findings from each study selected for meta-analysis. Depending on the study and the research question, outcome measures (referred to as the effect size of an individual study) could include numerical measures or categorical measures. For example, differences in scores on a questionnaire or differences in measurement levels such as scores on intelligence, personality traits, levels of adjustment, memory scales, and anxiety and depression measures, would be reported as a numerical mean.

Step 4: Doing analysis work—Take all precautions in conducting appropriate analyses of the collected information or data regarding individual studies in terms of their effect sizes. Here, attempts should be made to synthesize or integrate the effect sizes of individual studies. For doing this, assign appropriate weights to each, such that larger-scale studies are given more weight than smaller-scale studies.

Step 5. Conclusion drawing—Reach conclusions and offer suggestions for future research.

Significance and Importance of Meta-Analysis

Meta-analysis of several relevant studies, focused on answering a common research question related to one or the other clinical aspects, carries a wide significance and importance for clinical psychology researchers and practitioners. The results arrived at through meta-analysis technique are more trustworthy and graspable on account of their broader numerical and statistical representation, besides being sufficiently objective and scientific in their procedure, in comparison to the results derived through other traditional means such as (i) relying on what is available in terms of findings of a single study for getting the answer to the research question, or (ii) relying on a review of several research study findings answering the same common research question.

Consequently, it is the results of meta-analysis in the field of clinical psychology and mental health that are considered the most trustworthy sources of evidence for clinical psychologists in their research pursuits and practices. The unique advantages derived from the meta-analysis of independent research studies have been supported by several research studies. Some examples include:

- The meta-analysis of 15 individual studies focused on evaluating the effectiveness of cognitive therapy for generalized anxiety disorder, helped in reaching the conclusion that overall, cognitive therapy was much more effective than no therapy, and at least slightly more effective than other kinds of therapy (Hanrahan et al., 2013).
- The meta-analysis carried out on the findings of 18 studies on remote cognitive behavioral treatment for obsessive-compulsive disorder (through video conference and other media) helped in concluding that the remote treatments were much more effective than control conditions, and equally as effective as face-to-face treatments (Wootton, 2016).

> **To Sum Up**
>
> In the use of the method of meta-analysis, researchers try to have an appropriate statistical analysis of the results of independent research studies for arriving at a single conclusion helpful in answering a specific research question. For realizing its mission in a proper way, researchers are advised to make use of the systematic steps named as (i) Formulating the research question and establish the testable hypotheses, (ii) Obtaining a representative study sample in the form of selecting studies for being meta-analyzed, (iii) Extracting summary data or outcomes/findings from each study selected for meta-analysis, (iv) Doing analysis work, and (v) Deriving conclusions.

Ethical Issues in Clinical Psychology Research

It is hoped as well as expected from researchers in all fields of knowledge to be sufficiently ethical in their research pursuit by following all the norms and values as needed on their part in this concern. Such need and expectations are more intensified in the cases of researchers carrying out investigation or research work in clinical psychology, where human behavior under distress is the focus and human beings are the subjects of the research study. In general, in this concern, the researchers in clinical psychology are required to pay attention to the ethical issues like:

(i)   The prior consent of the individuals participating as the subjects of the study in the research.
(ii)   The maintenance of the privacy of what has been disclosed or being transacted between them and the researcher.
(iii) The consideration that the subjects of the study are not put to any harm—physical or psychological—in any way.
(iv)   Debriefing of the participants in case deception (misleading of the participants) has been employed in the study.
(v)   Being sufficiently objective, truthful, impartial, and judicious in collecting data from the subjects in making use of one or the other research methods.
(vi)   Being honest and truthful in data compilation, analysis, and drawing conclusions of the study.
(vii) Sharing the results of the study with the participants of the study.

For addressing all such ethical issues, researchers in clinical psychology are required to focus on things such as:

1. *Seeking voluntary participation:* They should always try to seek voluntary participation of individuals in their study by making the purpose of their study clear and then winning their willingly cooperation in this study. In no case should there be any coercion or excessive inducement for this purpose.
2. *Seeking formal consent about their role:* The participants of the study should be told about their role in the study. What type of information will be collected from them? What type of experiment is going to be performed on them? The participants should not only be properly aware about it, but they should also agree to it by providing their formal consent.
3. *Maintaining confidentiality and privacy:* The participants of the study should be assured fully that what they say and do in response to their role in the study will be a matter of

confidentiality. Their privacy related to answering their private or social life will not be disclosed and they should not have any fear or hesitation on this account. The commitment made by the participants should then be fully complied on the part of the researcher.

4. *Maintaining fairness in collecting, compiling, analyzing, and concluding about the study:* The researchers should follow all the needed rules and principles for being properly ethical in respect of all these aspects or elements of the research. They should never show subjectivity and partiality in recording the things they observe, and never resort to false cooking of the data, or interpret them in their own way for deriving their own conclusions. They should avoid the copying of the other's research efforts and remain away from acts of piracy.

5. *Debriefing the participants at the end of the study/experiment:* It is the duty as well as moral responsibility of researchers to do the task of debriefing—explaining to the participants of the study, at the end of the study/experiment, its true purpose and exactly what transpired during the study/experiment and why. It is most needed in the case when the researchers in their study makes use of deception—misleading participants about the true purpose of a study or events that would be actually happening during the experiment/study.

6. *Sharing the Findings of the Study with the Participants:* In socio-psychological research, the researchers aim to study about one or the other attributes or behavioral functioning of the participants. It is therefore quite natural for participants to be seriously interested in the findings of the research study for knowing about them. They are found to be eagerly waiting for the same, and the researcher should never disappoint them on this account. He should definitely reappear on the scene after having the conclusions of his study with him. With his deliberate efforts of meeting participants in person or contacting them through phone or by online meeting, he should thank them for their cooperation in the conduct of the study and tell them about what has resulted from the study.

In this way, researchers in clinical psychology should feel the necessity of taking the needed precautions and following the rules and principles for addressing one or the other ethical issues in conducting inquiry and research for answering their research questions. The guidelines provided as well as measures adopted by the Indian Government funding as well as research governing agencies such as the Indian Council of Social Science research (ICSSR) and University Grants Commission (UGC), as well as the respective Central and State Universities in this concern, may also help researchers in this task.

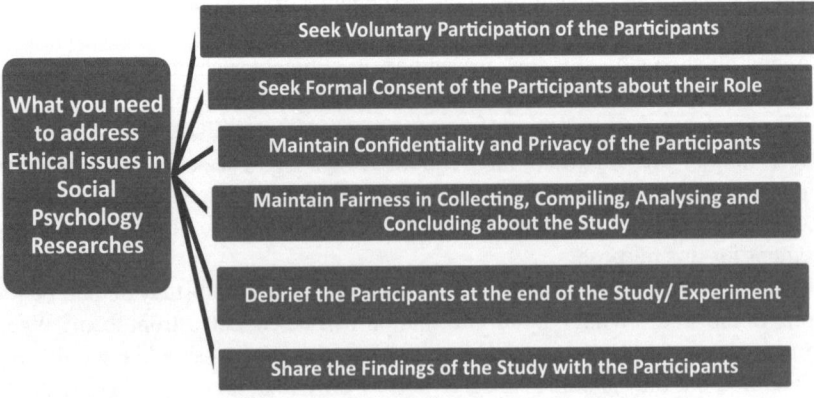

Figure 4.2 Addressing Ethical Issues in Clinical Psychology Research

At the international level, they may learn much in this direction, from the ethical guidelines issued by some of the eminent professional organizations such as The American Psychological Association for being followed by researchers in Psychology and its branches, including clinical psychology. In the Table 3.1 we are providing to our readers an adapted version of the some of the major ethical principles emphasized by the APA from time to time in the form of its prescribed Code of Ethics (APA, 2002, 2017).

Table 4.1 Ethical Principles for Researchers (Including those Working in Clinical Psychology)

- Researchers should obtain the needed consent from prospective participants in terms of their willingness to participate by providing them due information regarding the purpose, expected duration, and procedure of the study.
- Researchers should not in any way coerce participation by offering excessive or inappropriate rewards (financial or otherwise).
- Researchers should avoid using deception in their studies unless the prospective value of the research justifies its use and non-deceptive methods are not feasible. If deception is used, the researcher should explain it fully to participants as soon as possible and allow them to withdraw their data if they choose.
- Researchers should take all precaution to see that no participant included in the study is harmed during the procedure of the study, in case if it happens in some ways, then researcher should take responsibility for compensating or curing the harmed participant.
- Researcher should assure the participants about the confidentiality of any information they give to the researcher during the course of the study. In this regard he should feel a primary obligation and take reasonable precautions for the safeguard of the confidential information stored in any medium. It should not be revealed to any body without the consent or approval of the concerned participant.
- Researchers should always seek to promote accuracy, honesty, and truthfulness in conducting their research study. They should never fabricate or falsify their research data. They also need to refrain themselves from the evil of plagiarism, i.e., never presenting portions of another's work or data as their own.
- Researchers provide a prompt opportunity for participants to obtain appropriate information about the nature, results, and conclusion of the research after the end of the study.
- Researchers should share their data with other competent researchers who intend to reanalyze it for verification.

Source: Adapted from the code of ethics emphasized by American Psychology Association (APA).

To Sum Up

It is hoped as well as expected that researchers in psychology be sufficiently ethical in their research pursuit by following all the norms and values as needed on their part as per direction issued by their own university and agencies such as UGC, ICSSR, and professional organizations working on the national and international levels. In general, in this concern they are required to focus on aspects such as:

- Seeking voluntary participation of the subjects and seeking formal consent about their role
- Assuring the participants of the study about maintaining confidentiality and privacy

- Maintaining fairness in collecting, compiling, analyzing, and concluding about the study
- Debriefing or explaining the participants at the end about the purpose of the study and exactly what transpired during the study/experiment and why
- Sharing the findings of the study with the participants.

Review Questions

1. What do you understand by the term research or investigation as used in the field of clinical psychology? Point out the goals of such research or inquiry work undertaken in clinical psychology.
2. Name the different methods of investigation used by researchers for conducting research in the field of clinical psychology and discuss any one of them in detail
3. What is the experimental method of research? How is it utilized by researchers in clinical psychology research? Discuss.
4. What is the systematic or naturalistic observation method of research? Explain in detail, how is it utilized by the researchers in the clinical psychology research?
5. What is the survey method of investigation? Throw light on its nature and discuss how it is utilized by clinical psychology researchers in their research work.
6. What is the correlation method of investigation? How is it used by researchers in the field of clinical psychology for conducting their research work? Explain.
7. What is the case study method of research? Describe the type of investigation it is used for by researchers in clinical psychology.
8. What is ethnography? For what type of research is ethnography utilized as a method by researchers in clinical psychology and how?
9. What are documents or archives? Throw light on the mechanism of using documentary or archival analysis as a method of investigation in clinical psychology. Tell in what ways it proves helpful to researchers in their clinical psychology research.
10. What do you understand by the terms data and data analysis? How the tasks, related to quantitative and qualitative data analysis, are carried out in clinical psychology research or investigation? Discuss.
11. What are the different ethical issues coming out in the way of conducting researches in the field of Clinical Psychology? How can these be addressed? Discuss.

References

American Psychological Association (2002), Ethical principles of psychologists and code of conduct, *American Psychologist*, 57: 1060–1073.

APA (2017), Ethical principles of psychologists and code of conduct, retrieved on 5 February 2022 from www.apa.org›code›ethics-code-2017

Best, J. W., & Kahn, J. V. (2006), *Research in education* (10th ed.), New Delhi: Prentice Hall of India.

Campbell, D. T., & Stanley, J. C. (1963), *Experimental and quasi-experimental designs for research*, Chicago, IL: Rand McNally.

Cohen, L., Lawrence, M., & Morrison, K. (2000), *Research methods in education*, London: Routledge.

Durlak, J. A. (2003), Basic principles of meta-analysis, In M. C. Roberts & S. S. Ilardi (Eds.), *Handbook of research methods in clinical psychology* (pp. 196–209), Malden, MA: Blackwell.

Field, A. P. (2013), Meta-analysis in clinical psychology research, In J. S. Comer & P. C. Kendall (Eds.), *The Oxford handbook of research strategies for clinical psychology* (pp. 317–335), New York, NY: Oxford University Press.

Gove, P. B. (1966), *Webster's seventh new collegiate dictionary*, Springfield, MA: G&C Merriam Company Publishers.

Gravetter, N. E., & Forzano, L.-A. B. (2003), *Research methods for the behavioural sciences*, Belmont, CA: Thomson.

Hanrahan, F., Field, A. P., Jones, F. W., & Davey, G. C. (2013), A meta-analysis of cognitive therapy for worry in generalized anxiety disorder, *Clinical Psychology Review*, 33(1), 120–132.

Hedges, L. V., & Citkowicz, M. (2015), Metaanalysis, In R. L. Cautin & S. O. Lilienfeld (Eds.), *The encyclopedia of clinical psychology* (pp. 1803–1809), Chichester: Wiley Blackwell.

Hitchcock, G., & Hughes, D. (1995), *Research and the teacher* (2nd ed.), London: Routledge.

Hornby, A. S. (Eds.), (1952), *The advanced learner's dictionary of current English*, London: Oxford University Press.

Kothari, C. R. (1990), *Research methodology: Methods and techniques* (2nd ed.), New Delhi: Vishwa Prakashan.

Simsek, Z., & Veiga, Z. F. (2001), A primer on internet organized surveys, *Organizational Research Methods*, 4: 218–235.

Wampold, B. E., Mondin, G. W., Moody, M., Stich, I., Benson, K., & Ahn, H. (1997), A meta-analysis of outcome studies comparing bona fide psychotherapies: Empirically "all must have prizes", *Psychological Bulletin*, 122, 203–215.

Wootton, B. M. (2016), Remote cognitive-behavior therapy for obsessive compulsive symptoms: A meta-analysis, *Clinical Psychology Review*, 43, 103–113.

Young, P. V. (1966), *Scientific social surveys and research*, Hoboken, NJ: Prentice Hall.

Chapter 5

Mental Health, Hygiene and Clinical Psychologists

Learning Objectives

After going through this chapter you will be able to:

- Discuss the meaning of the term mental hygiene.
- Point out the aims and purposes of mental hygiene.
- Provide the meaning of the term mental health.
- Develop an understanding about the concept of mental health.
- Elucidate the characteristics of a mentally healthy individual/signs of good mental health.
- Elucidate the characteristics of a mentally unhealthy individual/symptoms of poor mental health.
- Discuss the importance of mental health.
- Throw light on the principles helpful in the maintenance of proper mental health.
- Tell about the role of clinical psychologists in the maintenance of mental health.

Meaning of the Term Mental Hygiene

Mental Hygiene, as the name suggests, is that branch of hygiene that deals with the mental health of individuals in the same way as physical hygiene is concerned with their physical health. In the subject of physical hygiene, we study the causes of physical ailments or diseases. Their prevention and curative measures are discussed in order to save individuals from the

> **Mental Hygiene**
>
> A science helpful in recommending useful principles and techniques for the preservation and promotion of mental health along with the prevention and treatment of mental disorders and diseases.

hazards of physical illness and ailments. In addition to this, the principles and techniques for maintaining proper physical health, with a healthy body and desirable working habits, are also suggested. Similarly, mental hygiene takes care of the prevention as well as treatment of mental illness, disorder, and maladjustment. It also suggests ways and means of maintaining proper mental health and efficiency and therefore helps in the mental or intellectual growth

DOI: 10.4324/9781003398325-5

and development of an individual. The meaning of the term Mental Hygiene can be made clear by the following definitions:

American Psychological Association (2022): Mental hygiene refers to "a general approach aimed at maintaining mental health and preventing mental disorder."

American Psychiatric Association: Mental Hygiene consists of measures to reduce the incidence of mental illness through prevention and early treatment and to promote mental health (Singh and Tiwari, 1971:434).

D.B. Klein (1965:2): Mental Hygiene, as its name suggests, is concerned with the realization and the maintenance of the mind's health and efficiency.

Drever (1952:167): Mental Hygiene means investigation of the laws of mental health, and the taking or advocacy of measures for its preservation.

Crow and Crow (1951:4): Mental Hygiene is a science that deals with human welfare and pervades all fields of human relationship.

Crow and Crow (1969:199): As conceived today, mental hygiene may be defined as the prevention of mental illness, the preservation of mental health, and the cure of mental illness.

From these definitions, we can conclude that *Mental Hygiene is a science that attempts to develop and apply principles and techniques for the preservation and promotion of mental health as well as for the prevention and treatment of mental disorders, diseases, and other abnormalities, ultimately leading to an adequate adjustment and balanced development of one's personality.*

Aims and Purposes of Mental Hygiene

Mental Hygiene, as we have seen previously, does not merely limit itself to the prevention and treatment of mental disorders or illnesses. It also takes into account the preservation and promotion of one's mental health. In this way, we

---

Mental Hygiene

* To suggest preventive measures against falling victim to mental illness and disorders.
* To suggest possible measures for the preservation and promotion of mental health.
* To suggest needed measures for the cure and treatment of mental illness and disorders.

---

can identify three important aspects or approaches in mental hygiene: preventive, preservative, and curative approaches. These aspects can be utilized for studying the aims and purposes of mental hygiene Crow and Crow (1951:4), as follows:

1. The prevention of mental disorders through an understanding of the relationship that exists between wholesome personality development and life experiences;
2. The preservation of mental health of both the individual and the group; and
3. The discovery and utilization of therapeutic measures to cure mental illnesses.

In the first phase, mental hygiene aims at suggesting preventive measures to save us from the dreadful clutches of conditions and situations that lead to mental illness, maladjustment, and disorders. In this direction it aims:

* To list various causes of maladjustment–personal as well as social.

- To furnish the knowledge of drives, needs, motives, conflicts of motives, frustrations, tensions, and so on.
- To suggest ways and means of achieving emotional and social adjustment.
- To suggest solutions for inner conflicts and frustrations, with the aim of relieving tensions, anxieties, and emotional disturbances.

The second broader aim of mental hygiene relates to the possible measures of preserving and promoting mental health. With this goal, mental hygiene aims to:

- Develop the total potentialities of an individual;
- Attain emotional maturity and stability;
- Achieve personal and social security as well as adequacy;
- Develop healthy human relationships and group interactions.

The third end of mental hygiene is related to treatment and curative measures. In this direction, mental hygiene may aim to:

- Furnish the individual with the necessary knowledge regarding types of mental illnesses, disorders, and diseases;
- Suggest various forms of therapy for the treatment and cure of specific mental illness and disorders, and
- Suggest means for the rehabilitation and readjustment of maladjusted, mentally disturbed, and mentally ill persons.

In these aspects, mental hygiene aims at achieving proper mental health and efficiency. But the aim of the development of sound mental health is not an end in itself; it is rather a platform to achieve greater ends. Mentally healthy persons acquire certain essential abilities and capacities that are helpful in their development as socially adequate and emotionally stable, well-balanced personalities. They can get along well with themselves and thus lead a contented, happy life free from unnecessary anxieties, conflicts, and frustrations. In this way, the ultimate aim of mental hygiene as Shaffer (1936:435) put it, *"is to assist every individual in the attainment of fuller, happier, more harmonious and more effective existence."*

To Sum Up

Mental hygiene is the branch of hygiene that deals with the mental health of individuals, in the same way as physical hygiene is concerned with their physical health. Accordingly, it aims for the prevention as well as treatment of mental illness, disorder, and maladjustment, and also suggests ways and means of maintaining proper mental health and efficiency.

Mental hygiene aims (i) to suggest preventive measures for saving us from mental illness, maladjustment, and disorders; (ii) to find out the ways and means of preserving and promoting our mental health; and (iii) to provide ways and means for the cure and treatment of mental illness, maladjustment, and disorders—ultimately helping us in the attainment of fuller, happier, more harmonious and effective existences.

Meaning of the Term Mental Health

Mental health stands for the health of the mind, as Carter V. Good in The Dictionary of Education (1959:263) has termed it as *"The wholesomeness of the mind"*–analogous to the wholesomeness of the body implicit in physical health. Accordingly, mental health is concerned with the health of one's mind and its functioning in the same way as the physical health is concerned with the health of one's physical organs and their functioning. To understand the nature and meaning of the term mental health, let us look at some of the well-known definitions.

> **Mental Health**
>
> Health of one's mind indicative of one's level of adjustment to their self and environment.

Waltin, J.E.W. (1951:41): Mental health concerns with the development of "wholesome" balanced personality, one who does not comfort himself like a series of compartmentalized selves—honest on Sunday, dishonest on Monday, generous today, crabbed tomorrow, reasonable and logical at times, at other times confused and inconsistent.

J.A. Hadfield (1952:1–2): Mental health is the full and harmonious functioning of the whole personality.

P.B. Lewkan (1949:68): A mentally healthy person is one who is happy, lives peacefully with his neighbors, makes his children healthy citizens and after fulfilling such basic responsibilities is still empowered with sufficient strength to serve the cause of the society in any way.

K.A. Menninger (1930:46): Let us define mental health as the adjustment of human beings to the world and each other with a maximum of effectiveness and happiness. It is the ability to maintain even temper, an alert intelligence, socially considerate behavior and a happy disposition.

Cutts and Moslay (1941:4): Mental health is the ability which helps us to seek adjustment in the difficult situations of our life.

Let us analyze these definitions one by one.

- The first two definitions given by Waltin and Hadfield consider mental health as the means and measure for the development and functioning of a wholesome, well-balanced, and integrated personality. Considered this way, mental health has a wider scope than physical health. It concerns the all-around development of the personality, and not merely the development of one's physical or bodily aspects. Moreover, it aims at the balanced personality—a personality that is able to stand firmly in the midst of stress and strain and who can exhibit adequate emotional maturity and balance between needs and circumstances. For this, a person should behave as an integrated personality and not a split personality or a mind torn between various courses of action or inconsistent behavior patterns. Truly speaking, for passing judgment about one's mental health, we may safely take the consistency of this behavior as one of the sound criteria. Individuals who can make proper judgments and are consistent in their behavior can be said to enjoy good mental health in comparison to those who are in conflict and practice double standards in their behavior.
- The remaining three definitions suggested by Lewkan, Menninger, and Cutts as well as Moslay consider mental health as the state of one's peace of mind, happiness, and harmony

brought out by one's level of adjustment with their self and environment. Such a person is capable of successfully steering away from difficult situations involving stresses without losing balance or breaking and exhausting themself. Judging in this way, we can conclude that *mental health is the health of one's mind which can prove a potent determinant of one's integrated personality and balanced behavior identified on the basis of their level of adjustment to self, others, and their environment.*

Understanding the Concept of Mental Health

There are certain well-known characteristics and findings for understanding the true concept of mental health. They are mentioned briefly as follows:

1. There is **no such thing as perfect mental health:** It is difficult to see a person who is mentally healthy in all aspects. Truly speaking, perfect mental health is a fiction and not reality. Hence, it is always better to talk of optimum mental health in place of perfect mental health.
2. **Mental health is a dynamic concept:** Mental health denotes a state of balance or equilibrium of our mind. This balance is not static; it is quite dynamic. The circumstances in our life are never static and since they are changeable, so is our adjustment. The adjustments we have achieved at any point with ourselves and the environmental forces may not be helpful in the future, so one's mental health is always in a state of flux. For example, suggestibility at the age of two may be a normal trait of personality, but not so after attaining maturity.
3. **Mental health can't be achieved without physical health:** The saying that "a sound mind lives in a sound body" is quite true. For achieving an optimal level of mental health, one must first acquire adequate physical health.
4. **Mental health and efficiency are not the same things:** It is not necessarily essential for a successful and efficient person to be mentally healthy as well. One may be efficient and successful at their work or profession, but also be quite unhappy, full of anxiety, and other issues.
5. **Mental health and social ability are not the same things:** While a mentally healthy person is sociable, not every sociable or socially adaptable person is healthy minded. One may be sociable but extremely anxious to please everybody. Similarly, they may act amenable because of an inherent sense of insecurity or inferiority.
6. **Mental health differs from ethical standards:** Mental health differs from ethical standards. Morality does not guarantee mental health. There exist many individuals who are very moral but suffer from serious abnormalities like phobias or sexual perversions.

Characteristics of a Mentally Healthy Individual
(Symptoms of Good Mental Health)

A mentally healthy individual can be easily distinguished from others by their mode of living, behavior, and personality characteristics. In general, these features and characteristics can be summarized as follows:

1. They know themself well and are in a position to evaluate their strengths and weaknesses. Therefore, they tend to choose tasks of intermediate difficulty—neither too difficult nor too easy.
2. They have adequate ability to make adjustments in changing circumstances and situations.

3. They are emotionally mature and stable, are able to express emotions in a desirable way, and exercise proper control over them.

4. They are socially adjustable and possess an adequate ability to get along well with themself and others.

5. Their intellectual powers are adequately developed. They are able to think independently and take proper decisions at the proper time.

6. They live in the world of reality rather than that of imagination and fantasy.

7. They possess enough courage and resilience for facing failures in life. They do not worry about failures and mistakes.

8. They feel quite safe and secure in their respective groups and environment. They like others and are liked by them. They possess an adequate sense of belonging and loyalty toward the groups to which they belong.

9. Although they try to accomplish work as well as possible, they do not prove to be an extremist by becoming a perfectionist.

10. They are free from undesirable mental disturbances, disorders, conflicts, anxieties, frustrations, ailments, and diseases.

11. They possess desirable social and health habits. They are regular and punctual in performing duties and do not suffer from forgetfulness.

12. They are self-confident and optimistic. They do not exhibit undue fear and anxiety about newly assigned tasks.

13. They have a healthy sexual life and do not suffer from sex abnormalities or dissatisfaction.

14. They possess an adequate philosophy of life that governs their conduct and activities.

15. They possess socially desirable healthy interests and aptitudes.

16. They lead a well-balanced life of work, rest, and recreation.

17. They are satisfied with their profession or occupation.

This list of characteristics should not be taken as necessary conditions for the maintenance of proper mental health; the absence of one or the other characteristics does not necessarily mean the negation of mental health. Acquisition of perfect mental health, as reflected by these characteristics, is an ideal state, and therefore, although we should aim to reach close to this, we should not be unduly worried about achieving perfection regarding these traits and characteristics.

Characteristics of a Mentally Unhealthy Individual (Symptoms of Poor Mental Health)

With regard to the symptoms of poor mental health, we can make a list of all the opposite negative features and characteristics of one's behavior and personality characteristics in contradiction to what has been said above about the symptoms of good mental health. In brief, these symptoms may be outlined as:

- Emotionally unstable and easily upset
- Apprehensive, suspicious, and insecure
- Self-critical, empowered with a feeling of guilt
- Lacks self-confidence and willpower
- No adequate adjustment with the self and the environment—physical, social, and professional
- Failure in setting a proper level of aspiration

- Suffers from frustrations, unresolved conflicts, strains, and stresses
- Lacks enduring power and tolerance
- Lacks decision-making ability
- Poor self-concept and achievement motivation
- Unrealistic attitude toward life and people
- Suffers from mental disturbances, disorders, ailments, and diseases
- Always dissatisfied with their achievements and tries to seek perfection in their own work or others'
- Lives in their own world of imagination and fantasy.

To Sum Up

Mental health is concerned with the health of one's mind and its functioning in the same way as physical health is concerned with the health of one's physical organs and their functioning. A mentally healthy person is supposed to possess an integrated personality and balanced behavior identified on the basis of the level of one's adjustment to self, others, and their environment. However, there is no such thing as perfect mental health. Therefore, it is always better to strive for *optimum* mental health in place of *perfect* mental health. A mentally healthy individual can be distinguished from others easily through their mode of living, behavior, and personality characteristics typically associated with good mental health. We can also list the opposite negative features and characteristics of behavior indicative of good mental health to list the symptoms of one's poor mental health.

Importance of Mental Health

Health is rightly called wealth. It involves one's physical as well as mental health. As said earlier, mental health has a much wider scope than physical health, as it aims for the development of a wholesome, balanced and integrated personality. The acquisition of such a personality is indeed a great asset and privilege for a normal individual. They can be able to actualize themself, live life to their satisfaction and happiness, and strive as well as attain one's goals in tune with taking and giving to society. It is possible only when one enjoys good mental health and one can enjoy good mental health only when one is cautious about their mental health and knows its value and importance along with means and ways for achieving and maintaining it. For this, let us first discuss the importance or value of mental health:

1. **Helps in the development of a desirable personality:** Mental health helps in the development of a wholesome, well-balanced, and integrated personality. A mentally healthy individual maintains a proper balance between self and their environmental situation, their needs, and the needs of society, and embodies an example of an integrated personality instead of a splitting one.
2. **Helps in proper emotional development:** There is a close relationship between one's mental health and emotional behavior. Individuals who enjoy good mental health demonstrate emotional maturity in their behavior. On the other side, those who are tense, disintegrated, and mentally unhealthy demonstrate sudden emotional outbursts and emotional immaturity.

3. **Helps in proper social development:** One's mental health helps one in becoming sociable and establishing proper social relationships in society. One who is not in conflict with oneself has sufficient time and energy available for attending to others, which helps in one's proper social behavior and adequate social adjustment.

4. **Helps in proper moral development:** Individuals who enjoy sound mental health are usually found to behave as people of integrity and character by following the ethical standards of society. The proper functioning of their intellect guards them against immoral and unsocial behavior. They are able to exercise reasonable control over their emotions and channel their energy to noble tasks.

5. **Helps in proper aesthetic development:** Proper mental health helps the individual in the development of appropriate aesthetic sense, artistic taste, and refined temperament. A mind free of any tension, conflict, frustration, inferiority, guilt, or hostile feelings, may have a better chance of drifting toward aesthetic, artistic, and creative channels than the mind torn between complexities and conflicts.

6. **Helps in actualizing one's potentialities:** Every one of us has a fund of natural abilities and potentialities that can be actualized through proper efforts. Exercising such efforts and striving toward the actualization of one's potentialities depend, to a great extent, on the state of one's mental health. While people with good mental health can strive well for the actualization of their potentialities, mentally unhealthy ones fail to do so on account of the malfunctioning of their intellectual powers, disintegrated personalities, and maladapted behaviors.

7. **Helps in seeking proper adjustment:** A mentally healthy individual is an adjusted person. They are able to seek adequate adjustment of self and environment. They are able to adjust their needs as per the demands of the situation and the well-being of society. Hence, mental health helps the individual to build a harmonious relationship between self and environment.

8. **Helps in seeking goals in life:** Mental health helps the individual to strive properly for the realization of the goals in their life. These goals may differ from person to person depending upon their lifestyles and philosophy of life. But optimum mental health helps individuals to divert their energies in full capacity for the realization of these goals and live life to their satisfaction, aiming toward happiness for themselves and others.

9. **Helps in the progress of society:** Mental health helps individuals to develop as well-balanced, useful citizens who are conscious not only of their rights but also of their responsibilities. They take essentials from society for their proper development and living but are also ready to give something back to society for its progress and development. The prosperity and progress of a society are linked with the health, particularly the mental health, of its members. The desired peace, progress, and happiness of a society can only be possible when its members enjoy the same in terms of their sound mental health.

10. **Helps in the prevention of mental illness:** Mental health helps an individual in protecting themself against abnormalities of behavior, maladjustment, illness, and mental diseases in the same way as maintenance of physical health helps save them from physical illness, ailments, and diseases. A sound mind and balanced personality has enough resistance to fight against the odds of life and bear the accidental stresses and strains of life in comparison to those with impaired mental health. Therefore, adequate preservation of mental health by the individual and proper education about it may help in a big way in reducing cases of mental illness and diseases in society.

Principles of Mental Health

Achievement of proper physical health rests on the observation of the principles of physical health. Similarly, we can help ourselves and others achieve good mental health by acquainting ourselves with the principles of mental health. What these principles comprise is an issue that must be considered wisely.

It is an established fact that one enjoys mental health to the extent to which one is reasonably satisfied with one's self as well as one's environment. Consequently, we can roughly divide these principles into two categories, as follows:

A. Principles seeking adjustment with one's self.
B. Principles seeking adjustment with one's environment.

Principles Seeking Adjustment with One's Self

One can ensure good mental health if one remains adjusted with oneself. The following seven principles may work well in seeking such adjustment.

THE PRINCIPLE OF KNOWING THE SELF

One must be quite aware of themself, specifically in terms of one's strengths and limitations, so that one can accordingly shape one's behavior and direct one's attempts for the realization of goals in life.

THE PRINCIPLE OF ACCEPTING ONE'S SELF

One who accepts and respects oneself is likely to enjoy good mental health while someone who always complains about their inadequacy or the circumstances of their life, or blames others for their misfortunes, cannot be expected to lead a healthy mental life.

THE PRINCIPLE OF BALANCING THE LEVEL OF ASPIRATION

One should not set one's level of aspiration and achievement motivation either too high or too low but should try to set it at a proper level by keeping in view one's own capabilities and opportunities on one hand and their goals and objectives on the other. This can help one avoid unnecessary frustrations and failures.

THE PRINCIPLE OF BALANCING ONE'S DEVELOPMENT

Mental health aims for the development of a wholesome, well-balanced personality. Accordingly, one should seek and strive for the balanced, harmonious development of their personality in all dimensions—physical, mental, emotional, social, moral. and aesthetic.

THE PRINCIPLE OF INTEGRATING THE SELF

The self of the person should portray itself as an integrated whole and not as a split personality. One should not make oneself torn between opposing and conflicting desires and ambitions, and should not fall prey to unnecessary tensions and indecisiveness.

THE PRINCIPLE OF SELF-DRIVE AND SHAPING

It is quite wrong and contrary to the principles of mental health when a person is forced into a shape that is wished by others while completely ignoring their own wishes. Similarly, it is wrong to allow others to drive oneself contrary to one's own ideals and aspirations. The individual themselves must be their own driver and be allowed to freely shape their own destiny; then and only then can they move in the direction of satisfactory mental health.

THE PRINCIPLE OF SELF CONTROL

There is no need to exercise external control for disciplining an individual. Enforced discipline may lead to aggression or regression of one's behavior. The better way to help them in gaining good mental health is to guide them to exercise control over themself.

The Principles Seeking Adjustment with Environment

Besides seeking harmony with oneself, one must have a reasonable harmony and adjustment with the people, materials, and situations present in their environment. Ten principles helping in this task are discussed, as follows:

THE PRINCIPLE OF UNDERSTANDING OTHERS

One must not only understand themself but also try to understand others properly so that they can behave well with them according to their limitations and strengths, needs and desires, interests and attitudes, and taste and temperaments.

THE PRINCIPLE OF ACCEPTING AND RESPECTING OTHER'S INDIVIDUALITIES

Every person has his or her unique individuality, style of life, and personality traits. While seeking respect for ourselves we must not forget to pay due respect to others' selves and individualities. We might invite unnecessary quarrels, tensions, and conflicts by attacking their self and showing disrespect to their individuality and personality. We must also try to accept others as they are in terms of their existing strengths and limitations, and good or bad habits, for seeking proper adjustment with them.

THE PRINCIPLE OF SOCIALIZING ONE'S SELF

Individuals who are better in terms of social relationships, adjustments, and adaptation, are able to achieve good mental health in comparison to those who are unsocial, ego-centric, selfish, and lonely. Therefore, in achieving good mental health for children, it is important to seek proper socialization for them. They must be taught to harmonize their self with the self of others. They must realize that the true fulfillment of life lies in service, i.e., giving oneself to some extent to the need of others.

THE PRINCIPLE OF ADEQUATE SATISFACTION OF NEEDS

We as human beings have many needs categorized as organic and socio-psychological needs. These needs are as basic and fundamental as the need for oxygen, water, food, and so on, which are essential for our survival. Sex gratification and satisfaction of socio-psychological needs like the need for security, love and affection, freedom, companionship, recognition, and self-actualization are also essential for the proper growth, development, and happiness of human beings. Truly speaking, the level of one's mental health depends upon the level of the satisfaction of one's needs. One remains normal and enjoys satisfactory mental health as long as their needs are gratified or are on the way to gratification. In case one is deprived of the satisfaction of their needs, or these are thwarted and threatened, one becomes maladjusted and drifts toward impairment of their mental health.

Therefore, due care should be taken in the satisfaction and gratification of the needs of the individuals for making them mentally healthy.

THE PRINCIPLE OF TRAINING THE EMOTIONS

Emotional energy, if utilized properly, is a big asset for the progress and development of an individual. However, if it drifts away from its normal expression and gets out of control, it may spell disaster. The repression of this energy is also equally dangerous, as it may give birth to various problems of mental health. The best way is to have one's emotions trained so that the flow of emotional energy may be directed into constructive channels. Such training may be properly imparted by adopting the techniques of sublimation and catharsis.

THE PRINCIPLE OF ADJUSTMENT TO THE WORLD OF WORK

For enjoying normal mental health, one must be reasonably satisfied and adjusted with their work life. Those who are maladjusted with their work and profession cannot remain adjusted in their lives and consequently suffer from mental worries and problems. The right thing is to develop a positive attitude toward one's world of work by remembering the maxim "work is worship." Work that is done half-heartedly or with a negative outlook and rebellious attitude is likely to affect not only the quality of the work but also the mental health of the workers quite adversely. Therefore, one must try to seek proper adjustment to their work and profession for the proper safeguard of their mental health.

THE PRINCIPLE OF A POSITIVE ATTITUDE TOWARD LIFE

The state of one's mental health is greatly determined by one's attitude toward life. While the positive and optimistic outlook may keep one smiling by providing sufficient strength and patience in facing the realities of life, the negative and pessimistic attitude may drive them toward feelings of inferiority, hostility toward one's environment, frustration, and agonies of life. Therefore, it is better to learn the lessons of developing a positive attitude toward the activities of life by looking at each morning as a new day and not carrying the troubles of yesterday. It is in learning such lessons that individuals gain control in terms of better mental health.

THE PRINCIPLE OF BEARING THE STRESSES AND STRAINS OF LIFE

Life is not always a bed of roses. It often offers challenges, struggles, and problems that are to be faced with patience and courage. In addition to this, there are many incidents and accidents involving stresses and strains, the pressures of which must be borne by the individuals concerned. It is the duty of parents to teach their children to remain strong in times of stress and strain. They must set positive examples of resilience against the odds and eventualities of life. Those who make themselves trained and wise for the stresses and strains of life are able to preserve their mental health in a proper way in comparison to those who easily break in the storms of life.

THE PRINCIPLE OF GOOD PHYSICAL HEALTH

A healthy mind lives in a healthy body. Keeping one's body and physical health in a satisfactory, normal condition is the prime and most basic requirement for achieving and maintaining good mental health. How can we expect a physically, somatically weak man to keep his mind free from tension, worries, and other negative and depressive feelings? The health of one's nervous system, ductless glands, body systems, and organs are sure to affect one's mental functioning and personal and social adjustment, leading to good or poor mental health.

THE PRINCIPLE OF HAVING FAITH IN GOD AND NATURE

In this age of extreme materialism and degradation of human values, there has been a tremendous rise in the rate of cases of mental illness and mental diseases. Everywhere in the world there is cut throat competition to outperform each other and snatch others' shares for enhancing oneself. "Self is great" is the slogan of the present age and this extreme selfishness has resulted in the miseries and agonies of human beings. The results are obvious. Nobody cares for others. There is nothing like mutual trust, harmony, love, and affection left among human beings. Everybody is suspicious and jealous of others. Consequently, everybody is tense and facing mental worries and problems. The loss of faith calls for the imposition of faith. There must be something to provide a sense of security. The only one who can be trusted to show due affection is none other than the Almighty. The wounded human psyche needs a healing touch, and it can be provided by one's faith in God. The ultimate cure for keeping oneself free from mental worries and tension thus lies in having faith in God and Nature. One should aim at doing one's duties and sharing one's responsibilities as sincerely as one can without caring for the fruits of one's action, and leaving it to God and Nature. Such attitudes and actions can certainly prove very helpful in achieving and maintaining proper mental health.

Role of Clinical Psychologists in the Maintenance of People's Mental Health

Clinical psychology as a distinguished branch of the subject of psychology tries to integrate science, theory, and practice to understand, predict, and alleviate maladjustment, disabilities, and discomfort as well as to promote their needed adaptation and adjustment for contributing toward the maintenance of their mental health and well-being in a proper way. Equipped with the useful knowledge and skills of the subject of clinical psychology, professional clinical psychologists play a useful role in serving the required purpose of helping people in the maintenance of their mental health, in the manner discussed next.

Preservation and Promotion of Mental Health

Clinical psychologists, recognized as the main mental health professionals in the community, work in a significant way for the preservation and promotion of the community's mental health. The measures they employ for this purpose are as follows:

- Arousing consciousness among the people for the upkeep of their proper mental health by working along with community workers and other health professionals.

- Suggesting ways and means for the proper preservation and promotion of mental health in the community.
- Helping people to seek proper adjustment with their self and environment as adequately as possible.
- Providing adequate guidance and help to maladjusted individuals by going through the possible causes of their maladjustment.

Prevention of Mental Health Problems and Ailments

The knowledge and skills acquired by clinical psychologists through their study and training in clinical psychology help them in getting acquainted with the possible causes of mental health problems and ailments among the community. Equipped with such knowledge, they help people in taking the necessary preventive measures for the avoidance of falling victim to mental health problems and ailments, in the manner as follows:

- To remain cautious about the genetic inheritance of mental disorders.
- To take care of the causes and factors for which they themselves are responsible, such as their physical health and fitness, undesirable social and emotional behavior, unrealistic goals and aspirations, negative thinking, pessimism, antagonism, aggressive attitude, maladjustment with self and environment, and so on.
- The due precautions adopted on the part of parents, elders, teachers, and the community for preventing people in their younger years from getting haunted by ugly experiences resulting in one or the other types of mental disorders.

Identification and Diagnosis of Mental Health Problems and Disorders

Clinical psychologists are well equipped for carrying out the task of identifying and diagnosing mental health problems and disorders. In fact, they are the health professionals who are first reached by victims of mental health problems before consulting psychiatrists for this purpose. Activities like the following are usually undertaken by them for this purpose.

- Filing the reports of the patient and their family members or friends regarding the suffering related to their emotional, behavioral, and mental problems.
- Observing the symptoms and signs related to the reported problem.
- Making use of non-testing devices like the naturalistic method of observation, case history, and a clinical interview for the diagnosis of the problem.
- Making use of testing devices such as achievement tests, intelligence tests, personality inventories, objective specific psychological tests (e.g., measures of adjustment, depression, anxiety, and self-esteem), projective personality tests, and neuropsychological testing as a method of clinical assessment.
- Drawing conclusions about the nature of the mental health problem and assessing the capacities and adequacies of the client (the person with the mental health problem).
- Naming the mental health problem or disorder by matching their observations and diagnosis with the symptoms and diagnostic criteria provided by the APA and WHO in the DSM and ICD for the purpose of psychological treatment conducted by themselves or further referral to specialists, such as psychiatrists.

Treatment of Mental Health Problems and Disorders

After carrying out the necessary identification, diagnosis, and assessment of the nature of a client's mental health problem, along with an assessment of their capabilities and adequacies, the actual task of providing needed treatment to the client is carried out by clinical psychologists in the manner as follows:

- Chalking out a plan or strategy for the cure and treatment of their mental health problems.
- Working with the client for their needed treatment by planning, implementing, and following up using a suitable psychotherapeutic treatment plan.
- Cooperating with other mental health professionals including psychiatrists and other specialists in mental health for dealing effectively with the client's problem.
- Taking necessary steps for the after-treatment care and proper rehabilitation of the treated patients.

To Sum Up

Attainment of good mental health occupies a very important place in one's life. One's overall adjustment to themself and their environment is essential for leading a happy and contented life, and this depends upon the acquisition of good mental health. For the proper attainment of good mental health, one has to observe certain basic principles specifically meant for seeking adjustment with one's self and environment. Clinical psychologists are health professionals who can assist people on both fronts of the maintenance of their mental health—its preservation and promotion, as well as providing a remedy for its derailment in the form of identifying, diagnosing, and treating mental health problems and disorders.

Review Questions

1. Define the term mental hygiene and discuss its aims and purposes in detail.
2. Define the term mental health and throw light on this concept in detail.
3. Who are mentally healthy individuals? Throw light on the characteristics or signs of good mental health.
4. Point out the characteristics or symptoms associated with poor mental health.
5. What is mental health? Discuss its significance and importance for us.
6. Discuss in detail the principles helpful in the maintenance of one's proper mental health.
7. Throw light on the roles and activities undertaken by clinical psychologists for helping people in the proper maintenance of their mental health.

References

American Psychological Association (2022), Definition of mental hygiene, *APA Dictionary of Psychology*, retrieved from dictionary, apa.org/mental-hygiene

Crow, L. D., & Crow, A. (1951), *Mental hygiene*, New York, NY: McGraw-Hill Inc.

Crow, L. D., & Crow, A. (1969), *Child psychology*, New York, NY: Barnes & Noble, Inc.

Cutts, N. F., & Moslay, P. (1941), *Practical school discipline and mental hygiene*, Boston, MA: Houghton Mifflin.

Drever, J. (1952), *A dictionary of psychology*, Middlesex: Penguin Books.

Good, C. V. (1959), *Dictionary of education*, New York, NY: McGraw-Hill.

Hadfield, J. A. (1952), *Mental health and the psychoneurosis*, London: George Allen & Unwin.

Klein, D. B. (1965), *Mental hygiene* (Revised ed.), New York, NY: Henry Holt.

Lewkan, P. B. (1949), *Mental hygiene in public health*, New York, NY: McGraw-Hill.

Menninger, K. A. (1930), *Human mind*, New York, NY: The Literary Guild of America.

Shaffer, L. F. (1936), *The psychology of adjustment*, New York, NY: Houghton Mifflin.

Singh, L., & Tiwari, G. P. (1971), *Essentials of abnormal psychology*, Agra: Vinod Pustak Mandir.

Waltin, J. E. W. (1951), *Personality, maladjustment and mental hygiene* (3rd ed.), New York, NY: McGraw Hill.

Chapter 6

Normality and Abnormality of Behavior

Learning Objectives

After going through this chapter, you will be able to:

- Define normal and abnormal behavior.
- Know about the criteria for determining the normality or abnormality of people's behavior.
- Decide the appropriateness of criteria for determining abnormal behavior.
- Throw light on the various causes or factors responsible for abnormality of behavior.

Meaning of the Terms Normal and Abnormal Behavior

The term "normal" seems to be derived from the word "norma," which means a carpenter's square or rule. A norm, therefore, indicates a rule, pattern, or standard, and it was in this sense that the term "normal" was introduced into the English lexicon. The term "abnormal" with its prefix "ab" (away from) thus came to signify the deviance or variation from the normal. Anything not normal must, therefore, be abnormal. But there is some difficulty in deciding what is normal. In the basic or medical sciences, it is easy to decide what is normal. In examining the temperature of the body, blood pressure, the amount of sugar in the blood, and pulse rate, there exist standard universal norms. On a psychological front, however, we cannot have an ideal model behavior to be used as a standard norm. As a result, the problem of deciding what behavior is or is not normal has proved to be a difficult one. However, several attempts have been made for describing what is normal or abnormal in the form of laying down several criteria for deciding the normality or abnormality of behavior. Let us look into them.

Normality and Abnormality Criteria

The criterion used for defining normality and abnormality can be grouped into the following two broad categories, named (A) Descriptive criteria and (B) Explanatory criteria. They indicate the ways in which abnormal behavior differs from normal behavior; they tell us why some behavior is abnormal. Let us examine them.

The descriptive criteria may be further subdivided into two groups—statistical or non-statistical. Under the non-statistical criteria, we may place methods or approaches like the

DOI: 10.4324/9781003398325-6

ethical or moral viewpoint, social conformity, perfectionism, and the legal viewpoint, whereas under explanatory criteria, we may include aspects such as pathological or medical criteria and psychological criteria. This classification can be represented diagrammatically as follows:

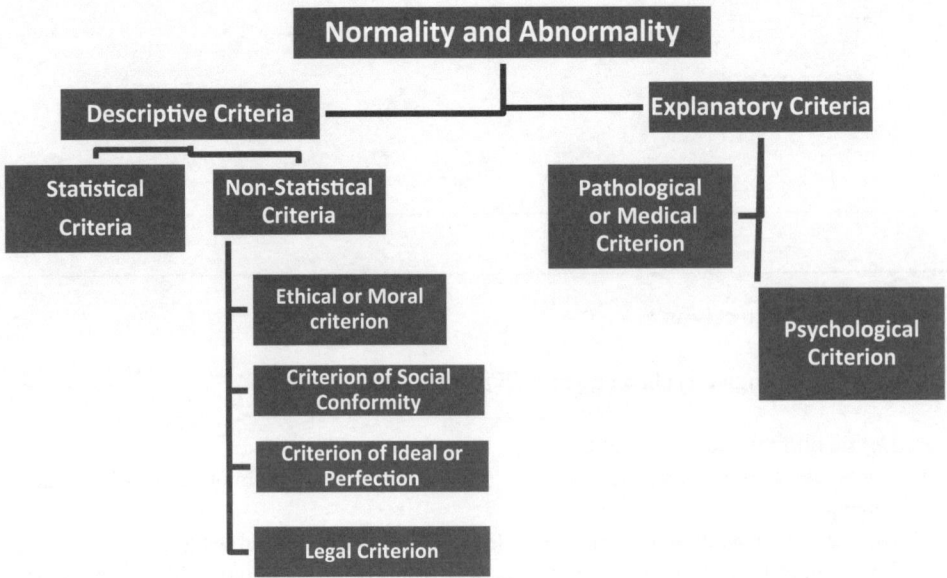

Figure 6.1 Diagrammatic representation of the criteria defining normality and abnormality

A. Descriptive Criteria

(a) Statistical criterion: According to this criterion, "average" is normal. A person is abnormal when he or she deviates from the "average." For example, there is an average height and an average weight for normal human beings, and those who come close to this average are considered normal while those who deviate from the average are considered abnormal. The statistical criterion may be properly explained through a normal distribution curve (See Figure 6.2).

Here the distribution of IQ in the general population is illustrated. The bell-shaped curve illustrates that the cases falling around the middle of the distribution are to be termed as normal and those at the extreme ends as abnormal.

Unfortunately, the statistical criterion is inadequate in several aspects described as follows:

First, according to this criterion, any deviation from the average or majority would be abnormal. A genius would be as abnormal as a mentally retarded person. The inadequacy of the Statistical criterion is self-evident, as we cannot label the people who deviate in a positive or favorable way as abnormal. They may be called "superior" or "above average" but not "abnormal."

Second, we are all deviant (or different) from one another in some aspects. No two individuals are alike in interests, abilities, or physical appearance. These are all potential dimensions of difference, and an individual may sometimes deviate seriously from the norms or averages set by us. If we take deviation from the average as the only criterion of abnormality, then perhaps Gandhi, Vivekanand, Christ, Prem Chand, Newton, and Pythagoras would surely be listed as abnormal.

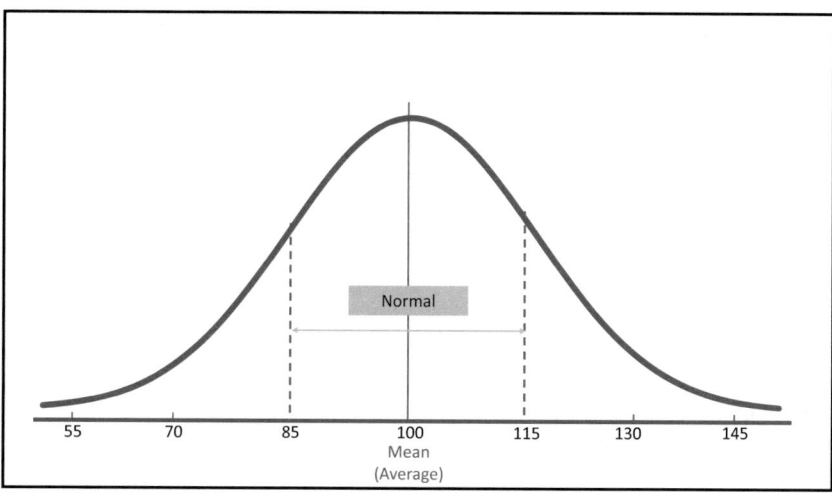

Figure 6.2 The distribution of IQ in the general population (IQ below 75 termed subnormal and those above 115 as above normal)

Third, to label something as abnormal we compare the deviance from the average, which may change from time to time or from group to group. Behaviors considered normal in a particular society or culture may be labeled abnormal in a different society or culture. What was considered abnormal in the 19th century may fit well in the current time (for example, widow remarriage, use of modem birth control measures, etc.). Therefore, abnormality is not simply a deviation from some average as advocated by the statistical criterion.

Fourth, the inadequacy of the statistical criterion also lies in its variability in the analysis of personality disturbance or mental illness. It becomes more pronounced when we come to know that these methods, however sophisticated they may be, hardly tell us why people become abnormal.

Statistical criteria is based on the false assumption that all personality traits and human variations can be expressed as quantitative deviations. But the difference between being disturbed or undisturbed is qualitative rather than quantitative. Not all maladjusted or affected people are high or low on a given dimension of behavior.

b. **Non-statistical criteria:** Under this broad category, we may include the criteria discussed ahead.

Ethical or moral criterion:

According to this criterion, a person is considered to be abnormal if he or she acts in an immoral manner. This criterion is solely based on value judgments made by people who observe behavior. For being taken as normal, the behavior should be appropriate and desirable from the viewpoint of ethics or morality. This description of normality and abnormality carries the following defects:

(i)   The major problem with this perspective is that morality is not an absolute concept. What is "moral" or "immoral" may change from place to place and from time to time.

(ii) A person who is known to have good morality may show signs of known behavioral disorders, while many people who are labeled as psychologically deviant may not exhibit any immoral behavior. To be affected by anxiety or depression cannot be labeled as immoral. Therefore, morality cannot be made a criterion for deciding one's behavior as normal or abnormal.

2. Criterion of social conformity:
   According to this criterion, those who conform to societal norms are considered normal and those who do not care for them are labeled abnormal. This view is based on the assumption that normality is what the majority of people approve of or follow. For example, if wearing short hair, tight jeans, or a sleeveless blouse gets social approval, it may be taken as normal or else it would be labeled abnormal. Hence, if we adopt social conformity as the sole criterion of deciding whether behavior is normal or abnormal, we will have to change our decision from place to place or culture to culture and in the same culture or place from time to time, as we cannot ignore the changes in attitude regarding what is socially acceptable and normal.

3. Criterion of ideal or perfection:
   According to this criterion, normal behavior is equated with perfect or ideal behavior. Very few persons attain a level of perfection unattained by the masses. They become ideals and serve as models for defining model behavior. A major flaw in this criterion lies in the fact that there exists no such thing as an absolute ideal or perfect person. This topic is purely subjective; for example, one may think the life and behavior of Gandhi as ideal, but for the activists and revolutionaries not he but Subhash Chandra Bose or Bhagat Singh may be the ideals. Besides, this approach is based on what ideal behavior ought to be and not what it is. The model of ideal behavior varies from situation to situation and, in a situation, from time to time. The behavior which is considered ideal for a particular age in a particular situation may altogether be labeled abnormal in a different age or a different situation.

4. Legal criterion:
   According to this criterion, a law-abiding citizen is normal but one who violates the law is labeled abnormal. Behaviors like murder, rape, burglary, or prostitution come from this legal definition arid are definitely labeled antisocial or abnormal. But what is legal or illegal is again a matter of controversy. In a dynamic society, laws change fast. Hence, they are not absolute, but change from society to society, place to place, and even from time to time. Therefore, the legal criterion cannot be made a reliable or valid criterion for the judgment of normality or abnormality.

B. Explanatory Criterion

The criterion falling into this broad category are discussed as follows.

(a) *Pathological or medical criterion*—According to this criterion, the normality or abnormality of one's behavior depends upon the functioning of the nervous system. In this way, all abnormal people are affected by some mental illness or disease. Consequently, they should be sent to mental hospitals as patients for treatment by persons who are trained to cure them. This view has a wide appeal and has been responsible for arousing a mass feeling that abnormal behavior is somehow an indication of an illness or disease.

However, the inadequacy of this criterion has now also been exposed. Most people who are found to be mentally disturbed do not suffer from "diseases" or "illnesses" in the usual sense of these terms. They show no signs of structural damage or dysfunction in their nervous systems. Therefore, it may be seen that the pathological or medical criterion cannot work as a reliable and valid criterion for the definition of normality or abnormality in all situations.

(b) *Psychological criterion:* According to this criterion, psychological functioning—whether defective or normal—is the deciding factor of abnormal versus normal behavior. Eysenck (1960) writes, "Abnormality then is not in terms of people suffering from mental diseases produced by definite causes; it is rather in terms of defective functioning of certain psychological systems."

On analyzing this criterion, it is seen that abnormality, whatever kind or form it may have, is linked with the malfunctioning of certain psychological systems. Abnormal people are psychologically handicapped individuals, but their behavior is not the exclusive product of psychological or sociological causes. In any case, biological and physiological factors may not be ruled out in the explanation of the behavior of abnormal people.

Conclusion Regarding Different Criteria

The different criteria discussed above represent the many ways and approaches for understanding "normal" and "abnormal" behavior. No criterion may be termed an absolute criterion for the complete description or explanation of normal versus abnormal behavior. One section of these views only describes and the other only explains which behavior is not normal or normal. As far as the criteria of morality, social conformity, perfection, or legality are concerned, they are purely subjective, and hence, no reliability or validity may be placed in their utility for the judgment of normal or abnormal behavior. The statistical criterion, which views deviation from the average as the deciding factor for abnormality, also suffers from serious defects. Human behavior which cannot be expressed as quantitative cannot be judged as normal or abnormal through this criterion. Moreover, deviation on any scale does not necessarily imply abnormality. On account of the theory of deviation, abnormal people have received social disapproval. The modern approach advocating the need for a healthy environment as a preventive and curative measure for the abnormal disregards the theory of deviation and replaces it with the concept of variance. According to Mahoney (1980:8), such modern views in this respect may be summarized as follows.

1. There are no thoughts, behaviors, or feelings which are inherently crazy or abnormal. The normality of any act or pattern is "relative" to many other factors, and it does not depend solely on the event itself.
2. All organisms vary in their thoughts, behaviors, and feelings. Presumed differences between normal and abnormal persons (or actions) have to do with the degree (and not of categories) of variance.

Empirical studies have now established that there are no "normal" people on one end of the scale and "abnormal" people on the other, as suggested by statistical criteria. Behavior, even in normal individuals, may fluctuate between normal and abnormal at times of stress. For example, a normal person may start drinking after an unhappy love affair, death of a spouse, or a loss in business. Therefore, it may be concluded that the statistical criterion does not give an adequate description and explanation for the normality and abnormality of one's behavior.

With regard to the effectiveness of other criteria known as the pathological or medical criterion and the psychological criterion, we may say that they both in their own ways possess a reasonable capacity for defining the normality and abnormality of one's behavior. They are also capable of providing satisfactory explanations for the abnormality or malfunctioning. They also possess a reasonable capacity of providing sufficient objectivity, reliability, and validity for diagnosing and assessing the level of abnormality and mental illness among affected individuals. However, we also cannot depend upon any of them exclusively in deciding whether a certain behavior is normal or abnormal. In some cases, the pathological or medical approach helps in the diagnosis and explanation of one's abnormality, while in others, the abnormality, in the absence of any organic cause, may be detected and explained through the malfunctioning of certain psychological systems. Therefore, it is wise and beneficial to make use of both these criteria for making decisions about the normality and abnormality of one's behavior.

To Sum Up

In its simple meaning the term normal stands for a set of rules, patterns, or standards, while abnormal indicates deviance or variance from the normal. For determining the abnormality of people's behavior, several criteria are in vogue, mainly divided into two broad categories known as Descriptive criteria and Explanatory criteria. In the category of descriptive criteria, we may place the statistical criterion and the non-statistical ones such as the Ethics or moral criterion, the Criterion of social conformity, the Criterion of ideal or perfection, and the Legal Criterion, while criteria like the Pathological or medical criterion and the Psychological criterion fall in the category of explanatory criteria. Among these so-described descriptive and explanatory criteria, a proper analysis of their functioning and usability reveals that the last two are more objective, reliable, and valid in providing explanations for and determining the abnormality of one's behavior in the context of the situation.

Causes or Factors Responsible for Abnormality in Behavior

The causes or factors responsible for abnormality in one's behavior may be broadly classified as (i) Heredity Factors, (ii) Biological Factors, (iii) Psychological Factors, and (iv) Sociological Factors. Let us look into these factors.

Hereditary Factors

Heredity consists of all that is transferred to offspring from the immediate parents in the form of genes and chromosomes at the time of conception when the fetus acquires 46 chromosomes, that is 23 pairs of chromosomes—one of each pair being derived from the mother and one from the father. Each chromosome contains genes numbering one to two thousand, each of which contributes to the transmission of hereditary characteristics.

The first 22 pairs of chromosomes are called autosomes. They determine physical characteristics. The remaining 23rd pair of chromosomes, called the sex-linked pair, determines the individual's sex and other sex-linked characteristics. In the male child, one member of the sex-linked pair is an X chromosome (usually large in size) contributed by the mother, and the other is a Y chromosome (comparatively smaller than X) contributed by the father. In the female child, both of these sex-linked chromosomes, one from each parent, are X chromosomes.

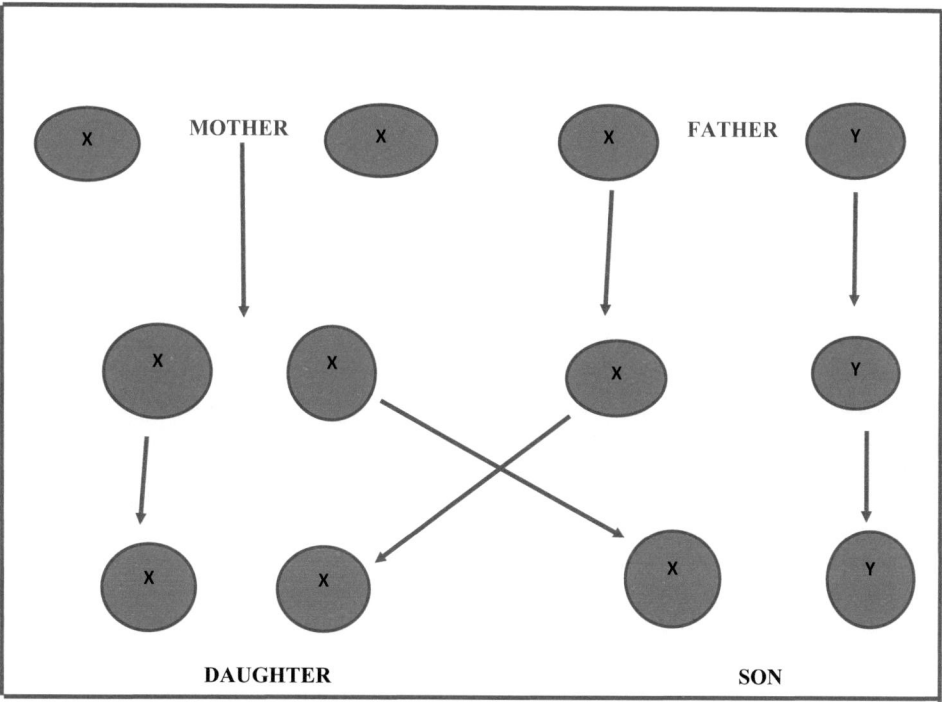

Figure 6.3 Son or daughter?

The Role of Chromosomes

Abnormalities are found to be transmitted both by the sex-linked chromosomes and the autosomes. A few examples are as follows.

1. One possible genetic anomaly is a missing sex chromosome. This abnormality, called Turner Syndrome, produces a person who has the superficial anatomical appearance of a female but usually has subsequent immature sexual development (all examples of this abnormality have been XO types and no YO types have been identified).
2. The presence of extra sex chromosomes also causes abnormality, diagnosed as Klinefelter Syndrome. Here the affected person has too many female chromosomes (XXY, XXXY, XXXXY, etc.) instead of the usual composition, XY. Such an individual has the superficial appearance of a male and usually a normal-sized penis, but very small testes, and may also possess many female characteristics, such as developed breasts, feminine face and voice, and little body hair. Such males are always sterile, usually suffer from emotional difficulties, and may show symptoms of psychosis and antisocial behavior.
3. The presence of extra chromosomes in any pair of the 22 autosomes (such as three instead of the usual two) has been found to cause Down syndrome, which can cause severe intellectual and developmental disability.

The Role of Genes

Genes, like chromosomes, occur in pairs. An individual derives a gene pair in one of the following forms:

- A dominant gene from one of the parents and a recessive gene from the other (Form Dr).
- Dominant genes from both the parents (Form DD).
- Recessive genes from both the parents (Form rr).

For purposes of distinction, where pure DD (completely dominant) or rr (completely recessive) gene pairs are called homo-zygotes, hybrid, Dr pairs are referred to as hetero-zygotes.

Defective genes transferred to offspring are often responsible for abnormalities. A child who receives defectively paired genes (dominant or recessive) from both parents runs a high risk of being affected with an abnormality. Figures 6.4 and 6.5 depict the transmission of genes.

A few notable examples of degenerative or hereditary diseases through the transmission of genes are cited as follows.

1. *Ataxia:* It causes a lack of coordination and an inability to maintain balance while standing or walking.
2. *Huntington's Chorea:* This degeneration is marked by speech impairment, intellectual impairment, and emotional disturbance.
3. *Idiopathic epilepsy.*
4. *Muscular Dystrophies:* A disorder involving paralysis of muscles.
5. *Neuralatrophy:* A disorder of peripheral nerves.
6. *Alzheimer's disease and Pick's disease*: Both relate to pre-senile psychosis in which atrophy of the cerebral cortex occurs. In Pick's disease, brain degeneration occurs in localized foci, mostly in the frontal areas, while in Alzheimer's disease, degeneration is diffused throughout the brain.

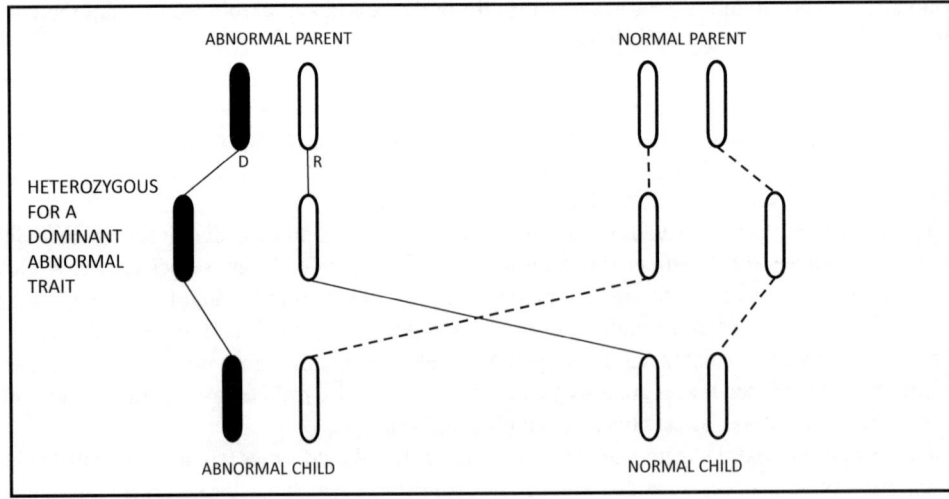

Figure 6.4 Mating of a normal person and an abnormal person

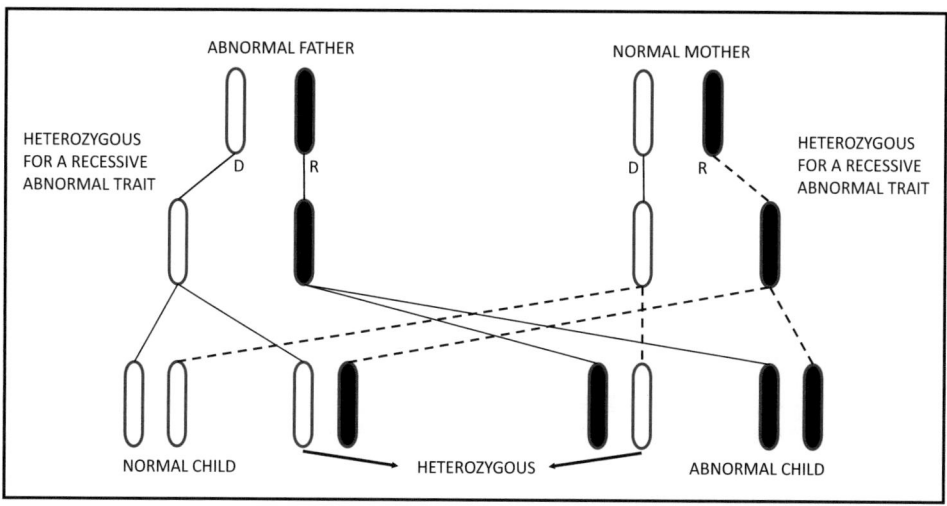

Figure 6.5 The mating from which the great majority of abnormal persons are born

7. *Schizophrenia:* A functional disorder in which heredity plays a strong part in the predisposing factors.
8. *Psychophysical disorders:* Certain psychophysical disorders like hyperthyroidism, peptic ulcers, and essential hypertension have been found to possess strong hereditary bases.

Physiological or Biological Factors

Several physiological or biological factors examined next play substantial roles in causing abnormality of behavior among people.

1. *Structure of the body (Physique):* In a normal course one should remain reasonably satisfied with their somatic structure or physique in order to adjust to oneself and one's environment. Any serious deviation from the norms, whether in terms of height, weight, body proportions, or appearance, may create a serious adjustment problem for the individual, and this in turn may develop malfunctioning or behavioral disorders.
2. *Endocrines:* Endocrines play an important role in the growth and development of the body and mind. Any defect in their functioning leads to significant physiological anomalies, which, in turn, provide fertile ground for the growth of

> **Physiological or Biological factors causing abnormality in behavior**
>
> - Structure of the body
> - Endocrines
> - Microorganisms
> - Toxic chemicals
> - Physical injury
> - Malnutrition
> - Deficiency of oxygen
> - Sleep deprivation

disorganized personalities. For example, overactivity of the secretion of adrenal glands may cause a woman to grow a beard and develop a masculine physique, and she may exhibit the physical and sexual maturity of an adult in a three- or four-year-old child. Similarly, pituitary gland imbalances may lead to an increase in height (seven to nine feet in height), dwarfism (two to four feet in height), a displeasing big size appearance or abnormal sex characteristics and behavior. The abnormalities so produced are liable to be made an object of ridicule, jest, social isolation, and harsh and unfair treatment, which, in turn, cause a variety of abnormalities in the behavior of the affected persons.

3. *Microorganisms:* Some disease-producing bacterial microorganisms may infect the brain along with the body, as in pneumonia, malaria, and syphilis, while others may affect the brain directly, as in meningitis.

4. *Toxic chemicals:* Chemicals such as lead, methyl alcohol, carbon monoxide, carbon tetrachloride, and intoxicating drugs and other materials produce toxicity. They affect the functioning of the brain and may result in behavioral disorders.

5. *Physical injury:* Physical injury and trauma may cause damage to the brain either directly or through interference with its blood supply and may thus result in brain disorders—structural or functional.

6. *Malnutrition:* Severe malnutrition during the early embryonic and infantile stages has been found to lower body resistance, and affect brain structure and growth of intelligence. Postmortem studies of malnourished infants have revealed the content of their brain cells to be sixty percent less than normal. Pellagra, a mental disorder, is found to be caused by vitamin deficiency. In the same manner, deficiencies of certain vitamins, glucose, and hormones have been found to cause many abnormalities—structural or functional.

7. *Deficiency of oxygen:* Anoxia—a deficiency of the oxygen supply to the tissues—has been found to cause many abnormalities. Human nerve cells are very sensitive to a lack of oxygen, and it may result in structural damage to the brain, lifelong mental deficiency, or difficulty with complex mental functions such as immediate memory.

8. *Sleep deprivation:* Sleep deprivation is considered an important biological factor causing abnormality under stress. Prolonged sleep deprivation brings abnormal symptoms in behavior, such as irritability, feelings of persecution, inability to concentrate, periods of disorientation and misperceptions, illusions, and hallucinations. In some cases, it may also bring about certain neurological changes and autonomic nervous system effects.

Psychological Factors

Besides hereditary and biological factors, psychological factors often cause the development of abnormal behavior and mental illness. All types of frustrations, conflicts, stresses, and pressures brought about by faulty psychological development, upbringing, and childhood socialization may result in disorganized personality and abnormal behavior. Truly speaking, in the satisfaction of needs, there lies the welfare

---

Psychological factors causing Abnormality in Behavior

- Psychological deprivations of the early ages (such as oral, parental, and anal deprivation)
- Faulty learning and horrible experiences
- Defective family environment and parental attitude
- Psychological stresses and self-devaluation

of the individual. When one feels frustrated in the satisfaction of their psychological needs, their behavioral reactions turn into maladaptation and abnormalities. Let us see how this happens.

1. *Psychological deprivations at an early age:* Psychological deprivation during infancy and early childhood contributes significantly toward causing abnormality of behavior in the manner discussed as follows.

   (i) Oral deprivation: Individuals who are deprived of the opportunity of seeking gratification from sucking behavior in infancy may be become emotionally unstable and disturbed at later stages.

   (ii) Parental deprivation: Loss of parental affection has been found to play a very significant role in the development of maladjustment and abnormality. The loss of the father or mother or both has a very damaging effect on the well-being of the child, who does not get adequate love and affection, attention, and care they should normally get. In such situations, the child feels insecure, develops neurotic or psychotic tendencies, and thus becomes susceptible to stressful situations in later life. The condition is more damaging in the case of separation, desertion, or divorce between the parents. Here the child cannot get the appropriate psychological environment for their development and consequently develops maladaptive reaction tendencies. Inadequate mothering, due to any reason in the form of indifference, rejection, and overprotection may cause tense, unsatisfied, and negativistic behavior on the part of children, which may develop into deviant behavior at a later stage.

   (iii) Anal deprivation: Anal frustrations on account of the early and rigorous toilet training of early years are reported to cause emotional difficulties and behavioral problems in later life. Accordingly, the children whose parents remain too forceful and harsh in training them for the control of bowel movements, may become rebellion by deliberately retaining their bowel movements. At the grown up stage, it may turn them into an anal retention personality characterized with excessive orderliness, extreme meticulousness, reserve and suspiciousness.

2. Faulty learning and horrible experiences: Most of the patterns in our behavior are the results of our learning and experiences. When one learns healthy habits, attitudes, interests, and other acquired traits, as well as physical mental, emotional, and social competencies, this proper learning results in adjustment, whereas inadequate and faulty learning may create a number of difficulties and problems in one's adjustment.

   Let us take, for example, the learning of sexual behavior. The child may learn that sex is shameful or fearful. They may think that they are not fit for normal sexual behavior. Such faulty acquisition, misconceptions, and wrong understanding of sex-related information are found to contribute to learning maladaptive behaviors such as one or the other type of sexual deviation, inadequacy and withdrawal tendencies, which may further result in serious disorganization of the personality.

   Certain painful experiences, especially at early ages, are bound to leave psychological wounds that never completely heal. Sometimes experiences such as an encounter with a vicious dog or a bull, a sexual assault, or an experience with a gang of robbers, may be sufficient to establish a conditioned fear response, which may result in certain types of abnormality and mental illness.

3. Defective family environment and parental attitude: An uncongenial family environment full of conflicts and stressful situations prove a potent source for causing abnormal behavior. In this connection, the following adverse situations may be cited as examples.

   (i) Negative models: When parents and other senior members of the family are emotionally unstable, inconsistent, antisocial, and disturbed in their behavior, they set negative role models for their children.

(ii) Undesirable parental attitude: Parental attitudes toward the child may be defective and erroneous such as (a) rejection, (b) overprotection, (c) overindulgence, (d) perfectionism—unrealistic ambitions for the child, (e) excessive dominance or strictness and (f) excessive leniency or carelessness.

(iii) Unhappy conditions: The family environment may be uncongenial due to (a) broken homes as a result of death, divorce, desertion, or separation, (b) marital discord of the parents in the form of quarreling, bickering, nagging, and general tensions, (c) sibling rivalry amounting to the feeling in a child that their brother or sister is getting more parental affection and attention than himself, and (d) poor resources due to tough economic conditions and finances, cultural and social deprivation, lack of education of the parents, and bad reputation of the family.

In all such defective family situations, the child fails to get favorable conditions for adequate adjustment and development. They receive neither balanced love and affection, nor adequate safety, security, and resources for the satisfaction of their essential needs. They are therefore always starved of one or the other of their physical or emotional needs. Predisposed in this manner, unfortunate occurrences are bound to make the child's behavior and reaction patterns quite deviant from the norm, and thus they drift toward abnormality and mental illness.

4. *Maladjustment in adolescence:* Adolescence is a crucial age of storms and stresses. The varying physical and sociopsychological needs of this age must be satisfied for the adjustment moving between independence versus dependence, realism versus idealism, parental affection versus peer group norms, temptations versus social taboos, and so on. The adolescent must be made to satisfy themself reasonably with their body development, somatic variations and organic and psychophysical changes must be supported in the proper exercising of emotions and channeling the stream of their valuable energy. Adolescents are very sensitive and should therefore be treated and cared for adequately according to their needs and problems of their age. An attack on their situation may invite a host of problems. Their resentment, indifference, and hostility should not be chastised, but rather they should be helped to establish self-identity and meaningful standards of conduct to follow. But this is not always possible and there begins "the conflict between generations." Adolescents are then misunderstood; their problems are not cared for and their aspirations thwarted. This gives rise to conflicts, tensions, and frustrations among adolescents, and thus leads to abnormalities and mental disorders.

5. *Psychological stresses and self-devaluation:* Stress refers to a psychological condition of an individual subjected to constant failures, frustrations, tensions, conflicts, and pressures. Stresses, as we have noticed, constitute the precipitating causes that disintegrate the personality of the affected person. The stress tolerance capacity of an individual is an important deciding factor and depends upon early upbringing, psychological and biological makeup, and the present favorable or unfavorable environment and emotional state. Still, the outcome of severely stressful situations causing personality disorders cannot be questioned. The central factor causing maladjustment and disorders in stressful situations is the feeling of self-devaluation. One loses faith in one's integrity, abilities, and capacities, and thinks themself unworthy, unwanted, and good-for-nothing. Some self-devaluing and devastating stressful situations may be cited as follows:

(i) *Personal limitations and shortcomings:* For their adequate adjustment, an individual should learn to be reasonably satisfied with their own limitations and shortcomings.

No one is perfect in this world; in addition to one's assets, one should know one's limitations and accept them so as not to cause damage to oneself. The person who plans their ambitions well within their own capacities avoids the risk of undesirable frustrations, while those who aim to reach the stars with no firm footing on the earth are destined to suffer from self-devaluation. Much of our unhappiness and feelings of self-devaluation are the result of our ignorance and failure to appreciate our assets, and unnecessary condemnation of our perceived limitations such as a big nose, short statute, dark complexion and poor vision etc.

(ii) *Failures and losses:* Repeated failures and accidental losses can lead to strong feelings of inferiority and self-devaluation to the extent that one may "go to pieces." A schoolboy may attempt suicide as a result of his successive failures, or an unemployed youth may turn into a split personality on account of his repeated failures to get a job and the subsequent sufferings. The losses relating to human or material resources can be painful and frustrating in their effects, especially on account of the fact that there is nothing one can do about them once they have occurred. As a result of an appreciable financial loss, damage to one's property, loss of social status, loss of friendship and companionship of our dearest loved ones, one may feel frustrated, even to the extent of losing the will to live.

(iii) *Guilt feelings:* Feelings of guilt leading to self-devaluation are associated with abnormal behavior and mental disorders. The lady who washes her hands constantly under compulsive neurosis reactions does so on account of some inherent guilt feelings. Similarly, early sexual experiences and tragedies may lead to feelings of guilt, a sinful attitude, and self-devaluation, and thus cause abnormality of sexual behavior and other personality disorders.

(iv) *Unreasonable comparisons:* We are more sad, unhappy, and unworthy on account of the fact that we are in the habit of making unreasonable comparisons of our gains and status with other people of resources and capabilities. We seldom realize that in this world of great diversities and differences there are people who appear to enjoy more facilities than ours, but there are others also who are not fortunate enough to make both ends meet. Therefore, one must be content with a level suited to their own resources and capabilities. People who fail to develop a mature and reasonable outlook are bound to suffer from self-devaluation, feelings of inferiority and frustrations that lead them to abnormality.

(v) *Severe conflicts*: Many times conflicts in the form of what to do or what not to do, out of the given choices or alternatives, become sources of frustrations and stresses that ultimately lead to the development of abnormality and behavior disorders. The central idea behind any conflict—the choices to make—is the inability to determine what is good or bad, desirable or undesirable. Sometimes the conflicting situations are loaded with extreme anxiety, feeling of threat, insecurity, and uncertainty. Under such stresses one is likely to fall victim to abnormalities or mental disorders.

(vi) *Severe pressures:* Stressful situations affecting our behavior are often generated through severe pressures stemming from inner or outer sources. While mild pressures may be tolerated with or without strain, excessive and severe pressures may lead to the disorganization of behavior. Some common pressure- generating situations are cited here:

a. The desire to excel beyond others or reach the top in competitive endeavors.
b. The unreasonable and excessive demands of the work environment—educational or occupational.
c. The stressful demands of marital or family life.

    d. The stressful demands of living as an efficient and adjusted citizen in the complicated and demanding conditions of the modern age.

    e. The hazards and calamities of life.

Sociological Factors

It is difficult to separate sociological influences from psychological ones, as the sociological factors rooted in the social and cultural environment of an individual cast their impact on the behavior of an individual through the organic and psychological channels of one's personality and behavior. However, for the sake of convenience, we will survey some social and cultural factors and stress situations responsible for the faulty development and disorganization of one's personality and behavior.

An individual's social and cultural environment consists of all the external factors within his home, family, neighborhood, school and college, world of work, society and community, caste and religion, state, country, and so on. One's personality and behavior at any stage of their development is a product of the interaction of their biological and psychological makeup with their sociocultural environment.

It is true that much of our abnormal behavior is an acquired disposition or learned behavior. As a result of what an individual experiences or what they become conditioned to through formal and informal contacts in their sociocultural environment, their behavior patterns are fixed accordingly. Consequently, abnormalities and mental disorders are the results of defective and unfavorable sociocultural environments. Most of the maladaptive and abnormal behaviors such as antisocial behavior, alcoholism, drug addiction, sexual deviations and disorders, and neurotic and psychotic disorganizations, when analyzed, possess deep-rooted sociocultural causes. Let us cite a few devastating situations within our defective and pathogenic sociocultural environment for the growth and perpetuation of abnormal behavior.

1. *Problems related to earning a living:* The world of work often brings stressful situations to an individual. Particularly in developing countries like ours, the earning of one's living is a source of much frustration and stress. Millions of our youth face unemployment and underemployment. It is bound to push them into trouble, complications, and personality disorders. Frustration, coupled with strong urges for the satisfaction of one's basic needs, makes them either aggressive toward their sociocultural environment or turn their aggression inward for the development of suicidal tendencies and neurotic or psychotic splits of the personality. The increasing cases of corruption, nepotism, favoritism, provincialism, and day-to-day interference of political bosses are adding to occupational problems. Under these circumstances, it is no surprise to find the cases of mental illness and behavioral disorders among the frustrated employed as well as unemployed individuals. Such abnormalities of behavior are the result of emerging sociocultural conditions related to the earning of one's livelihood.

2. *Caste considerations and minority status:* The consciousness about minority status and socioeconomic factors related to caste considerations in our country may be said to be a major source of frustrations, conflicts, and stress. Linguistic, religious, and cultural minorities face a great deal of adjustment problems, particularly when majority groups are in the grip of linguistic, religious, or sectarian sentiments and divisive forces. In such a situation, their security and safety are threatened and their self-esteem injured. It leads them to un-adjusting defensive behavior resulting in malfunctioning of their behavior. The caste groups falling into specific lower categories in the hierarchy of castes, besides their low socioeconomic

status, are maltreated and become victims of apathy and even scorn from the upper caste groups. This creates in them feelings of inferiority, frustration, resentment, and other behavioral disorders.

A new dimension has been emerging from the problems created by caste considerations in our country. It concerns the reservation of seats for scheduled classes in educational institutions and career openings. The youth belonging to the upper castes are giving rise to peculiar frustrations, resentments, and feelings of self-devaluation on account of this policy of reservation. They become more disturbed in a situation when the facilities of reservation are enjoyed by the wards of more privileged and economically sound members of the lower castes.

3. *Effect of urbanization and modernization:* Heavy industrialization, increasing urbanization, and rapid modernization have disturbed our usual sociocultural patterns. The family structure has shrunk, the village culture is being trounced by urban ways, old cultural values are being lost, and the new generation has adopted the ways of western culture in the name of modernization. All this has created a new sociocultural environment without caring for its ill effects, which are obvious. The gulf between the poor and the rich, or the privileged and the unprivileged has widened. The village farmers have been forced to become factory workers and laborers and live in unhygienic and depressive conditions. Emotional feedback and feelings are missing today in our society. A next-door neighbor or even inmates of the same building are strangers to each other. Nobody is there to listen or sympathize with each other's sufferings and inadequacies. Parents have no time for their children, and sons have no time or resources to look after their aged parents. Urbanization, industrialization, and modernization have been the causes of insecurity, emotional cravings, self-devaluation, conflicts, and frustrations leading toward the disorganization of behavior and personality.

4. *Cultural and social evils:* Cultural setting profoundly and widely affects the development of personality and behavior. Every culture through its established norms of traits and behaviors provides a basic model of living. Cultural patterns like child-rearing practices, family organizations, sex practices, marital status, beliefs and traditions, restrictions and taboos, ways of treating the elders or youngsters, and superstitions differ from culture to culture. These patterns cause frustrations, complexes, feelings of guilt, and self-devaluation depending upon the emotional conflicts and stresses they generate. The social evils attached to our society like the dowry system, the preferential treatment of sons over daughters, the maltreatment of widows, superstitions and orthodox views, and unreasonable dominance of religions provide a precipitating factor for the development of abnormality and behavioral disorganizations.

5. *Marital discord and family instability:* Marital adjustment is a key to happiness. The reverse is also true. Marital discords, as may be witnessed in day-to-day happenings, are bound to result in utter disillusionment, self-devaluation, and severe psychological wounds. These situations are harmful not only to the well-being of the marriage partners but are destined to prove devastating to their children also. The stability of family life depends upon marital harmony. Divorce, separation, and desertion lead to destabilizing the equilibrium of mental peace. Similarly, the untimely death of a spouse brings severe stress situations to the other partner. Economic fluctuations and the absence of the father or mother on account of them earning a living may disrupt the usual family pattern. All such situations often prove detrimental to the parents and their dependents.

6. *Natural and national catastrophes:* Catastrophes like floods, fires, earthquakes, droughts, hailstorms, wars, economic depressions, and acute national crises create severe stress situations for affected groups or individuals. Huge losses of property, deaths, physical deformities, and disorganizations of social institutions brought out by such catastrophes disturb the

lives of unfortunate millions. These have far-reaching consequences, resulting in pathological sociocultural environments and the development of behavioral disorganizations.

To Sum Up

The factors responsible for developing psychological abnormalities or disorders may be broadly classified as Heredity factors (incorporating the roles of chromosomes and genes), Biological or physiological factors (e.g., body structure, endocrines, microorganisms, malnutrition, physical injury, sleep deprivation, etc.), Psychological factors (e.g., early age psychological deprivations, faulty learning and horrible experiences, defective family environment and parental attitude, psychological stresses and self-devaluation), and sociological factors (e.g., problems related to earning or living, caste considerations and minority status, effects of urbanization and modernization, cultural and social evils, marital discord and family instability, and natural and national calamities, etc.).

Review Questions

1. Explain, what do you understand by the terms normal and abnormal behavior?
2. What are the different criteria for deciding normality and abnormality of people's behavior? Discuss them in detail.
3. Provide your own evaluation about the different criteria used in assessing the normality or abnormality of one's behavior. Draw your conclusion about the use of one or the other criterion.
4. What are the various causes or factors responsible for abnormalities in behavior? Discuss them in detail.

References

Eysenck, H. J. (1960), *Handbook of abnormal psychology*, Oxford: Isaac Pitman & Sons Ltd.
Mahoney, M. J. (1980), *Abnormal psychology*, San Francisco, CA: Harper & Row.

Chapter 7

Classification of Mental Disorders

Learning Objectives

After going through this chapter, you will be able to:

- Discuss the attempts made for the development of systems of classifying mental disorders in the old era prior to those developed by the APA and WHO.
- Name the attempts made by the APA and WHO for classifying mental disorders.
- Name the different systems of classification brought out by the APA from time to time with their nomenclature, number of diagnosed disorders, and years.
- Tell in what ways the DSM-5 differs from previous ones.
- Describe the evolution and development of the ICDs over time.
- Elucidate the way in which the ICD-11 differs from the ICD-10.
- Describe the necessity and purposes of the classification of mental disorders.

Introduction

Behavioral abnormalities as described in the previous chapter may result in one or the other types of maladjustment, illness, or mental disorders. Here it may be seen that there is no limit to human variance, and as such abnormality in behavior and the resultant mental illness or disorders are also innumerable. However, for the sake of the diagnosis, prevention, and treatment of these disorders, it becomes essential to put them into some definite categories. Making attempts for the classification of mental disorders, abnormalities and diseases, therefore, must be quite essential, as well right steps for moving in this direction. Let us look into the attempts made in this concern by the world societies.

Development of the Classification System

A. The old era: The historical evidence of the classification of behavioral disorders takes us to the attempts made by Hippocrates, nearly 2,500 years ago. He divided behavioral disorders into three categories—mania, melancholia, and phrenesis—and developed a theoretical account of their appearance. In India too, the rishis, much earlier than Hippocrates' era, gave a reasonable classification of abnormal behavior in terms of disequilibrium in the three gunas (*Satguna, Rajoguna,* and *Tamoguna*).

DOI: 10.4324/9781003398325-7

However, the credit for giving a formal systematic classification of mental disorders that is prevalent today goes to the German psychiatrist Emile Kraepelin in the later part of the 19th century. He linked all forms of disorders and mental illness to hereditary and biological factors and provided a classification based on the causes, prognosis, and symptoms of mental diseases.

B. *The modern era:* The two world wars tore apart millions of families, social organizations, and individuals. With increased cases of mental disorders and diseases and the subsequent expansion of psychiatric services all over the world, the need for a standardized classification system was widely felt. The American Psychiatric Association in 1948 set up a committee to develop such a system for classifying mental disorders. This system was further refined and an official *Diagnostic and Statistical Manual of Mental Disorders-First Edition* (DSM-I) was published in 1952. It acknowledged three main groups of disorders, as indicated in Table 7.1.

The problems concerning the adequacy and universality of the DSM-I system created the need for modified systems. As a result, in 1965, the World Health Organization (WHO) brought out a classification system known as the International Classification of Diseases (ICD-8), containing Section V on behavior disorders.

Table 7.2 presents a summary of this section of the ICD.

Dissatisfied with their edition of the DSM-I, the American Psychiatric Association, in 1968, brought out a more comprehensive system of classification known as DSM-II. It gave ten major categories of mental disorders, instead of three given under DSM-I, as shown in Table 7.3.

In the years to follow, the ICD-8 and DSM-II were subjected to wide criticism on account of their specific limitations and shortcomings. To provide a more uniform pattern of classification and common terminology for the different countries of the world, the WHO brought out, toward the end of 1977, an improved classification known as the ICD-9.

Table 7.1 Diagnostic and Statistical Manual of Mental Disorders—First Edition *(DSM-I)*

A. Disorders of brain tissue function
a. Acute
b. Chronic
B. Mental deficiency
a. Familial or hereditary
b. Idiopathic
C. Disorders of psychogenic origin (no clearly defined physical cause)
a. Psychotic disorders
(i)   Involutional reactions
(ii) Affective reactions
(iii) Schizophrenic reactions
(iv) Paranoid reactions
(v) Other
b. Psychophysiologic disorders
c. Psychoneurotic disorders
d. Personality disorders
e. Transient situational personality disorders

Source: Adapted from American Psychiatric Association (1952), *Diagnostic and Statistical Manual of Mental Disorders*, Washington D.C.: American Psychiatric Association).

Table 7.2 Summary of ICD-8 (Section V) Classification

290–315	*Mental Disorders*
290–299 Psychoses	290. Senile and pre-senile dementia
	291. Alcoholic psychosis
	292. Psychosis associated with intracranial infection
	293. Psychosis associated with other cerebral condition
	294. Psychosis associated with other physical condition
	295. Schizophrenia
	296. Affective psychoses
	297. Paranoid states
	298. Other psychoses
	299. Unspecified psychoses
300–309	300. Neuroses
Neurosis	301. Personality disorders
Personality	302. Sexual deviations
Disorders, and	303. Alcoholism
Other non-	304. Drug dependence
psychotic mental	305. Physical disorders of presumably psychogenic origin
disorders	306. Specified symptoms
	307. Transient situational disturbances
	308. Behavior disorders in childhood
	309. Mental disorders not specified as psychotic associated with physical conditions.
310–315	310. Borderline mental retardation
Mental Retardation	311. Mild mental retardation
	312. Moderate mental retardation
	313. Severe mental retardation
	314. Profound mental retardation
	315. Unspecified mental retardation

Source: Adapted from WHO (1965), *International Classification of Diseases, 8th Revision, (ICD-8)*, Geneva: World Health Organization.

Table 7.3 Diagnostic and Statistical Manual of Mental Disorders—Second Edition (DSM-II)

1. Mental retardation
2. Organic brain syndromes
3. Psychoses
   a. Schizophrenia
   b. Major affective disorders
   c. Paranoid states
   d. Other psychoses.
4. Neuroses
5. Personality disorders
   a. Personality disorders
   b. Sexual deviations
   c. Alcoholism
   d. Drug dependence
6. Psycho-physiologic disorders
7. Special symptoms
8. Transient situational disturbances
9. Behavior disorders of childhood and adolescence
10. Conditions without manifest psychiatric disorder

Source: Adapted from: American Psychiatric Association (1968), *Diagnostic and Statistical Manual of Mental Disorders* (2nd ed.), DSM-II, Washington D.C.: American Psychiatric Association.

Table 7.4 gives a summary of Section V of the ICD-9 dealing with the classification of mental diseases.

Along the lines of the WHO, the American Psychiatric Association also tried to improve its DSM-II classification by setting up a new committee. It resulted in the emergence of DSM-III. The new system was named the "multiaxial classification system" because it allowed classification on five separate dimensions (axes) as shown in Table 7.5.

After the emergence of the classification systems known as the ICD-9 and DSM-III by the WHO and American Psychiatric Association, there have been continued efforts on the part of these two bodies for improving and bringing new classification systems. In this concern, whereas the WHO brought out the classification systems known as ICD-10 and ICD-11 in the years 2010 and 2019, respectively, the American Psychiatric Association published the classification systems known as the DSM III-R, DSM-IV, DSM IV-TR, DSM-5, and DSM 5-TR in the subsequent years 1987, 1994, 2000, 2013, and 2022, respectively. The different classification systems brought out by the American Psychiatric Association with their increased vision and years of publication have been presented below in Table 7.6.

We will now discuss the latest developed classification systems of the DSM, namely, DSM-IV-TR, DSM-5, and DSM-5-TR published in the years 2000, 2013, and 2022, respectively.

Table 7.4 Summary of ICD-9 (Section V)

290–319	*Mental disorders*
290–294 **Organic Psychotic Conditions**	290. Senile and pre-senile psychiatric conditions 291. Alcoholic psychosis 292. Drug psychosis 293. Transient organic psychotic condition 294. Other organic psychotic conditions (chronic)
295–299 **Other Psychoses**	295. Schizophrenia 296. Affective psychoses 297. Paranoid states 298. Other organic psychoses 299. Psychoses with origins specific to childhood
300–302 **Neurotic Personality and Other non-psychotic disorders**	300. Neurotic disorders 301. Personality disorders 302. Sexual deviations and disorders
303–305 **Psychoactive substance**	303. Alcohol dependence syndrome 304. Drug dependence 305. Non-dependence, abuse of drugs
306–311 **Other Mental Disorders (Primarily adult onset)**	306. Physiological malfunctioning arising from mental disorders 307. Special symptoms or syndromes not classified elsewhere 308. Acute reaction to stress 309. Adjustment reaction 310. Frontal lobe syndromes 311. Depressive disorders not classified elsewhere
312–316 **Mental Disorders Diagnosed in Childhood**	312. Disturbance of conduct not classified elsewhere 313. Disturbance of emotions specific to childhood and adolescence 314. Hyperkinetic syndrome of childhood
317–319 **Mental retardation**	315. Specific reading retardation 316. Specified arithmetical retardation

Source: Adapted from WHO (1977), *International Classification of Diseases, 9th revision, (ICD-9)*, Geneva: World Health Organization.

Table 7.5 Diagnostic and Statistical Manual of Mental Disorders—Third Edition (*DSM-III*)

Axis I	*Clinical psychiatric Syndrome(s) and other conditions*
	1. Organic mental disorders
	2. Drug use disorders
	3. Schizophrenic disorders
	4. Paranoid disorders
	5. Affective disorders
	6. Psychoses not elsewhere classified
	7. Anxiety disorders
	8. Factitious disorders
	9. Somatoform disorders
	10. Dissociative disorders
Axis II	*Adult personality disorders and specific developmental disorders*
	1. Personality disorders
	2. Psycho-sexual disorders
	3. Disorders usually arising in childhood or adolescence
	4. Reactive disorders not elsewhere classified
	5. Disorders of impulsive control not elsewhere classified
	6. Sleep disorders
	7. Other disorders and conditions
Axis III	*Non-mental medical disorders*
Axis IV	*Severity of psychosocial stressors*
Axis V	*Highest level of recent adaptive functioning*

Source: Adapted from American Psychiatric Association (1980), *Diagnostic and Statistical Manual of Mental Disorders*, (3rd ed.), DSM-III, Washington D.C.: American Psychiatric Association.

Table 7.6 The Evolution and Developments of the DSM

Nomenclature of DSM	Number of Mental Disorders for which Diagnoses have been provided	Year of Publication
DSM-I	128 disorders and diagnoses	1952
DSM-II	193 disorders and diagnoses	1968
DSM-III	228 disorders and diagnoses	1980
DSM-III-R	253 disorders and diagnoses	1987
DSM-IV	383 disorders and diagnoses	1994
DSM-IV-TR	383 disorders and diagnoses	2000
DSM-5	541 disorders and diagnoses	2013
DSM-5-TR	Revisions on more than 70 disorders from DSM-5	2022

DSM-IV-TR

The DSM-IV-TR was published in 2000. It consists of a total of five Axes. The first two, Axis I and Axis II, provide the necessary classification and diagnoses for 383 disorders. Among the other three, Axis III covers General Medical Conditions, Axis IV Psychosocial and Environmental Problems, and Axis V presents The Global Assessment of Functioning Scale (GAF Scale).

The classification of disorders provided in Axis-I and Axis-II is presented in Table 10.7.

Table 7.7 Diagnostic and Statistical Manual of Mental Disorders—Fourth Edition-Revision (DSM-IV-TR)

Axis I:

1. Disorders Usually First Diagnosed in Infancy, Childhood, and Adolescence

- *Learning Disorders (Reading Disorder, Mathematics Disorder, Disorder of Written Expression)*
- *Motor Skills Disorder (Developmental Coordination Disorder)*
- *Communication Disorders (Expressive Language Disorder, Mixed Receptive/Expressive Language Disorder, Phonological Disorder, Stuttering)*
- *Pervasive Developmental Disorders (Autistic, Rett's, Oppositional defiant and Asperger's Disorder)*
- *Attention-deficit and Disruptive Behavior Disorders (Attention-deficit/Hyperactivity Disorder*
- *Feeding and Eating Disorders of Infancy or Early Childhood*
- *Tic Disorders (Tourette's Disorder, Chronic Motor or Vocal Tic Disorder, Transient Tic Disorder)*
- *Elimination Disorders (Encopresis, Enurisis)*
- *Other Disorders of Childhood and Adolescence (Separation of Anxiety Disorder, Selective Mutism, Reactive Attachment Disorder of Infancy or Early Childhood, Stereotypic Movement Disorder)*

2. Delirium, Dementia, Amnestic, and Other Cognitive Disorders

3. Substance-Related Disorders

- *Alcohol-Induced Disorders*
- *Amphetamine-related Disorders*
- *Caffeine-related Disorders*
- *Cannabis-related Disorders*
- *Caffeine-related Disorders*
- *Cocaine-related Disorders*
- *Hallucinogen-related Disorders*
- *Inhalant-related Disorders*
- *Nicotine-related Disorders*
- *Opioid-related Disorders*
- *Phencyclidine-related Disorders*
- *Sedative, Hypnotic, or Anxiolytic-related Disorders*
- *Poly-substance-related Disorders*

4. Schizophrenia and Other Psychotic Disorders

- *Schizophrenia (Paranoid Type, Disorganized Type, Catatonic Type, Undifferentiated Type, Residual Type)*
- *Schizophreniform Disorder*
- *Schizoaffective Disorder*
- *Delusional Disorder*
- *Brief Psychotic Disorder*
- *Shared Psychotic Disorder*
- *Psychotic Disorder Due to a General Medical Condition*

5. **Mood Disorders** (Depressive, Bipolar, Mood Disorder due to a General Medical Condition and Substance-Induced Mood Disorder)
6. **Anxiety Disorders**
   - Panic Disorder
   - Agoraphobia without History of Panic Disorder
   - Specific Phobia
   - Social Phobia (Social Anxiety Disorder)
   - Obsessive-Compulsive Disorder
   - Posttraumatic Stress Disorder
   - Acute Stress Disorder
   - Generalized Anxiety Disorder
   - Anxiety Disorder Due to a General Medical Condition
   - Substance-Induced Anxiety Disorder
7. **Somatoform Disorders** (Somatization, Conversion, Hypochondriasis, Body Dysmorphic, and Pain Disorders)
8. **Factitious Disorders**
9. **Dissociative Disorders** (Amnesia, Fugue, Identity orMultiple Personality Disorder)
10. **Sexual and Gender Identity Disorders**

   Sexual Dysfunctions (Sexual Desire Disorders: Hypoactive Sexual Desire Disorder, Sexual Aversion Disorder; Sexual Arousal Disorder: Female Sexual Arousal Disorders: Male Erectile Disorder, Orgasmic Disorder: Female Orgasmic Disorder, Male Orgasmic Disorder, Premature Ejaculation, Sexual Pain Disorder, Sexual Dysfunction due to a General Medical Condition, Substance-Induced Sexual Dysfunction.)

   Paraphilias (Exhibitionism, Fetishism, Frotteurism, Pedophilia, Sexual Masochism, Sexual Sadism, Voyeurism, Transvestic Fetishism)

   Gender Identity Disorders (Gender Identity Disorder: in children, adolescents, and adults)

11. **Eating Disorders** (Anorexia Nervosa, Bulimia Nervosa and Eating Disorders Not Otherwise Specified
12. **Sleep Disorders**
13. **Impulse Control Disorders Not Elsewhere Classified**

   Axis II

   1. **Mental Retardation**
   2. **Personality Disorders** (Paranoid, Schizoid, Schizotypal, Antisocial, Borderline, Histrionic, Narcissistic, Avoidant, Dependent and Obsessive-Compulsive Personality Disorder)
   3. **Other Conditions that may be a Focus of Clinical Attention**

Source: Adapted from American Psychiatric Association (2000), *The Diagnostic and Statistical Manual of Mental Disorders*, Washington D.C.: American Psychiatric Association.

Diagnostic and Statistical Manual of Mental Disorders—Fifth Edition (DSM-5)

The DSM-5 represents a version of the Diagnostic and Statistical Manual of Mental Disorders brought out by the American Psychiatric Association (APA) in 2013. It is a 947-page manual that lists 541 diagnoses. The classification of mental disorders provided in the DSM-5 is presented in brief in the Table 7.8.

The ways in which the classification system of the DSM-5 stand distinguished from the previous ones may be briefly summarized as follows:

A. Nomenclatures for certain categories have been changed in DSM-5

New Name given in DSM-5	*Old Name*
Intellectual Disability	Mental Retardation
Major Neuro-cognitive Disorder	Dementia
Illness Anxiety Disorder	Hypochondriasis
Delayed Ejaculation	Male Orgasmic Disorder
Gender Dysphoria	Gender Identity Disorder

B. A few categories appearing in previous DSMs have been dropped in DSM-5

(i)   Dissociative fugue (sub-category of Dissociative Disorders in DSM-IV-TR)

(ii) Asperger's Disorder (sub-category of Pervasive Developmental Disorder in DSM-IV-TR)

(iii) Sexual Aversion Disorder (sub-category of Sexual Dysfunctions in DSM-IV-TR)

(iv) Substance Abuse and Substance Dependence (Both of them previously categorized separately have been submerged in the category of Substance Use Disorder in the DSM-5.)

C. A few new categories (not appearing in previous DSMs) have been added in the DSM-5:

(i)   Hoarding Disorder (a conscious, ongoing urge to accumulate possessions, as well as corresponding feelings of anxiety or mental anguish whenever those possessions get thrown away)

(ii)   Excoriation Disorder (repeated picking at one's own skin which results in skin lesions and causes significant disruption in one's life)

(iii) Persistent Depressive Disorder (a consolidation of DSM-IV-defined chronic major depressive disorder and dysthymic disorder)

(iv)   Premenstrual Dysphoric Disorder (a severe form of pre-menstrual syndrome)

(v)   Disruptive Mood Dysregulation Disorder (a childhood condition of extreme irritability, anger, and frequent, intense temper outbursts)

(vi)   Somatic Symptom Disorder (characterized with distressing somatic symptoms along with abnormal thoughts, feelings, and behaviors in response to these symptoms).

(vii) Binge Eating Disorder (Recurrent and persistent episodes of binge eating)

(viii) Mild Neurocognitive Disorder (characterized by modest declines in memory or other cognitive functions)

DSM-5-TR (Diagnostic and Statistical Manual, Fifth Edition-Text Revised)

The DSM-5-TR is the latest version of the Diagnostic and Statistical Manual of Mental Disorders brought out by the American Psychiatric Association (APA) in 2022.

Table 7.8 DSM-5: Classification of Mental Disorders

Axis I:
10. Disorders Usually First Diagnosed in Infancy, Childhood and Adolescence
- *Learning Disorders* (Reading Disorder, Mathematics Disorder, Disorder of Written Expression)
- *Motor Skill Disorder* (Developmental Coordination Disorder)
- *Communication Disorders* (Expressive Language Disorder, Mixed Receptive/Expressive Language Disorder, Phonological Disorder, Stuttering)
- *Pervasive Developmental Disorders* (Autistic, Rett's, Oppositional defiant and Asperger's Disorder)
- *Attention-deficit and Disruptive Behavior Disorders* (Attention-deficit/Hyperactivity Disorder
- *Feeding and Eating Disorders of Infancy or Early Childhood*
- *Tic Disorders* (Tourette's Disorder, Chronic Motor or Vocal Tic Disorder, Transient Tic Disorder)
- *Elimination Disorders* (Encopresis, Enurisis)
- *Other Disorders of Childhood and Adolescence* (Separation of Anxiety Disorder, Selective Mutism, Reactive Attachment Disorder of Infancy or Early Childhood, Stereotypic Movement Disorder)

11. Delirium, Dementia, and Amnestic and Other Cognitive Disorders
12. Substance-Related Disorders
- *Alcohol-Induced Disorders*
- *Amphetamine-related Disorders*
- *Caffeine-related Disorders*
- *Cannabis-related Disorders*
- *Caffeine-related Disorders*
- *Cocaine-related Disorders*
- *Hallucinogen-related Disorders*
- *Inhalant-related Disorders*
- *Nicotine-related Disorders*
- *Opioid-related Disorders*
- *Phencyclidine-related Disorders*
- *Sedative, Hypnotic, or Anxiolytic-related Disorders*
- *Poly-substance-related Disorders*

13. Schizophrenia and Other Psychotic Disorders
- *Schizophrenia* (Paranoid Type, Disorganized Type, Catatonic Type, Undifferentiated Type, Residual Type)
- *Schizophreniform Disorder*
- *Schizoaffective Disorder*
- *Delusional Disorder*
- *Brief Psychotic Disorder*
- *Shared Psychotic Disorder*
- *Psychotic Disorder due to a General Medical Condition*

14. **Mood Disorders (***Depressive, Bipolar, Mood Disorder due to a General Medical Condition, and Substance-Induced Mood Disorder*)

15. Anxiety Disorders
- *Panic Disorder*
- *Agoraphobia without History of Panic Disorder*
- *Specific Phobia*
- *Social Phobia (Social Anxiety Disorder)*
- *Obsessive-Compulsive Disorder*
- *Posttraumatic Stress Disorder*
- *Acute Stress Disorder*
- *Generalized Anxiety Disorder*
- *Anxiety Disorder due to a General Medical Condition*
- *Substance-Induced Anxiety Disorder*

(Continued)

Table 7.8 (Continue)

16. **Somatoform Disorders (***Somatization, Conversion, Hypochondriasis, Body Dysmorphic, and Pain Disorders)*
17. **Factitious Disorders**
18. **Dissociative Disorders (***Amnesia, Fugue, Identity orMultiple Personality Disorder)*
10. **Sexual and Gender Identity Disorders**
    Sexual Dysfunctions (Sexual Desire Disorders: Hypoactive Sexual Desire Disorder, Sexual Aversion Disorder, Sexual Arousal Disorder: Female Sexual Arousal Disorders: Male Erectile Disorder, Orgasmic Disorder: Female Orgasmic Disorder, Male Orgasmic Disorder, Premature Ejaculation, Sexual Pain Disorder, Sexual Dysfunction due to a General Medical Condition, Substance-Induced Sexual Dysfunction.)
    Paraphilias (Exhibitionism, Fetishism, Frotteurism, Pedophilia, Sexual Masochism, Sexual Sadism, Voyeurism, Transvestic Fetishism)
    Gender Identity Disorders (Gender Identity Disorder: In children, in adolescents and adults)
14. **Eating Disorders (***Anorexia Nervosa, Bulimia Nervosa and Eating Disorders Not Otherwise Specified*
15. **Sleep Disorders**
16. **Impulse Control Disorders Not Elsewhere Classified**
    Axis II
    4. Mental Retardation
    5. Personality Disorders (*Paranoid, Schizoid, Schizotypal, Antisocial, Borderline, Histrionic, Narcissistic, Avoidant, Dependent, and Obsessive-Compulsive Personality Disorder)*
    6. Other Conditions that may be a Focus of Clinical Attention

Source: Adapted from American Psychiatric Association (2000), *The Diagnostic and Statistical Manual of Mental Disorders*, Washington D.C.: American Psychiatric Association.

The classification of mental disorders provided in the DSM-5-TR is presented in brief in Table 7.9.

Table 7.9 Classification of Mental Disorders in DSM-5-TR (Summarized)

1. **Neurodevelopmental Disorders (***Intellectual Development Disorder*; Communication Disorders; Autism Spectrum Disorder; Attention-Deficit/Hyperactivity Disorder; Specific Learning Disorder; Motor Disorder; and Other Neurodevelopmental Disorders)
2. **Schizophrenia Spectrum Psychotic Disorders** (Schizotypal-Personality Disorder; Delusional Disorder; Brief Psychotic Disorder; Schizophreniform Disorder; Schizophrenia—Bipolar and Depressive type; Substance/Medication-Induced Psychotic Disorder; Psychotic Disorder due to Another Medical Condition—with delusion or with hallucinations; Catatonia Associated with Another Mental Disorder; Catatonic Disorder due to Another Medical Condition; Unspecified Catatonia; Other Specified Schizophrenia Spectrum and Other Psychotic Disorder; Unspecified Schizophrenia Spectrum and Other Psychotic Disorders)
3. **Bipolar & Related Disorders** (Bipolar and Related Disorders—with manic, hypomanic, or mixed features; Other specified or unspecified bipolar and Related Disorders)
4. **Depressive Disorders** (Disruptive Mood Dysregulation Disorder; *Persistent Depressive Disorder*; Permanent Dysphoric disorder; Depressive Disorder due to Another Medical Condition; Other Specified or Unspecified Depressive Disorder)
5. **Anxiety Disorders** (Separation Anxiety Disorder; Selective Mutism; Specific Phobia; *Social Anxiety Disorder*; Panic Disorder, Agoraphobia; Generalized Anxiety Disorder; Anxiety Disorder due to Another Medical Condition; Other Specified or Unspecified Anxiety Disorder)

Table 7.9 (Continued)

6. **Obsessive-Compulsive Disorders (**Obsessive Compulsive Disorder: Body Dysmorphic Disorder; Hoarding Disorder; Trichotillomania; Excoriation (Skin Picking) Disorder; Substance/Medication-Induced Obsessive-Compulsive and Related Disorder; Obsessive-Compulsive and Related Disorder due to another medical condition; Other Specified Obsessive-Compulsive and Related Disorder (including Olfactory Reference Disorder); Unspecified Obsessive-Compulsive and Related Disorders)

7. **Trauma and Stressor Related Disorders** (Reactive Attachment Disorder; Disinhibited Social Engagement Disorder; Posttraumatic Stress Disorder; Acute Stress Disorder—with Depressive mood or anxiety, with disturbance of conduct or emotions or both, unspecified; Prolonged Grief Disorder; Other Specified or Unspecified Trauma and Stressor-Related Disorder

8. **Dissociative Disorders** (Dissociative Identity Disorder; Dissociative Amnesia; Depersonalization/Derealization Disorder; Other Specified or Unspecified Dissociative Disorder)

9. **Somatic Symptoms and Related Disorders** (Somatic Symptom Disorder; Illness Anxiety Disorder; Functional Neurological Symptom Disorder/Conversion Disorder; Psychological Factors Affecting Other Medical Conditions; Factitious Disorder; Other Specified or Unspecified Somatic Symptom and Related Disorder)

10. **Feeding and Eating Disorders (**Pica in Children or Adults; Rumination Disorder; Avoidant/Restrictive Food Intake Disorder; Anorexia Nervosa; Bulimia Nervosa; Binge Eating Disorder; Other Specified or Unspecified Feeding or Eating Disorder)

11. **Elimination Disorders** (Enuresis; Encopresis; Other Specified or Unspecified Elimination Disorder—with Urinary or Fecal symptoms)

12. **Sleep-Wake Disorders** (Insomnia Disorder; Hypersomnolence Disorder; Narcolepsy; Breathing-Related Sleep Disorders; Parasomnias—Sleepwalking, Sleep Terror, Nightmare, Rapid Eye Movement Sleep Behavior Disorder, Restless Legs Syndrome; Substance/Medication-Induced Sleep Disorder; Other Specified or Unspecified Insomnia Disorder; Other Specified or Unspecified Hypersomnolence Disorder; Other Specified or Unspecified Sleep-Wake Disorder)

13. **Sexual Dysfunctions** (Delayed Ejaculation; Erectile Disorder; Female Orgasmic Disorder; Female Sexual Interest/Arousal Disorder; Genito-Pelvic Pain/Penetration Disorder; Male Hypoactive Sexual Desire Disorder; Premature Ejaculation; Substance/Medication-Induced Sexual Dysfunction; Other Specified or Unspecified Sexual Dysfunction)

14. **Gender Dysphoria** (Gender Dysphoria in Children or Adolescence and Adults; Other Specified or Unspecified Gender Dysphoria)

15. **Disruptive, Impulse-Control and Conduct Disorders** (Oppositional Defiant Disorder; Intermittent Explosive Disorder; Conduct Disorder; Antisocial Personality Disorder; Pyromania; Kleptomania; Other Specified or Unspecified Disruptive, Impulse-Control, and Conduct Disorder)

16. **Substance-Related and Addictive Disorders** (Alcohol-Related Disorders; Caffeine-Related Disorders; Cannabis-Related Disorders; Hallucinogen-Related Disorders; Inhalant-Related Disorders; Opioid-Related Disorders; Sedative, Hypnotic or Anxiolytic-related Disorders; Stimulant-Related Disorders; Tobacco-Related Disorders; Other or Unknown Substance-Related Disorders; and Non-Substance- Related Disorders)

17. **Neurocognitive Disorders** (Delirium; Major or Mild Neurocognitive Disorder due to Alzheimer's Disease; Major or Mild Frontotemporal Neurocognitive Disorder; Major or Mild Neurocognitive Disorder with Lewy Bodies; Major or Mild Vascular Neurocognitive Disorder; Major or Mild Neurocognitive Disorder due to Traumatic Brain Injury; Major or Mild Neurocognitive Disorder due to HIV Infection; Major or Mild Neurocognitive Disorder due to Parkinson's Disease; Major or Mild Neurocognitive Disorder due to Huntington's Disease; Major or Mild Neurocognitive Disorder due to Another Medical Condition; Major or Mild Neurocognitive Disorder due to Multiple Etiologies; Stimulant-induced major or mild neurocognitive disorder and Unspecified Neurocognitive Disorders)

(Continued)

Table 7.9 (Continued)

18. **Personality Disorders** ((i) Cluster A Personality Disorders—Paranoid, Schizoid and Schizotypal Disorders; (ii) Cluster B Personality Disorders—Antisocial, Borderline, Histrionic, and Narcissistic Personality Disorders; (iii) Other Personality Disorders— Personality Change due to Another Medical Condition, Other Specified and Unspecified Personality Disorder)
19. **Paraphilic Disorders** (Voyeuristic Disorder; Exhibitionistic Disorder; Frotteuristic Disorder; Sexual Masochism Disorder; Sexual Sadism Disorder; Pedophilic Disorder; Fetishistic Disorder; Transvestic Disorder; Other Specified or Unspecified Paraphilic Disorder)
20. **Other Mental Disorders:** (Other Specified Mental Disorder due to another Medical Condition; *Unspecified Mood Disorder*; Unspecified Mental Disorder due to Another Medical Condition; and Other Specified or Unspecified Mental Disorder); Medication-Induced Movement Disorders and Other Adverse effects of Medication; Neuroleptic-Induced Parkinsonism; Other Medication-Induced Parkinsonism; Neuroleptic Malignant Syndrome; Medication-Induced Acute Akathisia; Tardive Dyskinesia; Tardive Dystonia; TardivAkathisia; Medication-Induced Postrul Tremor; Other Medication-Induced Movement Disorder; Antidepressant Discontinuation Syndrome; and Other Adverse Effects of Medication)
21. **Other Conditions that may be a Focus of Clinical Attention** (Problems related to Family Upbringing; Other Problems Related to Family, the Primary Support Group; Child Physical Abuse; Child Sexual Abuse; Child Neglect, Child Psychological Abuse; Spouse or Partner Violence—Physical; Spouse or Partner Violence—Sexual; Spouse or Partner Violence—Psychological; Adult Abuse by Non-Spouse or Non-Partner; *Suicidal behavior and non-suicidal self-injury (NSSI)*; Educational and Occupational Problems; Housing and Economic Problems; Other Problems Related to the Social Environment; Problems Related to Crime or Interaction with the Legal System; Other Health Service Encounters for Counseling and Medical Advice; Problems Related to Other Psychosocial, Personal, and Environmental Circumstances; Other Circumstances of Personal History; Problems Related to Access to Medical and Other Health Care; and Non-Adherence to Medical Treatment)

Notes: (i) The changes from the DSM-5 to the DSM-5-TR here are shown in italics.
(ii) ICD-10-CM codes given to the classified mental disorders are not shown here.
Source: Adapted from American Psychiatric Association (2022), *Diagnostic and statistical manual of mental disorders: DSM-5-TR*, Washington, DC: American Psychiatric Association Publishing.

The Ways in which Classification System of the DSM-5-TR Stands Distinguished from the DSM-5

A. **Addition of new disorders or specific categories:**

(i) In the broad class of "Trauma and Related Stressors," a new disorder named *Prolonged Grief Disorder* has been added. It has been defined as intense yearning or longing for the deceased (often with intense sorrow and emotional pain), and preoccupied with thoughts or memories of the deceased

(ii) The category named stimulant-induced major or mild neurocognitive disorder has been added in the broad class named as *Neurocognitive Disorders*.

(iii) In the broad class "*Other Conditions That May Be a Focus of Clinical Attention,*" a new category of disorder in the name of *Suicidal behavior and Nonsuicidal Self-Injury (NSSI)* has been added.

(iv) The category of "Unspecified Mood Disorder" that was excluded in the DSM-5 has been restored.

B. **Changes in the Nomenclatures of certain disorders:** In addition to the appearance of new disorders or specific categories, **a**ll disorders previously appearing in the DSM-5 have been retained in the DSM-5-TR except some minor changes in the nomenclature of a few such as:

(i) The disorder named as "Intellectual disability" appearing in the broad class of *Neurodevelopmental Disorders* of the DSM-5 has been renamed as "Intellectual Developmental Disorder."

(ii) The disorder named as "Persistent depressive disorder-dysthymia" appearing in the broad class *Depressive Disorders* of the DSM-5 has been renamed as "Persistent depressive disorder" by removing the parenthesis "dysthymia."

(iii) The disorder named as "Social anxiety disorder—social phobia" in the broad class *Anxiety Disorders* of the DSM-5 has been renamed as "Social anxiety disorder" by removing the phrase "social phobia."

(iv) The disorder named as "Conversion Disorder—Functional Neurological Symptom Disorder" has been renamed as the "Functional Neurological Symptom Disorder—Conversion Disorder.

(v) The disorder named as "Olfactory reference disorder" was added as an example of presentations that can be specified under an "other specified" designation in the "other specified obsessive-compulsive and related disorder" category.

C. **Other significant changes reflected in the DSM-5-TR:**

(i) There have been significant changes in the terminology used in the discussion about the category *Gender Dysphoria*. Here the terms mentioned in the DSM-5 have been replaced, such as replacement of the term "desired gender" with "experienced gender"; "natal sex" to "birth-assigned gender"; "natal male/natal female" with "individual assigned male/female at birth"; and "cross-sex treatment regimen" with "gender-affirming treatment regimen."

(ii) There has been a commendable effort for appropriate modifications in the diagnostic criteria or specifier definitions of a number of disorders numbering more than 70.

(iii) For coding of all the mentioned disorders in the DSM-5-TR, only ICD-10-CM (International Classification of Diseases, 10th Edition, Clinical Modification) codes have been used.

ICD-10 Classification of Mental and Behavioral Disorders

ICD-10 is the Tenth Revision of the International Statistical Classification of Diseases and Related Health Problems brought out in the year 1994 by the WHO. It includes in its Chapter V a detailed classification of over 300 mental and behavioral disorders. The ICD-10 is available in its two main versions (i) *Clinical Descriptions and Diagnostic Guidelines* and (ii) *Diagnostic Criteria for Research*.

The former provides clinical descriptions detailing the principal signs and symptoms of each disorder, together with other important but less specific associated features, as well as comprehensive guidelines for their diagnosis. The latter version is intended to help those researching specific disorders to maximize the homogeneity of study groups. To this end, it sets out criteria that allows the selection of individuals with clearly similar symptoms and other characteristics.

Here we present the classes or main categories of mental disorders specified in the ICD-10 in Table 7.10.

Table 7.10 Classification of Mental Disorders in the ICD-10

Broad Class	Categories included
F00 to F09 **Organic, Including Symptomatic Mental Disorders**	F00 Dementia in Alzheimer's Disease F01 Vascular Dementia F02 Dementia in other diseases classified elsewhere F03 Unspecified Dementia F04 Organic amnestic syndromes, not induced by alcohol and other psychoactive substances F05 Delirium, not induced by alcohol and other psychotic substances F06 Other mental disorders due to brain damage and dysfunction and to physical disease F07 Personality and behavioral disorders due to brain disease, damage and dysfunction F08 Unassigned F09 Unspecified organic or symptomatic mental disorder
F10 to F19 **Mental and Behavioral disorders due to Psychoactive substances use**	F10 Mental and Behavioral Disorder due to the use of Alcohol F11 Mental and Behavioral Disorder due to the use of Opioids F12 Mental and Behavioral Disorder due to the use of Cannabinoids F13 Mental and Behavioral Disorder due to the use of Sedatives or Hypnotics F14 Mental and Behavioral Disorder due to the use of Cocaine F15 Mental and Behavioral Disorder due to the use of other stimulants including Caffeine F16 Mental and Behavioral Disorder due to the use of Hallucinogens F17 Mental and Behavioral Disorder due to the use of Tobacco F18 Mental and Behavioral Disorder due to the use of Volatile solvents F19 Mental and Behavioral Disorder due to the use of multiple drug and of other psychoactive substances
F20 to F29 **Schizophrenia, Schizotypal, and Delusional Disorders**	F20 Schizophrenia F21 Schizotypal disorder F22 Persistent delusional disorders F23 Acute and transient psychotic disorders F24 Induced delusional disorder F25 Schizoaffective disorders F26 Unassigned F27 Unassigned F28 Other non-organic psychotic disorders F29 Unspecified non-organic psychosis

F30 to F39
Mood (affective) Disorders

F30 Manic episode
F31 Bipolar affective disorder
F32 Depressive episode
F33 Recurrent depressive disorder
F34 Persistent mood (affective) disorders
F35 Unassigned
F36 Unassigned
F37 Unassigned
F38 Other mood (affective) disorders
F39 Unspecified mood (affective) disorders

F40 to F49
Neurotic, Stress-related, and Somatoform Disorders

F40 Phobic anxiety disorders
F41 Other anxiety disorders
F42 Obsessive-Compulsive disorders
F43 Reaction to severe stress and adjustment disorders
F44 Dissociative (Conversion) disorders
F45 Somatoform disorders
F46 Unassigned
F47 Unassigned
F48 Other Neurotic disorders
F49 Unassigned

F50 to F59
Behavioral syndromes Associated with Psychophysical disturbances and Physical factors

F50 Eating disorders
F51 Non-organic sleep disorders
F52 Sexual dysfunction, not caused by organic disorder and disease
F53 Mental and behavioral disorders associated with the puerperium, not elsewhere classified
F54 Psychological and behavioral factors associated with disorders or diseases classified elsewhere
F55 Abuse of non-dependence producing substances such as vitamins, steroids or hormones and antidepressants
F56 Unassigned
F57 Unassigned
F58 Unassigned
F59 Unspecified behavioral syndromes associated with psychological disturbances and physical factors

(Continued)

Table 7.10 (Continued)

Broad Class	Categories included
F60 to F69 **Disorders of Adult Personality and Behavior**	F60 Specific personality disorders—paranoid, schizoid, dissocial personality disorder F61 Mixed or other personality disorders F62 Enduring personality changes, not attributable to brain damage and disease F63 Habit and Impulsive disorders such as pathological gambling, pathological stealing (Kleptomania) F64 Gender Identity disorders such as Trans-sexualism F65 Disorders of sexual preferences such as fetishism, exhibitionism F66 Psychological and behavioral disorders associated with sexual development and orientation such as sexual relationship disorders F67 Unassigned F68 Other disorders of adult personality and behaviors F69 Unspecified disorder of adult personality and behavior
F70 to F79 **Mental Retardation**	F70 Mild F71 Moderate F72 Severe F73 Profound F74 Unassigned F75 Unassigned F76 Unassigned F77 Unassigned F78 Other Mental retardation F79 Unspecified Mental retardation
F80 to F89 **Disorders of Psychological Development**	F80 Specific developmental disorders of speech and language F81 Specific developmental disorder of scholastic skills F82 Specific developmental disorders of motor function F83 Mixed specific developmental disorder F84 Pervasive developmental disorders F85 Unassigned F86 Unassigned F87 Unassigned F88 Other disorders of psychological development F89 Unspecified disorder of psychological development

F90 to F98
Behavioral and Emotional
Disorders with Onset usually
Occurring in Childhood and
Adolescence
F-99
Unspecified
Mental Disorders

F90 Hyperkinetic Disorders
F91 Conduct disorders
F92 Mixed disorders of conduct and emotions
F93 Emotional disorders with onset specific to childhood such as separation anxiety, sibling
    rivalry
F94 Disorders of social functioning with onset specific to childhood and adolescence
F95 Tic disorders such as chronic motor or vocal tic disorders
F96 Unassigned
F97 Unassigned
F98 Other behavioral and emotional disorders with onset usually
    occurring in childhood and adolescence such as stammering, feeding disorders
F99 Unspecified mental disorders, not otherwise specified

Source: Adapted from World Health Organization (2010), *The ICD-10 Classification of Mental and Behavioural Disorders: Clinical Descriptions and Diagnostic Guidelines,* 10th ed. Geneva: World Health Organization.

ICD-11 Classification of Mental and Behavioral Disorders

The ICD-11 is the latest version of the WHO classification system meant for bringing needed improvement in the diagnosis and classifications of mental diseases, mental and behavioral disorders, and health problems on the global basis. In this concern, a final draft of the ICD-11 system was endorsed by the 72nd World Health Assembly in 2019 and came into effect on 1st January 2022.

The overall significance of ICD-11 over the existing ICD-10 may be briefed as follows:

- ICD-11 is much easier and simpler in its use than ICD-10
- It is more clinically relevant on account of the systematic reliance on the use of code combinations and extension codes
- It is multilingual, existing in 43 languages in electronic versions
- It is capable of providing description of each disease entity (category) in clear terms, aiming to help users in understanding the meaning of the category in comprehensible terms. It is a significant development of ICD-10, which had only title headings. We present the classes or main categories of mental disorders specified in ICD-11 in Table 7.11.

To Sum Up

Attempts for the classification of mental disorders may be studied in terms of the old era and the modern era. Among the attempts made in the old era, notable ones include Hippocrates' classification (mania, melancholia, and phrenesis), the Indian classification (Satguna, Rajoguna, and Tamoguna), and Kraepelin's classification. However, these are of purely historical interest. The modern era witnesses the well-organized attempts made for this purpose on the part of two important agencies—the American Psychiatric Association and the WHO. The systems developed by the former are named the DSM (Diagnostic and Statistical Manual of Mental Disorders) and by the latter, the ICD (International Classification of Diseases). Up to this time, the American Psychiatric Association has published a number of manuals in the names of the DSM-I, DSM-II, DSM-III, DSM III-R, DSM-IV, DSM IV-TR, DSM-5, and DSM-5-TR, from the years 1952 through 2022. In comparison to the use of the DSMs, the ICDs developed by the WHO are in wide usage throughout the world on the part of clinicians, practitioners, health workers, students, and researchers in the field. The contemporary position witnesses the development and use of the DSM-5-TR and ICD-11 (both were updated in 2022) for the classification, diagnosis, and treatment of mental and behavioral disorders.

The Necessity and Purposes of Classification

The classification of mental disorders or diseases is based on the following similarities.

(i)   Similarity of the symptoms and syndromes.
(ii) Similarity of the treatment techniques.
(iii) Similarity of the possibilities of improvement.

In light of this, the commonly recognized functions or purposes of the classification of mental disorders or diseases may be summarized as follows.

Table 7.11 Classification of Mental Disorders in ICD-11 (Summarized)

Broad Class or Block	Categories Included
Neurodevelopmental disorders (6A00 to 6A06 & 6A0Y, 6A0Z)	6A00: Disorders of intellectual development 6A01: Developmental speech or language disorders 6A02: Autism spectrum disorder 6A03: Developmental learning disorder 6A04: Developmental motor coordination disorder 6A05: Attention deficit hyperactivity disorder 6A06: Stereotyped movement disorder 6A0Y: Other specified Neurodevelopmental Disorders 6A0Z: Neurodevelopmental disorders, unspecified
Schizophrenia or other primary psychotic disorders (6A20 to 6A25 & 6A2Y, 6A2Z)	6A20: Schizophrenia 6A21: Schizoaffective disorder 6A22: Schizotypal disorder 6A23: Acute and transient psychotic disorder 6A24: Delusional disorder 6A25: Symptomatic manifestations of primary psychotic disorders 6A2Y: Other specified primary psychotic disorders 6A2Z: Primary psychotic disorders, unspecified
Catatonia (6A40 to6A41 & 6A4Z)	6A40: Catatonia associated with another mental disorder 6A41: Catatonia induced by substances or medications 6A4Z: Catatonia, unspecified
Mood disorders- Bipolar and Depressive disorders (6A60 to 6A62; 6A70 to 6A72; 6A80; 6A8Y & 6A8Z)	6A60: Bipolar type I disorder 6A61: Bipolar type II disorder 6A62: Cyclothymic disorder 6A70: Single episode depressive disorder 6A71: Recurrent depressive disorder 6A72: Dysthymic disorder 6A80: Symptomatic and course presentations for mood episodes in mood disorders 6A8Y: Other specified mood disorders 6A8Z: Mood disorders, unspecified

(Continued)

Table 7.11 (Continued)

Broad Class or Block	Categories Included
Anxiety or fear-related disorders (6B00 to 6B06; 6B0Y & 6B0Z)	6B00: Generalised anxiety disorder 6B01: Panic disorder 6B02: Agoraphobia 6B03: Specific phobia 6B04: Social anxiety disorder 6B05: Separation anxiety disorder 6B06: Selective mutism 6B0Y: Other specified anxiety or fear-related disorders 6B0Z: Anxiety or fear-related disorders, unspecified
Obsessive-compulsive or related disorders (6B20 to 6B25; 6B2Y & 6B2Z)	6B20: Obsessive-compulsive disorder 6B21: Body dysmorphic disorder 6B22: Olfactory reference disorder 6B23: Hypochondriasis 6B24: Hoarding disorder 6B25: Body-focused repetitive behavior disorders 6B2Y: Other specified obsessive-compulsive or related disorders 6B2Z: Obsessive-compulsive or related disorders, unspecified
Disorders specifically associated with stress (6B40 to 6B45; 6B4Y &6B4Z)	6B40: Posttraumatic stress disorder 6B41: Complex posttraumatic stress disorder 6B42: Prolonged grief disorder 6B43: Adjustment disorder 6B44: Reactive attachment disorder 6B45: Disinhibited social engagement disorder 6B4Y: Other specified disorders specifically associated with stress 6B4Z: Disorders specifically associated with stress, unspecified
Dissociative disorders (6B60 to 6B66; 6B6Y& 6B6Z)	6B60: Dissociative neurological symptom disorder 6B61: Dissociative amnesia 6B62: Trance disorder 6B63: Possession trance disorder 6B64: Dissociative identity disorder 6B65: Partial dissociative identity disorder 6B66: Depersonalization-derealization disorder 6B6Y: Other specified dissociative disorders 6B6Z: Dissociative disorders, unspecified

Feeding or eating disorders
(6B80 to 6B85; 6B8Y & 6B8Z)

6B80: Anorexia Nervosa
6B81: Bulimia Nervosa
6B82: Binge eating disorder
6B83: Avoidant-restrictive food intake disorder
6B84: Pica
6B85: Rumination-regurgitation disorder
6B8Y: Other specified feeding or eating disorders
6B8Z: Feeding or eating disorders, unspecified

Elimination disorders
(6C00 to 6C01; & 6C0Z)

6C00: Enuresis
6C01: Encopresis
6C0Z: Elimination disorders, unspecified

Disorders of bodily distress or bodily experience
(6C20 to 6C21;6C2Y & 6C2Z)

6C20: Bodily distress disorder
6C21: Body integrity dysphoria
6C2Y: Other specified disorders of bodily distress or bodily experience
6C2Z: Disorders of bodily distress or bodily experience, unspecified

Disorders due to substance use or addictive behaviors
(6C40 to 6C49; 6C4A to 6CAH; 6C4Y & 6C4Z; 6C50, 6C51; 6C5Y & 6C5Z)

6C40: Disorders due to use of alcohol
6C41: Disorders due to use of cannabis
6C42: Disorders due to use of synthetic cannabinoids
6C43: Disorders due to use of opioids
6C44: Disorders due to use of sedatives, hypnotics or anxiolytics
6C45: Disorders due to use of cocaine
6C46: Disorders due to use of stimulants including amphetamines, methamphetamine or methcathinone
6C47: Disorders due to use of synthetic cathinones
6C48: Disorders due to use of caffeine
6C49: Disorders due to use of hallucinogens
6C4A: Disorders due to use of nicotine
6C4B: Disorders due to use of volatile inhalants
6C4C: Disorders due to use of MDMA or related drugs, including MDA
6C4D: Disorders due to use of dissociative drugs including ketamine and phencyclidine [PCP]
6C4E: Disorders due to use of other specified psychoactive substances, including medications
6C4F: Disorders due to use of multiple specified psychoactive substances, including medications
6C4G: Disorders due to use of unknown or unspecified psychoactive substances
6C4H: Disorders due to use of non-psychoactive substances
6C4Y: Other specified disorders due to substance use

(Continued)

Table 7.11 (Continued)

Broad Class or Block	Categories Included
	6C4Z: Disorders due to substance use, unspecified
Impulse control disorders (6C70 to 6C70;6C7Y & 6C7Z)	6C50: Gambling disorder
	6C51: Gaming disorder
	6C5Y: Other specified disorders due to addictive behaviors
	6C5Z: Disorders due to addictive behaviors, unspecified
	6C70: Pyromania
	6C71: Kleptomania
	6C72: Compulsive sexual behavior disorder
	6C73: Intermittent explosive disorder
	6C7Y: Other specified impulse control disorders
	6C7Z: Impulse control disorders, unspecified
Disruptive behavior or dissocial disorders (6C90 to 6C91; 6C9Y & 6C9Z)	6C90: Oppositional defiant disorder
	6C91: Conduct-dissocial disorder
	6C9Y: Other specified disruptive behavior or dissocial disorders
	6C9Z: Disruptive behavior or dissocial disorders, unspecified
Personality disorders and related traits (6D10 & 6D11)	6D10: Personality disorder
	6D11: Prominent personality traits or patterns
Paraphilic disorders (6D30 to 6D36; 6D3Z)	6D30: Exhibitionistic disorder
	6D31: Voyeuristic disorder
	6D32: Pedophilic disorder
	6D33: Coercive sexual sadism disorder
	6D34: Frotteuristic disorder
	6D35: Other paraphilic disorder involving non-consenting individuals
	6D36: Paraphilic disorder involving solitary behavior or consenting individuals
	6D3Z: Paraphilic disorders, unspecified
Factitious disorders (6D50 to 6D51; 6D5Z)	6D50: Factitious disorder imposed on self
	6D51: Factitious disorder imposed on another
	6D5Z: Factitious disorders, unspecified

Neurocognitive disorders
(6D70 to 6D72; 6D80 to
   6D85;6E0Y &6E0Z)

6D70: Delirium
6D71: Mild neurocognitive disorder
6D72: Amnestic disorder
6D80: Dementia due to Alzheimer disease
6D81: Dementia due to cerebrovascular disease
6D82: Dementia due to Lewy body disease
6D83: Frontotemporal dementia
6D84: Dementia due to psychoactive substances including medications
6D85: Dementia due to diseases classified elsewhere
6E0Y: Other specified neurocognitive disorders
6E0Z: Neurocognitive disorders, unspecified

Mental or behavioral disorders associated with pregnancy, childbirth or the puerperium
(6E20 to 6E20; 6E2Z)

6E20: Mental or behavioral disorders associated with pregnancy, childbirth or the puerperium, without psychotic symptoms
6E21: Mental or behavioral disorders associated with pregnancy, childbirth or the puerperium, with psychotic symptoms
6E2Z: Mental or behavioral disorders associated with pregnancy, childbirth or the puerperium, unspecified

Secondary mental or behavioral syndromes associated with disorders or diseases classified elsewhere
(6E60 to 6E69)

6E60: Secondary neurodevelopmental syndrome
6E61: Secondary psychotic syndrome
6E62: Secondary mood syndrome
6E63: Secondary anxiety syndrome
6E64: Secondary obsessive-compulsive or related syndrome
6E65: Secondary dissociative syndrome
6E66: Secondary impulse control syndrome
6E67: Secondary neurocognitive syndrome
6E68: Secondary personality change
6E69: Secondary catatonia syndrome

Sleep-Awake Disorders
(a) Insomnia disorders
(7A00 to 7A01; 7A0Z)

7A00: Chronic insomnia
7A01: Short-term insomnia
7A0Z: Insomnia disorders, unspecified

(Continued)

Table 7.11 (Continued)

Broad Class or Block	Categories Included
(b) Hypersomnolence disorders (7A20 to7A26;7A2Y & 7A2Z)	7A20: Narcolepsy 7A21: Idiopathic hypersomnia 7A22: Kleine-Levin syndrome 7A23: Hypersomnia due to a medical condition 7A24: Hypersomnia due to a medication or substance 7A25: Hypersomnia associated with a mental disorder 7A26: Insufficient sleep syndrome 7A2Y: Other specified hypersomnolence disorders 7A2Z: Hypersomnolence disorders, unspecified
(c) Sleep-related breathing disorders (7A40 to7A42;7A4Y & 7A4Z)	7A40: Central sleep apneas 7A41: Obstructive sleep apnoea 7A42: Sleep-related hypoventilation or hypoxemia disorders 7A4Y: Other specified sleep-related breathing disorders 7A4Z: Sleep-related breathing disorders, unspecified
(d) Circadian rhythm sleep-wake disorders (7A60 to 7A60;7A6Z)	7A60: Delayed sleep-wake phase disorder 7A61: Advanced sleep-wake phase disorder 7A62: Irregular sleep-wake rhythm disorder 7A63: Non-24 hour sleep-wake rhythm disorder 7A64: Circadian rhythm sleep-wake disorder, shift work type **7A65:** Circadian rhythm sleep-wake disorder, jet lag type 7A6Z: Circadian rhythm sleep-wake disorders, unspecified
(e) Sleep-related movement disorders (7A80 to 7A88;7A8Y &7A8Z)	7A80: Restless legs syndrome 7A81: Periodic limb movement disorder 7A82: Sleep-related leg cramps 7A83: Sleep-related bruxism 7A84: Sleep-related rhythmic movement disorder 7A85: Benign sleep myoclonus of infancy 7A86: Propriospinal myoclonus at sleep onset 7A87: Sleep-related movement disorder due to a medical condition 7A88: Sleep-related movement disorder due to a medication or substance 7A8Y: Other specified sleep-related movement disorders 7A8Z: Sleep-related movement disorders, unspecified

(f) Parasomnia disorders
(7B00 to 7B02;7B0Y &7B0Z)

7B00: Disorders of arousal from non-REM sleep
7B01: Parasomnias related to REM sleep
7B02: Other parasomnias
7B0Y: Other specified parasomnia disorders
7B0Z: Parasomnia disorders, unspecified

Sexual dysfunctions
(HA00 to HA03; HA0Y & HA0Z)

HA00: Hypoactive sexual desire dysfunction
HA01: Sexual arousal dysfunctions
HA02: Orgasmic dysfunctions
HA03: Ejaculatory dysfunctions
HA0Y: Other specified sexual dysfunctions
HA0Z: Sexual dysfunctions, unspecified

Source: World Health Organization (WHO), *ICD-11 for Mortality and Morbidity Statistics* (version: 02/ 2022), downloaded from https://icd.who.int/ browse11/l-m/en

1. *Diagnosis purposes:* The classification of mental disorders helps with diagnosis on the following grounds.

   (i) Symptoms and syndromes related to the specific class can be properly investigated.
   (ii) The possible factors contributing to the development or maintenance of the disorder can be identified.

2. *Treatment purposes:* Classification of mental disorders renders valuable help in the treatment task in relation to the following.

   (i) It suggests appropriate therapeutic techniques and other treatments.
   (ii) It helps in the prediction of the affected person's chances of improvement (a) without treatment and (b) with various treatments.
   (iii) It helps in evaluating the improvement or change in the behavior of the affected person during a course of treatment or with the passage of time.

3. *Descriptive and communicative purposes:* The knowledge that a particular mental disorder lies in a particular class or category helps in describing the disorders in terms of some general or specific behavior patterns. What is the nature of that mental disorder? How can the affected person react? How can they be helped in seeking adjustment, and up to what extent? In short, the categorization tries to communicate a brief but meaningful summary of the problem or problems of the affected person to the concerned professional persons.

   The why and how of the classification of mental disorders may be further explained in light of the following examples.

Case 1: Bimla, a housewife, was terrified by lizards. Despite being aware that she could not be harmed by them, the mere sight of a lizard was enough to make her tremble with fear.

Case 2: Surendra, a young man of 30 years, feared that he would not be able to swallow. The severe and overwhelming anxiety sometimes escalated to a panic attack leading him to believe that his heart would stop beating and he would die. While knowing the absurdity of his fear and anxiety, he had no control over his feelings.

Case 3: Savita, a college student 22 years of age living in the college hostel developed a belief that she would soon be poisoned. She was unable to explain who would poison her and why. Her fear and anxiety developed to the extent that she stopped taking anything from the mess and began to cook her food herself and even make her food purchases herself.

Case 4: Prem Singh, a retired army personnel, believed that the British government was after him, as he had been in association with Azad Hind Fauze. He believed the government of free India should now take full responsibility for protecting him from being kidnapped and killed by people in police uniform spying for the British government. He wrote to the D.I.G. police for appropriate screening of the district police to identify the British spies. He also wrote to the Prime Minister and President of India, requesting them for his adequate protection. Gradually, his anxiety and fear became so intense that he confined himself in a locked room closing all the windows and ventilators so that none could get at him.

Case 5: Ramesh Chandra, 23 years of age, reported for psychiatric help. He believed that he would be unable to perform normal sexual acts, as he was impotent, and therefore, his fiancée should not suffer unnecessarily on account of him. He insisted on her forgetting him and marrying someone else. On medical examination, it was found that there was nothing wrong with his sex organs and his fear had no organic cause.

All the five cases cited above are obviously the cases of mental disorders. Their diagnosis, understanding, and treatment definitely requires some classification since it would be futile to group them into a broad category—mental disorders. The cases have some similarities and also dissimilarities. Let us classify them on this basis.

The symptoms of fear and anxiety are common to all. In the cases of Savita and Prem Singh, the disorder is in the thought process (delusion or hallucination). They have beliefs that are irrational and baseless. There is a gross distortion or misrepresentation of external reality in both these cases, which is significantly absent in the remaining three cases. These two cases may then be classified as psychotics.

The other three cases show neurotic symptoms but the last one typically differs in some characteristics with the cases of Bimla and Surendra. The behavior patterns in the case of Ramesh Chandra are significantly attached to his sexual behavior. In the absence of any organic cause, his problem is concerned with psychic impotence—a common psycho-physiological disorder associated with sex. The remaining two cases of Bimla and Surendra may then be classified as neurotics.

On further classification, we may differentiate the cases of Bimla and Surendra by distinguishing the particular type of neurosis. Similarly, the psychotic cases of Savita and Prem Singh may also be further differentiated.

The problem of differentiation and classification is a typical one in any attempt of the diagnosis and treatment of mental diseases and disorders. The symptoms often overlap. Even different diagnoses may have symptoms in common. Take the case of schizophrenia. Here a particular patient may have delusions and hallucinations, but along with these psychotic symptoms, neurotic symptoms like excessive fear, anxiety, hysteria, depression, and obsessive-compulsive reactions may also be present. Typically, anxiety symptoms may occur in all cases of mental disorders.

Therefore, a mere diagnosis of anxiety reactions will not serve any useful purpose for classification. The other symptoms related to the similarities and differences typical to a particular class or category of mental disorders must therefore be searched for an appropriate classification.

To Sum Up

The classification of mental disorders or diseases is needed for serving three main purposes: Diagnosis purposes, Treatment purposes, and Descriptive and Communicative purposes. In this concern, whichever the symptoms and syndromes exhibited on the part of the patient, their problem is classified in the name of a particular category of mental disorder (on the basis of it being defined as such in the latest DSM or ICD). This facilitates mental health professionals in their diagnosis process and treatment task. Besides this, another big help rendered with the classification of mental disorders is concerned with its ability to provide a brief but meaningful summary of the problem of the patient for its description and communication to concerned professionals.

Review Questions

1. Discuss in brief the attempts made for the development of systems for classifying mental disorders in the old era prior to those developed by the APA and WHO.
2. Provide a description of the attempts made by the APA and WHO from time to time for classifying mental disorders.

3. Name the different systems of classification brought out by the APA from time to time with their nomenclature, number of diagnosed disorders, and years.
4. Explain in what ways (i) the DSM-5 differed from previous ones, and (ii) the present DSM-5-TR differs from the DSM-5?
5. Discuss in brief the evolution and development of the ICDs over time, published by the WHO.
6. Throw light on the ways in which the ICD-11 differs from the ICD-10.
7. Describe in detail the necessity and purposes served by the classification of mental disorders.

References

American Psychiatric Association (1952), *Diagnostic and statistical manual of mental disorders*, Washington, DC: American Psychiatric Association.

American Psychiatric Association (1968), *Diagnostic and statistical manual of mental disorders, DSM-II* (2nd ed.), Washington, DC: American Psychiatric Association.

American Psychiatric Association (1980), *Diagnostic and statistical manual of mental disorders, DSM-III* (3rd ed.), Washington, DC: American Psychiatric Association.

American Psychiatric Association (1994), *Diagnostic and statistical manual of mental disorders, DSM-IV* (4th ed.), Washington, DC: American Psychiatric Association.

American Psychiatric Association (2000), *The diagnostic and statistical manual of mental disorders, DSM IV-TR*, Washington, DC: American Psychiatric Association.

American Psychiatric Association (2013), *Diagnostic and statistical manual of mental disorders* (5th ed.), Washington, DC: American Psychiatric Association.

American Psychiatric Association (2022), *Diagnostic and statistical manual of mental disorders: DSM-5-TR*, Washington, DC: American Psychiatric Association.

WHO (1965), *International classification of diseases* (8th revision, ICD-8), Geneva: World Health Organization.

WHO (1977), *International classification of diseases* (9th revision, ICD-9), Geneva: World Health Organization.

WHO (2010), *The ICD-10 classification of mental and behavioural disorders: clinical descriptions and diagnostic guidelines* (10th ed.), Geneva: World Health Organization.

WHO (2022), *ICD-11 for mortality and morbidity statistics* (version: 02/2022), retrieved from https://icd.who.int/browse11/l-m/en

Chapter 8

Psycho-Physiological or Psychosomatic Disorders

Learning Objectives

After going through this chapter, you will be able to:

- Define the term psycho-physiological disorders.
- Understand the meaning and characteristics of psycho-physiological disorders.
- Discuss the nature and occurrence of psycho-physiological disorders like Respiratory, Cardio-vascular, Gastrointestinal, Genito-urinary, skin, Endocrine, Hemic and Lymphatic, and Musculoskeletal disorders.
- Know and tell about the psycho-physiological disorders, newly appearing in the DSM-5 such as Somatic Symptom Disorder, Illness Anxiety, Conversion, and Factitious disorders.
- Describe in detail the causes underlying psycho-physiological disorders.
- Throw light on the measures taken for the prevention and treatment of psycho-physiological disorders.

What are Psycho-Physiological or Psychosomatic Disorders?

Psycho-physiological disorders are also known as psychosomatic disorders, which implies that the mind (psyche) determines the disease or disorders of the body (soma).

According to the American Psychiatric Association publication DSM II (1968:46),

> psycho-physiological disorders are characterized by physical symptoms that are caused by emotional factors and involve a single organ system, usually under autonomic nervous system intervention. The physiological changes involved are those that normally accompany certain emotional states, but in these disorders the changes are more intense and sustained.

This definition leads us to the following characteristics of psycho-physiological disorders:

- Psycho-physiological disorders exhibit physical symptoms like pain, vomiting, difficulty in breathing, diarrhea, and so on. It is the severity of the distress caused by these symptoms that usually compels the individual to seek medical help.
- Although the physical symptoms developed on account of psycho-physiological disorders appear similar to those reflected in certain emotional states (anxiety, anger etc.), the visceral

DOI: 10.4324/9781003398325-8

effects of emotional conflict in these disorders are so pronounced that actual and irreversible damage may be done to the body's structure. In this way, a so-called psychological illness or disorder turns into "a real" illness or disorder with identifiable tissue pathology.

- In psycho-physiological disorders the emotional conflicts affect the viscera through the autonomic nervous system, which has two main divisions, known as the sympathetic and parasympathetic systems. These two systems of the autonomic nervous system are controlled by the brain in such a way that in normal conditions the effects of the two systems are kept in approximate balance. These disorders result in the predominance of either sympathetic or parasympathetic activity flooding a single organ system—respiratory, circulatory, and so on.
- The psycho-physiological disorders are neither exclusively caused by psychological factors nor by organic factors, but are brought about by an interaction of psychological and organic factors.

To Sum Up

Psycho-Physiological or Psychosomatic Disorders represent the type of disorders in which people are found to show and feel one or the other types of physical symptoms of an ailment or disease on account of psychological difficulties with no trace of a specific physical or biological cause. The symptoms present similarly to a specific physical disease, and their pain or suffering on this account is also real and may last for several years, but their cure and treatment are psychological rather than medical.

The Main Psycho-Physiological or Psychosomatic Disorders

Based on the different types of psychosomatic disorders mentioned in the classification systems provided by the American Psychiatric Association prior to the evolvement of the DSM-5, we are providing an essential discussion about some of the main psycho-physiological or psychosomatic disorders, as follows.

1. Respiratory disorders: Respiratory disorders are concerned with the malfunctioning or dysfunction of the respiratory system. A few common psycho-physiological disorders include:

   (a) *Asthma:* The main symptom involves difficulty in breathing (wheezing) and a sense of constriction of the chest. In psycho-physiological cases of asthma, the muscles in the walls of the bronchi (tubes in the lungs) contract because of the relative underactivity of the sympathetic system or the relative overactivity of the parasympathetic system.

   (b) *Common cold:* It consists of the inflammation of the muscular membranes of the nose and throat with profuse discharge.

   (c) *Rhinitis:* It involves non-infectious inflammation and swelling of the nasal mucosa with itching, sneezing, and profuse watery secretion from the nose.

   (d) *Hay fever:* It concerns some sort of allergic reaction in which the mucous membranes of the nose become inflamed.

   (e) *Hyperventilation:* It means "over breathing." It consists of episodes of fairly deep breathing with the mouth open or rapid shallow breathing and results in the sensations of dizziness, chest pain, blurred vision, and tingling or numbness in the extremities.

2. **Cardiovascular disorders:** Today, cases of disorders and diseases of the heart and vascular system are on the increase. The major cardiovascular disorders with psycho-physiological factors are hypertension, angina pectoris, migraine, and coronary disease.

   a) *Hypertension:* It is a chronic state of high blood pressure. It may have organic causes in the form of interference with the circulatory function of the kidneys. When no such organic cause can be found, the condition is referred to as essential hypertension, indicating that it is caused by emotional factors.

   b) *Angina pectoris:* It is severe pain in the chest. In the form of organic cause, it is related to an insufficient supply of oxygen to the heart muscles. But in many cases, the individuals experiencing angina feel pain and a sensation of being stabbed in the heart, yet usually do not show any signs of organic disturbances, indicating that they may be caused by psychological factors.

   c) *Migraine:* It involves extremely painful headaches. The pain usually occurs on the side of the head. Sometimes it is associated with nausea and blurred vision. The attack rarely lasts more than twenty-four hours and is often much briefer. It is generally caused by sympathetically innervated contraction, followed by dilation of blood vessels in the brain. Emotional disturbance, early psychological experiences, and genetic influences may be the causes of migraine disorders, in addition to or in absence of the known bodily causes.

   d) *Coronary diseases:* Diseases of the heart like clotting of blood (thrombosis) blocking one of the vessels serving the heart involve both physiological and psychological factors. In cases of psychologically stressful situations, the rate of blood clotting may increase. Anxiety, anger, and excitement result in an increase of heart palpitation, which in turn increases resistance to the flow of blood and speeds up blood clotting. The presence of such psychological factors, thus, may work as predisposing or precipitating causes for coronary diseases or heart disorders.

3. **Gastrointestinal disorders:** According to Mahoney (1980:243), disorders of the gastrointestinal system may be roughly divided into three types (a) anorexia nervosa, (b) digestive problems, and (c) peptic ulcer and colitis.

   (a) *Anorexia nervosa:* Loss of appetite is known as anorexia. In the absence of an organic disorder, when it is caused by emotional factors, it is referred to as anorexia nervosa. The more severe cases of anorexia nervosa are characterized by weight loss to the point of emaciation. According to some writers, anorexia nervosa is often related to sexual events in the patient's life history—the onset of puberty, guilt felt in connection with sexual activity or fantasy, and so on. Other psychological factors contributing toward this malfunctioning of the gastrointestinal system may include: a desire to remain undeveloped and being a favored child, rather than a responsible adult; an unconscious association of food with impregnation; continuation of childhood negativism created by parents over the child's health and nourishment. We will be discussing this disorder in detail in this text.

   (b) *Disorders related to digestive problems:* Emotional factors are responsible for the serious alteration of a delicate balance of digestive enzymes and acids in our body, which in turn, as Mahoney (1980:245) observes, give rise to the following digestive problems.

      (i) Diarrhea—frequent liquid bowel movements.
      (ii) Constipation—infrequent and occasionally painful bowel movements.
      (iii) Nausea—loss of appetite and feeling of imminent vomiting.
      (iv) Gastritis—an inflammation of the lining of the stomach often associated with an excess stomach acid and a burning sensation.

(c) *Peptic ulcer and colitis:* Peptic ulcer and colitis represent the disorders associated with structural damage to the stomach and intestines. A peptic ulcer is an open sore (an inflamed wound) on the lining of the stomach, or more frequently in the duodenum (the upper portion of the small intestine). An important symptom is pain that a person experiences after meals, and that can be eased only by eating. There may be nausea or vomiting along with pain. There is bleeding in severe cases. It is caused by the corrosive action of the overactivity and excessive secretion of digestive acids on the protective mucous membranes of the stomach and small intestine. Ulcers arise from a complex interplay of emotional and organic factors. Emotional states are closely related to the physiological factors responsible for the cause of an ulcer. A strong and sustained conflict evokes a chronic emotional response, usually of hostility or anxiety. The inability to reduce the emotional tension in some harmless ways (like defense mechanisms or proper channelization) causes the stomach or duodenum to be susceptible to injury by its own acid secretions. It has often been found that the persistent emotional stress and resulting autonomic nervous system activities are responsible for the overactivity and excessive secretion of digestive acids. They cause an ulcer by weakening the mucous membranes and breaking down the digestive tissues. It is also significant to note that people with higher achievement motivation, aggressive nature, and levels of anxiety and resentment are more susceptible to ulcers. This supports the role of emotional tensions and stresses in the development of ulcers.

Colitis is an inflammation of the colon (large intestine). Its first sign is often the presence of mucus in the stools. If the inflammation continues over a long period of time, the colon may suffer structural damage in the form of lesions developing into ulcerative colitis. This psycho-physiological disorder has been recognized to correspond with a strong emotional episode, such as the death of a dear one, separation or divorce, and loss of a job or property. Similarly, anger, hostility, strong resentment, and lack of emotional maturity have also been found to play a decisive role in the development of colitis.

4. **Genito-urinary disorders:** A number of psycho-physiological disorders are connected with the genito-urinary system of our body. Some of them are urinary disorders, menstrual disorders, and disorders associated with sex.

   (a) *Urinary disorders:* The frequency of urination is known to increase in a state of anxiety or nervousness. Similarly, under psychological stress, bladder function in some persons is inhibited. The urinary tract is connected with autonomic fibers, and therefore, it is quite possible that emotional difficulties prove an important causative factor of urinary disorders. Psychological conflict and aggravated emotional states in children have been found to be the main factors in many cases of enuresis (bed wetting), the most common urinary disorder of childhood.

   (b) *Menstrual disorders:* Menstrual disorders in women are often caused by emotional factors. Dysmenorrhea or painful menstruation is one such disorder that may have an autonomic basis. Similarly, amenorrhea, related to the failure of menstruation for several months, may be caused by psychological factors like an intense desire for pregnancy, a bodily defense against sexuality, emotional shocks, and tension created by marital discord or sexual conflicts.

   (c) *Disorders associated with sex:* Two of the major psychosomatic disorders connected with sex are impotence in men and frigidity in women. Only a few cases of these disorders are found to have an organic cause, while in most cases, psychological factors play a key role. Hostility toward one's partner, anxiety and fear of disease, injury, pregnancy, and guilty feelings concerning sex are the major sources of such disorders. As a result, the impotent male is unable to perform the sexual act and derive pleasure from it. Similarly, in the frigid female, there is either a pathological lack of sexual desire or a diminished desire for sex. In chronic cases, it leads to dyspareunia (painful intercourse), in which the establishment of normal heterosexual relationships becomes difficult or impossible on account of the local neuromuscular reaction in the form of vaginal spasms.

5. **Skin disorders**: In day-to-day life, our skin may be seen as a mirror of our many emotions. States of embarrassment, anger, tension, and stress may exhibit some typical signs on our skin. The skin, in fact, is so richly supplied with small blood vessels controlled by the autonomic nervous system that it becomes a sensitive indicator of emotional behavior, and consequently, psychological factors may successfully lead to various skin disorders. Some of the most common skin disorders are the following.

- *Acne:* It is a disorder in which oily secretions clog pores or form pimples.
- *Dermatitis or eczema (allergic):* It involves inflammation of the skin often associated with an itching sensation. In neuro-dermatitis, there is specific inflammation of the skin with causes of emotional origins.
- *Hives:* It is an allergic reaction in which affected skin areas may become inflamed and itchy.
- *Dandruff:* It involves an accumulation of greasy scales in the hair.
- *Herpes simplex:* In this disorder, there are inflamed blisters (cold sores) usually around the mouth.
- *Hyperhidrosis:* It involves excessive perspiration, which is sometimes accompanied by blisters, rash, or infection.

All these skin disorders may have organic as well as psychological causes. Emotional disturbances and stressful events are observed to cause various skin disorders. For example, high-stress situations may lead to typical emotionally linked sweat responses (hyperhidrosis), quite different from heat-related perspiration. Similarly, acne and eczema disorders may be precipitated or increased substantially during emotional strains and stresses. It has been also observed that skin disorders can be learned, like other autonomic and visceral symptoms. Commenting on this aspect, Kisker (1964:222–223) writes,

> Disorders of the skin usually cannot be hidden. The evidence of the sufferer's distress is quite evident to everyone. For this reason, there are immediate and considerable expressions, of attention and concern from friends, family members and physicians. Environment support is strong, and if the person affected perceives the symptoms as being rewarding in any way, they are reinforced and autonomic learning occurs.

6. *Endocrine disorders* are related to disorders of glandular functioning. The functioning of these glands has a close relation with the autonomic nervous system; disturbance or deviations from the normal conditions in one automatically upsets the other. This is why emotional stresses have been found to cause overactivity or underactivity of the endocrine glands (for example, excessive activity of the thyroid gland in hyperthyroid disorder). On the other hand, glandular dysfunction caused by hereditary, biological, or environmental factors may lead to emotional problems and behavioral disorders.

7. *Hemic and lymphatic disorders* are related to disorders of the blood and lymph systems. Psychological factors are found to play a substantial role in these disorders. For example, anemia is known to be caused or precipitated by emotional disturbances and stressful events.

8. *Musculoskeletal disorders* are associated with the bones and voluntary muscles. Some of the important psycho-physiological disorders of this type are backache, muscle cramps, psychogenic rheumatism, and arthritis. In these disorders of emotional origin, the individual experiences pain localized in the bones or voluntary muscles of the back, or the rest of the body. For example, in arthritis (pain due to inflammation of a joint), emotional factors play their part through the autonomic system by inducing the blood supply to the affected part.

All types of psycho-physiological or psychosomatic disorders mentioned previously have been put under the broad classification category of Somatic symptom disorder (SSD) in the classification systems of the DSM-5 and DSM-TR provided by the American Psychiatric Association.

To Sum Up

There are several types of psycho-physiological or psychosomatic disorders that have been named in the classification systems provided by the APA and WHO. They include: (i) Respiratory disorders (e.g., asthma, common cold, rhinitis, hyperventilation, hay fever, etc.) involving malfunctioning of the respiratory system, (ii) Cardiovascular disorders (e.g., hypertension, angina pectoris, migraine and coronary disease) referred to as the disorders of the heart and vascular system, (iii) Gastrointestinal disorders (e.g., anorexia nervosa, digestive problems, peptic ulcer and colitis, etc.), known as the disorders of the gastrointestinal system, (iv) Genito-urinary disorders—disorders of the Genito-urinary system, including urinary, menstrual, and sexual disorders, (v) Skin disorders, including acne and eczema (allergic), (vi) Endocrine disorders—disorders of the glandular functioning, (vii) Hemic and lymphatic disorders—the disorders of the blood and lymph systems, and (viii) Musculoskeletal disorders, associated with the bones and voluntary muscles of the body such as backache, muscle cramps, and arthritis.

The Other Psychosomatic Related Disorders Appearing in the DSM-5 and DSM-TR

There are several types of the other somatic-related disorders such as Somatic Symptom Disorder, Illness Anxiety Disorder, Conversion Disorder, and Factitious Disorder, newly appearing in the latest DSM-5 (APA, 2013) and DSM-5-TR (APA,2022). Let us look into them.

Somatic Symptom Disorder

Somatic symptom disorder, in accordance with its naming, is characterized by multiple somatic symptoms present in the affected individuals at one time. The symptoms can be localized (i.e., in one spot) or diffused (i.e., the entire body), and can be specific or nonspecific (e.g., fatigue). Individuals with somatic symptom disorder often report excessive thoughts, feelings, or behaviors surrounding their somatic symptoms. Moreover, their interpretation of symptoms is often viewed as threatening, harmful, or troublesome (APA, 2022). As a result, in a generalized way, people suffering from somatic symptoms are found to exhibit a lot of worry about their illness and remain in a grip of fear that their medical status is more serious than it typically is. The presence of somatic symptoms along with their wrongful interpretation on the part of individuals is found to adversely affect their daily life adjustment and functioning related to their family obligations, schooling, and professional work.

Illness Anxiety Disorder

People with this type of somatic disorder are persistently worried and preoccupied with a concern that they have or will be affected by a serious illness or disease. Here, their concern about their supposed illness and health is so great that cannot think beyond it. The topic of their conversation and interaction with people always hangs around their illness. They are often frustrated when medical examinations are negative and feel convinced that the doctors have erred. Their concern about their health and the resulting anxiety is so high that a minor body complaint or appearance of a somatic symptom such as a slight headache may be adjudged and believed on their part as a sign of a brain tumour. Not only this, but they may also be gripped with excessive anxiety when they read, listen to, or come across information about the illness of others. They begin to assume that they are also most likely to suffer from the same in a short while. The diagnosis and advice of doctors do not rid them of their anxiety and fear about their health and illness.

A question may arise about the difference between somatic symptom disorder and illness anxiety disorder, as the affected persons in both these disorders are found to be anxious and concerned about their health and illness. The difference lies in the way this concern is expressed. In somatic symptom disorder, one expresses their concern by worrying about the somatic symptoms related to some health problem or illness. On the other hand, in illness anxiety disorder, it is some or other types of illness present or assumed to be coming in the future that becomes the focus of one's anxiety, quite greater in its intensity and frequency. Moreover, where in somatic symptom disorder, the presence of somatic symptoms is a must, in illness anxiety disorder, somatic symptoms are not present, or if present, are only mild in intensity.

Conversion Disorder

This type of somatic disorder is reflected and diagnosed through one or the other types of functional neurological symptoms visible in behavior with no satisfactory medical explanation available for them. These symptoms may include conditions like (i) Weakness or paralysis, (ii) Abnormal movements (such as tremors, unsteady gait, or seizures), (iii) Blindness, (iv) Deafness, (v) Difficulty in walking or standing, and (vi) Loss of sensation or numbness.

The affected person is found to show such symptoms all of a sudden, mostly on account of being exposed to a stressful situation. Regarding their ill effects, the symptoms or deficits associated with conversion disorder are found to cause a great degree of clinically significant distress or impairment in social, occupational, or other important areas of functioning of the affected people.

Factitious Disorder

The term factitious disorder stands for the type of disorder that is artificially created or developed on the part of the affected individual, with no valid medical or organic cause available for it. It is in this sense a deceptive behavior and a self-imposed disorder in which the affected people themselves create or build symptoms for an illness or injury.

The diagnostic criteria for Factitious Disorder noted in the DSM 5 are:

- Falsification of physical or psychological signs or symptoms, or induction of injury or disease.
- The individual presents himself or herself to others as ill, impaired, or injured.
- The deceptive behavior is evident even in the absence of obvious external rewards.
- The behavior is not better explained by another mental disorder, such as delusional disorder or another psychotic disorder.

To Sum Up

The other related disorders in the category of Somatic symptom-related disorders in the DSM-5 and DSM-TR are known as (a) Somatic Symptom Disorder (the presence of somatic symptoms along with their wrongful interpretation as threatening, harmful, or troublesome on the part of individuals), (b) Illness Anxiety Disorder (where the affected people are persistently worried and preoccupied with a concern that they have or will be affected by a serious illness or disease), (c) Conversion Disorder (one or the other types of functional neurological symptoms such as blindness or deafness visible in the behavior, with no satisfactory medical explanation) and (d) Factitious Disorder (a self-imposed disorder in which the affected people themselves build symptoms of one or the other illness).

Causes Underlying the Psycho-Physiological Disorders

In all types of psycho-physiological disorders discussed in this chapter, we have found a close association between psychological and bodily factors affecting each other. Truly speaking, these disorders are always the result of a close interaction between organic (genetic and other biological factors) and psychological factors. Psychological factors sometimes work as predisposing causes. and at other times, as strong precipitating ones. The role of causative factors may be analyzed through the case studies of a few disorders.

Case 1 (A case of asthma): Kavita, a young woman of 22 years of age, was reported for the treatment of asthma. The patient was the only child of a happy marriage. She had a history of asthma since the age of six. Her mother was a patient of asthma and her father and other members of the family were very sympathetic and attentive to her mother. The patient was severely handicapped by the disease until she was 14 years. This attack then ceased until her honeymoon, which was her first night away from her parents. In the subsequent year, her condition became serious. In an interview, she revealed that interaction with her husband had become very strained and that she often experienced difficulty breathing when confronted with her domestic unhappiness.

Case 2 (A case of peptic ulcer): A young man was admitted for the treatment of peptic ulcer. As a child, he was quite submissive and was always in the company and protection of his brother, who was five years older than him, and his parents, who provided him much attention. When he was 13, his brother died, and about two years later he lost his father. Following the death of his father, his mother became psychologically dependent on him, consulting him about important problems and requiring him generally to substitute for both his older brother and his father, a situation for which he was completely unprepared intellectually and otherwise. While maintaining a secure outer appearance, he was aroused emotionally and his emotional reactions were repeatedly intensified by the excessive expectations of his mother. At the age of 18, he experienced a short period of stomach discomfort which was followed by the initial hemorrhaging of a duodenal ulcer (adapted from Davison and Neale, 1978).

Case 3 (A case of anorexia nervosa): Kamini, a young girl 25 years of age, reported for medical help. She was an emaciated girl weighing 28 kg at a height of five feet. She was depressed and seemed to be totally preoccupied with not becoming fat and her parents could not reason with her about her diet. Historically she was traced to be normal until she was 21 years of age. With an occasional remark from her friends and family members, she began to feel that she was too fat and not as attractive as her friends. Her parents were in search of a good match for her. Her belief about her figure became more pronounced after going through a few matrimonial interviews. She rigorously started to slim down and became fussy about her diet. Her periods stopped after a year and gradually she became weak and thin. For the last six months, she had been too emaciated to work and felt difficulty carrying out her daily routine.

Case 4 (A case of frigidity): Kanchan, a woman 30 years of age, complained to a lady doctor that she derived no satisfaction from the sexual act. After examination, it was found that she did not have any organic cause for it (any mental or physical abnormality). Her husband was also found to be normal. It was revealed that the patient had an affair before marriage from which she had derived some pleasure. Her parents found out about the affair and made life impossible for her lover, who left the area. At the age of 22, she married a teacher who was obsessive and rigid in all matters. She got no pleasure from intercourse throughout her marriage of eight years, and often objected to his mechanical approach. Intercourse took place two or three times per month at his insistence. She certainly never made any advances. There were no children.

Case 5 (A case of skin disorder): Kamla, a married woman 22 years of age, reported for treatment. At the age of three, she had developed eczema on both arms and hands. This condition remained problematic for two years, then cleared up at the age of seven, when her mother was pregnant. Her hands and arms again had eczema with the onset of her first menstruation for a period of three months. Recently she had a severe skin eruption associated with the impending absence of her husband. As the date of his departure approached, her symptoms gradually worsened and eventually, she was hospitalized.

Case 6 (illustrating the impact of stresses): Richard Nixon, the President of America, suffered repeated attacks of phlebitis in 1974, soon after his resignation on account of the Watergate scandal. He developed a number of blood clots in his left leg and one large clot required emergency surgery to prevent further complications. Historically, it was revealed that President Nixon suffered his first phlebitis attack in 1965. Predisposed to such a disorder, his phlebitis was probably aggravated by the stressful situation of his sudden loss of power, position, and prestige on account of his forced resignation.

(Adapted from: G.W, Kisker, 1964)

An analysis of these cases reveals the following facts:

1. Genetic or hereditary factors may play some part in the development of psycho-physiological disorders.
2. Body structure, its chemical functioning, allergies, and infections may initiate and precipitate many disorders.

Apart from these organic factors, psychological factors, by all means, initiate, control, precipitate, and determine the severity and occurrence of these disorders. Many psycho-physiological disorders can be caused through conditioning and reinforcement. For example, a child who is repeatedly allowed to stay home from school when he has an upset stomach may learn to be rewarded for chronic indigestion. Similarly, a housewife may suffer chronic backache or asthma on account of her conditioning to get sympathy and attention due to her illness.

Emotional factors and psychological stresses have always been found to play a significant role in all types of psycho-physiological disorders. They may relate to the patient's childhood experiences, behavior, and treatment by the parents, as well as early inconveniences, deprivation, and accidents in one's life, an uncongenial familial environment, unhealthy parent-child relationships, and unhappy family life. All of these prove to be great predisposing factors for these disorders. The newly emerging demands and perplexities of an adolescent's life and many of the stresses and strains of adulthood pose problems and conflict situations for the perpetuation of psycho-physiological disorders. These stressful situations have been found to contribute toward psycho-physiological disorders in the following ways:

- By affecting unfavorably the autonomic nervous system and thus the body chemistry and metabolism.
- By reducing the fighting capacity of an individual against viruses and bacteria.
- By creating a precipitating and immediate cause to the already predisposed individual. In such cases, the physical damage is said to be triggered by the intense emotional stress of the life events.
- By providing a means of escape through developing and intensifying a desire to be ill.

Prevention and Treatment of the Psycho-Physiological Disorders

The psycho-physiological disorders are caused by the interaction of organic and psychological factors. Therefore, prevention and treatment of these disorders lay in caring for these factors.

As far as genetic influences are concerned, they are beyond one's control. Hence, their presence as a predisposing factor can never be ruled out. For the other biological factors and psychological factors we may adopt a good number of preventive measures in the form of the provision of better environmental facilities and education for good physical and mental health and satisfactory living. Regarding the treatment of these disorders, various approaches have been suggested in the following manner:

1. *Biomedical measures:* In psycho-physiological disorders, the illness is real and not apparent. There are real organic problems, disturbances in the body, which require medical-cum-biological treatment. Depending on the therapist's specific beliefs and diagnosis, the treatment may range from surgery to medication. In many cases of psycho-physiological disorders, such as heart diseases, bleeding ulcers, and severe urinary disorders, emergency medical treatment is urgently required; while in other cases, it becomes desirable at a certain stage when various types of drugs and medicines are used to control the severity of the disease. Sometimes physical health is restored by changing the diet, modifying the environment, and removing unfavorable biological conditions that cause the growth of viruses and bacteria.
2. *Psychoanalytic measures:* From the psychoanalytic point of view, a painful and health-damaging psycho-physiological symptom may represent some sort of symbolic aggression or self-punishment for unacceptable impulses associated with unconscious conflicts. Therefore, in psychoanalytic treatment, the patient is helped to confront and resolve the unconscious conflict that lies at the root of the symptom.
3. *Behavior modification measures: Psycho-physiological* disorders are also caused by the learning of maladaptive behavior. In behavior modification therapy, attempts are made to unlearn the unfavorable learning through extinction and differential reinforcement. For example, there was a case of a child who happened to exhibit symptoms of asthma (heavy coughing and wheezing) at bedtime. The parents were prepared to induce behavior therapy in the following two ways:

   (i) To ignore systematically (extinguish) the child's asthmatic response.
   (ii) To reward more normal breathing with some incentive (love and affection, good food, and sometimes, money).

The results were encouraging, as the child gradually got rid of the maladaptive response.

4. *Psychotherapy measures:* Emotional factors and psychological stresses prove to be predisposing as well as precipitating causes for the psycho-physiological disorders. A proper training of the emotions and helping the patient to learn adaptive ways to cope with their conflict and stressful situations may bring favorable results. As far as possible, attempts should be made to improve the patient's life situations by modifying their environment so as to reduce daily stress. Measures like short-term psychotherapy may also help the patient for the release of tension, anxiety, and similar factors making them unhappy. These measures prove helpful at least in decreasing the patient's vulnerability to subsequent stress and improving their mental health.

5. *Biofeedback measures:* Recently, biofeedback measures have been studied to control many of the psycho-physiological disorders, such as headaches, backaches, irregular heartbeats, asthma, muscular spasms, teeth grinding, epilepsy, and sexual impotency. Biofeedback refers to procedures in which selected biological processes, such as heart rate and muscle tension, are amplified via special instruments so that the individual may be made aware of them (in the form of signals such as lights or sounds) and then may be trained to control their occurrence. For example, blood pressure or pulse rate can be measured and amplified so that the person knows them through suitable signaling. By getting training in lowering the frequency of such signals, the person may learn to exercise voluntary control over these functions, and thus may be helped in the treatment of related disorders.

To Sum Up

The causes related to Psycho-physiological disorders are the outcomes of close interaction of genetic and other biological factors (such as body structure, its chemical functioning, allergies, and infections) and psychological factors (such as conditioning and reinforcement, early deprivations, emotional problems, and psychological stress). For their prevention, it is therefore necessary to take care of all these three types of factors. In the case of genetic factors, it can be said that genetic influences are beyond one's control. However, reasonable control may be exercised over biological and other psychological factors for their prevention. In the case of thinking about taking measures for the treatment of these disorders, we may see that there are measures like biomedical, psychoanalytic, behavior modification, psychotherapies, and biofeedback, that can be successfully employed as per the need of the situation and nature of the problem.

Review Questions

1. What are the psycho-physiological disorders? Throw light on their meaning and characteristic features.
2. Name the different disorders appearing in the Diagnostic Statistics Manuals (DSMs) developed by the APA and discuss any three of them in detail.
3. Throw light on the nature and occurrence of any four psycho-physiological disorders among the following:
   (i) Respiratory disorders, (ii) Cardio-vascular disorders, (iii) Gastrointestinal disorders, (iv) Genito-urinary disorders, (v) Skin disorders, (vi) Endocrine disorders, (vii) Hemic and Lymphatic disorders, and (viii) Musculoskeletal disorders.

4. Discuss in detail the psycho-physiological disorders newly appearing in the DSM-5 and DSM-5-TR known as Somatic Symptom disorder, Illness Anxiety disorder, Conversion disorder, and Factitious disorder.
5. Describe in detail the causes underlying the psycho-physiological disorders.
6. Throw light on the measures taken for the prevention and treatment of the psycho-physiological disorders.

References

American Psychiatric Association (1968), *DSM-II, quoted by Mahoney, Michael J. (1980), abnormal psychology*, San Francisco, CA: Harper & Row.

American Psychiatric Association (2013), *Diagnostic and statistical manual of mental disorders* (5th ed.), Washington, DC: American Psychiatric Association.

American Psychiatric Association (2022), *Diagnostic and statistical manual of mental disorders-5th edition revised* (DSM-5-TR), Washington, DC: American Psychiatric Association.

Davison, G. C., & Neale, J. M. (1978), *Abnormal psychology* (2nd ed.), New York, NY: John Wiley & Sons.

Kisker, G. W. (1964), *The disorganized personality* (3rd International Students ed.), New York, NY: McGraw-Hill.

Mahoney, M. J. (1980), *Abnormal psychology*, San Francisco, CA: Harper & Row.

Chapter 9

Neuroses or Psychoneurotic Disorders

Learning Objectives

After going through this chapter, you will be able to:

- Define the term neuroses or psychoneurotic disorders.
- Tell about the meaning and nature of psychoneurotic disorders.
- Distinguish neurotic behavior from psychotic behavior.
- Name the specific forms or types of neuroses or psychoneurotic disorders.
- Describe the nature of anxiety disorders along with the symptoms displayed by the individuals suffering from anxiety disorders.
- Discuss the meaning, nature, and impact of the anxiety disorders known as generalized anxiety disorder, panic disorder, separation anxiety disorder, and social anxiety disorder.
- Throw light on the meaning, nature, and types of phobias along with the underlying causes.
- Tell about the nature, types, and impact of trauma and stressor related disorders.
- Define the term Posttraumatic Stress Disorder (PTSD) along with the underlying symptoms.
- Discuss the nature and characteristic symptoms of the disorders known as acute stress disorder, adjustment disorder, and prolonged grief disorder.
- Throw light on the meaning, nature, and impact of obsessive-compulsive behavior along with its causation.
- Understand the nature and impact of certain new varieties of obsessive-compulsive behavior known as Hoarding disorder, Trichotillomania (Hair pulling disorder), Excoriation (Skin picking disorder), and Body dysmorphic disorder.
- Tell about the meaning, nature, and impact of the depressive disorders.
- Throw light on the meaning and nature of the conversion disorders along with the symptoms (sensory and motor) visible among affected persons.
- Understand the meaning, nature, and types of the dissociative disorders.
- Discuss the nature and impacts of the various types of dissociative disorders, known as dissociative identity disorder, dissociative amnesia, and depersonalization/de-realization disorder.
- Throw light on the causation and treatment of the psychoneurotic disorders.

DOI: 10.4324/9781003398325-9

Neuroses or Psychoneurotic Disorders—Meaning and Definition

Neuroses or Psychoneurotic disorders are purely psychological disorders. There is no relevant organic pathology present in these disorders of behavior and thus, they may be clearly distinguished from the psychosomatic disorders, which are known as the disorders of the psyche as well as the body. The illness of any nature diagnosed in psychosomatic disorders is more real than the apparent one visible in the case of psychoneurotic or psychotic disorders. That is why a psychoneurotic patient is not labeled as suffering from some bodily illness or disease.

In the sequence of the disorders of behavior, neurosis falls midway between minor emotional maladjustment and psychotic disorders. Consequently, it is known as more serious than a minor emotional maladjustment and less serious than a psychotic disorder. Neurotic disorders in a real sense represent the Typical ways of dealing with frustrations or conflicts and anxiety (such as demonstration of phobic, and obsessive-compulsive behavior).

"Anxiety," as described in DSM-II (1968:39), "is the chief characteristic of neuroses. It may be felt and expressed directly, or it may be controlled unconsciously." It is in this context that George W. Kisker (1977:194) has defined neurosis as "a pattern of maladaptive behavior in which a person responds to life stress with persistent anxiety or other behavior representing attempts to control the anxiety."

Anxiety is closely linked to an individual's needs and motives. If the essential needs linked with affection, security, self-esteem, achievement, and freedom are not satisfactorily gratified, it may give rise to feelings of excessive anxiety or guilt, which in turn results in neurotic behavior. But it should not be concluded that every anxiety reaction leads to neurotic behavior. We are occasionally quite anxious, irritable, down, or restless, but it does not mean that we are neurotic. It is only when the anxiety behavior patterns become persistent and interfere with our ability to lead a normal life, and thus qualify as "breakdowns" in the adjustment mechanism, that they are usually labeled "neuroses."

Distinguishing Neurotic Behavior from Psychotic Behavior

Despite displaying extreme anxiety, neurotic behavior is neither disorganized nor is the neurotic personality a split personality. It can be safely distinguished from the psychotic behavior or personality in the manner discussed ahead.

- The relation of a neurotic person to reality is not defective. He talks rationally and does not show marked distortion of external reality. He perceives his environment well within the normal range. Since he is not affected by bizarre ideas, hallucinations, or illusions, it is not difficult to follow his train of thought.
- In neuroses, there are no deep and lasting disturbances of effect. In other words, emotional distortions in neuroses are mild and not as severe as in psychoses. For example, a neurotic may at times be depressed, but his depression is not so severe as to affect seriously his thought processes and general behavior, as in the case of a psychotic personality. Characteristics like severe agitation and stupor are not found in neurotic depression.
- The cognitive distortion is relatively mild in neuroses. The intellectual potentialities in a neurotic personality more or less remain unaffected, whereas in psychotic behavior the cognitive distortion is severe and causes impairment of intellectual functioning.
- The social relations in neurotic behavior are not as disturbed as in cases of psychotic behavior. A neurotic, although disturbed and confused, does not live in some other world as a psychotic does. He is not much handicapped by his behavior pattern as to make his social adjustment impossible.

- In neuroses no severe disorganization of personality, as in psychoses, is found. A neurotic therefore remains relatively well integrated. In comparison to a psychotic, the neurotic proves less harmful to others and the symptoms of his behavior deviation are not severe to cause anxiety to others. The need for care and attention in a mental hospital is not usually felt in the case of neurotics as it is for psychotics.

To Sum up

Psychoneurotic disorders or neuroses are purely psychological disorders. There is no relevant organic pathology present and the illness is more apparent than real as in the case of psycho-physiological disorders. Among psychological disorders, they are more serious than minor emotional maladjustment and less serious than a psychotic disorder. The feeling of excessive anxiety or guilt makes the central core of neurotic behavior. However, this behavior is not disorganized and a neurotic personality is not a split personality, as in the case of psychosis.

Specific Forms or Types of Neuroses or Psychoneurotic Disorders

The major types of neuroses listed in the classification systems provided by the American Psychiatric Association and the WHO are as follows:

1. Anxiety Disorders
2. Phobic Disorders
3. Trauma and Stressor-Related Disorders
4. Obsessive-Compulsive and Related Disorders
5. Depressive Disorders
6. Conversion Disorders
7. Dissociative Disorders

Let us look into all these disorders grouped as Neuroses or Psychoneurotic disorders.

Anxiety Disorders

Anxiety neurosis represents a behavior dominated by anxiety reactions that interfere with the individual's personal and social adjustment. The anxiety involved here is a free-floating anxiety characterized by the following:

(i) It is irrational in the sense that no relevant or justified explanations can be given by the individual for his anxiety reactions.
(ii) Quite often, a very minute danger or stress situation gives rise to disproportionately strong anxiety reactions in the individual.
(iii) In anxiety neurosis, unlike other neuroses, the anxiety is experienced directly and not indirectly in the form of phobias or compulsions.

According to the DSM and ICD, the anxiety disorders may be classified as (i) Generalized Anxiety Disorder, (ii) Panic disorder, (iii) Separation anxiety disorder, (iv) Social anxiety disorder, and (v) Phobic disorder or Phobias. We will next examine the latter four, leaving the discussion about phobias to a later stage.

Generalized Anxiety Disorder refers to a type of anxiety disorder in which one's thinking and feeling related to one's anxiety is so generalized that it may lead him to prolonged, vague, unexplained, and intense fears not necessarily attached to any particular object. He fears, worries, and has an intensive apprehension for one or the other things with no reason attached to his fear or apprehension. The length to which he may go for finding things to worry about his concerns is remarkable. As soon as one cause for worry is removed, he finds another until his kith and kin lose patience with him.

Panic Disorder: This type of anxiety disorder is more severe than generalized anxiety disorder in the sense that here, the anxiety reactions are more intense, frequent, and damaging in their nature and consequences. The range of triggers that could cause panic is quite wide. One may demonstrate signs or symptoms of the state of panic reactions for a host of things and situations, characterized by symptoms like losing sense of thought, losing control over motor responses, suffering from shortness of breath, chest pain, dizziness, trembling, and choking, to the extent of utter helplessness in protecting himself from the danger faced.

Separation Anxiety Disorder: This type of anxiety disorder is developed among children on account of an intense fear of getting separated from their near and dear to which they are closely attached, such as mothers, caretakers, or to whom they are dependent on the satisfaction of their physical and psychological needs. Children suffering from this disorder show a lot of anxiety, restlessness, and apprehensions around getting separated from their attachment figures even for a short duration. They need them everywhere for their protection and care, and cry and show resentment regarding their separation in one or the other situations.

Social anxiety disorder (social phobia): Social anxiety disorder or social phobia is related to the type of abnormal anxiety experienced on one's part in his or her participation in specific social situations. In the DSM-5 and ICD-11, it has been defined and characterized as follows.

- It is marked with an excessive fear or anxiety that consistently occurs in social situations such as social interactions (e.g., having a conversation), doing something while feeling observed (e.g., eating or drinking in the presence of others), or performing in front of others (e.g., giving a speech).
- The individual is concerned that he or she will act in a way, or show anxiety symptoms, that will be negatively evaluated by others. On account of this assumption, he consistently avoids the relevant social situations or else experiences intense fear or anxiety.
- The excessive anxiety shown by the individual in this concern is quite out of proportion to the encountering situation and is not liable to be better explained by a medical condition, medication, substance abuse, or other mental disorder.
- It is quite detrimental to the individual, resulting in significant distress or significant impairment in his personal, family, social, educational, occupational, or other important areas of functioning.

The Overall Symptoms Displayed in the Anxiety Disorders

An individual suffering from anxiety neurosis, may exhibit the following symptoms for no apparent reason:

(a) *Physiological*

    (i) Mild nausea, loss of appetite, and loss of weight.

(ii) Heart palpitations, feeling of heartburn, elevated blood pressure, increased pulse rate, and difficulty breathing.

(iii) Cold sweat, headaches, muscle tension or pain, dryness of the mouth, trembling of hands and lips, and frequent sighing.

(iv) Speech disorder, sleep disturbances, and sexual dissatisfaction.

(v) Inappropriate eating habits, chronic mild diarrhea, frequent urination, and digestion difficulties.

(vi) The excessive use of alcohol, tranquilizing drugs, or sleeping pills.

(b) *Psychological:*

(i) Disturbances in thinking: Neurotically anxious individuals often complain of a lack of concentration in work and a lack of interest in life. They are always uncertain and fearful of making mistakes. As a result, they prefer making no decision than making a wrong one.

(ii) Disturbances in feeling: Anxiety neurosis is characterized by extreme and generalized apprehension and feelings of helplessness and resentment. Anxious neurotics are likely to have pronounced feelings of dread and apprehension, no matter how well things seem to be going. They are convinced of something terrible happening but cannot tell what it will be or even why it should happen. The length to which they go to find things to worry about is remarkable. As soon as one cause for worry is removed, they find another until their kith and kin lose patience with them. Similarly, while suffering from the feeling of helplessness, an anxious neurotic does not know which way to turn. He is sure that anything he attempts will result in failure. He is likely to be dependent on others, which he does not like to do. So, resentment wells up within him and ultimately results in aggression toward the self, as he does not possess enough courage to attack those upon whom he is dependent.

Examples of Anxiety Neurosis

Case 1: A married working woman, 37 years of age, reported for help. She was unable to go out on her own and always felt frightened. She felt uneasy at work and anxious if left alone at home by her husband. She usually worked with a tense feeling and occasionally had a sense of doom. Medical examination revealed that she had no physical disease. Her pulse rate was 100 per minute at rest and she was extremely tense and fearful. Her case history revealed that she was the second of five siblings. Her parents had frequent quarreling when she was a child. She was married at the age of 20 and had a girl child at the age of 22. She reported that illness came on at the age of 24. She reported that intercourse had been reduced since her daughter's birth. It occurred two or three times in a year and then without orgasm. Her husband, a busy businessman, reported that she had been ill for some time, possibly two or three years, but she had become worse in the past few months, when at times she developed a cancer phobia. Before that, she worried over everything—"You name it, she worries about it. I can't understand it. At times she's nasty but I understand that and put up with it." He was completely self-contained and introverted.

Case 2: An engineer, 50 years of age, sought help for his problem. He was anxious, frightened, tense, and sweating. He began to worry about his heart, which had sped up to a rate of 102 beats per minute. At times he felt as if he was choking. He had diarrhea. His hands trembled and his mouth was dry. He had a deformed penis. The case history revealed that he had been married for 26 years, but had never been capable of sexual intercourse. His wife and he had an almost continuous life of clubs, parties, and theatres together, and they had been perfectly happy. Two months ago he had been bypassed for promotion. He became concerned and he and his wife stopped going to social functions and theatres (adapted from *Psychiatric Investigation*, J.H. Price, London: Butter Worth, 1972:18–21).

Case 3: An 18-year-old girl was referred to a psychiatric clinic. She first came to the attention of the authorities eight months earlier, when she attempted suicide. At the time of the interview, she was found to be under considerable tension. The anxiety lessened somewhat in the face of repeated encouragement and reassurance. Eventually, she told a story that revolved for the most part around her father. She said that he had told her that her mother had frustrated him sexually. At another time, he kissed her, but she denied any further advances. She admitted having frequent dreams and nightmares most of which involved the father. Her anxiety became so great that she insisted that her mother should sleep with her. Before going to bed, she went through a ritual of barricading the bedroom door. She could sleep as long as her mother kept an arm over her. At the same time, she was afraid of the mother, and occasionally hesitated to eat anything she had prepared, and was sometimes so fearful that she remained awake all night in order to watch her mother. The problem got intensified by the father's advances when he attempted to molest her and by the mother's passive reaction to the situation. The girl had deeply ambivalent feelings about both her father and her mother. Despite her repeated expressions of fear and hatred for the father, she was found to be preoccupied with thoughts of him both in her waking anxieties and her dream life (adapted from Kisker, 1977:197).

To Sum Up

Anxiety disorders represent the type of psychological disorders in which people are found to demonstrate a behavior dominated by anxiety reactions that interfere with the individual's personal and social adjustment. The anxiety involved here is a free-floating anxiety characterized by the exhibition of one or the other typical physiological symptoms. There are many types of anxiety disorders, such as (i) Generalized Anxiety Disorder (an intensive fear or apprehension for one or the other things with no reason attached to it), (ii) Panic Disorder (showing more intense, frequent, and damaging anxiety reactions), and (iii) Separation Anxiety Disorder (severe anxiety shown on account of an intense fear of getting separated from the object of attachment).

Phobic Disorders

The term "phobia" comes from the Greek word *"phobos,"* which means panic, flight, or fear. In this sense, the term phobic neurosis may be defined as a disorder of the behavior in which a person experiences persistent, intense, irrational fear of a specific situation or object. Despite his rational knowledge that his fear is unrealistic and overwhelming, he is forced to experience great apprehension and anxiety symptoms while in contact with the phobic object or situation. In a natural sense, fear reactions are very common to every one of us. It is normal and indeed adaptive to be fearful of situations that pose real danger. Fear does not become a phobia unless it is irrational. It turns into a neurotic disorder when it becomes so intense as to interfere with the person's normal activities and to affect his mental health. Some of the common phobias with their technical names and inherent meaning are listed as follows:

Acrophobia—fear of high places.
Agoraphobia—fear of open places.

Aichmophobia—fear of short and pointed objects
Algophobia—fear of pain
Astraphobia—fear of storms, thunder and lightning
Claustrophobia—fear of closed spaces or confinement
Hematophobia—fear of the sight of the blood
Hydrophobia—fear of water
Lalophobia—fear of (public) speaking
Mysophobia—fear of dirt or contamination
Nyctophobia—fear of darkness
Ochlophobia—fear of crowds
Pathophobia—fear of disease or illness
Photophobia—fear of intense light
Pyrophobia—fear of fire
Thanatophobia—fear of death
Toxophobia—fear of being poisoned
Xenophobia—fear of strangers
Zoophobia—fear of animals or some particular animal

In this way, it is clear that phobias may involve any situation or object surrounding one's life. More-over, they have no respect for age, intellectual level or social position. King Henry III of France had a peculiar phobia concerning eggs and became terrified at the sight of them. Schopenhauer, the German philosopher, had a fear of razors and thereby preferred to singe his beard rather than shave it.

Phobias are essentially morbid fears. The nature, symptoms, and causation of phobic neuroses may be understood through some of the following illustrations:

Case 1: A young woman had *ochlophobia—fear of crowds*. Whenever there were many people around her, she was afraid that she would be crushed or killed by suffocation. Despite the knowledge that her fear was irrational, she was not able to travel by train or bus, go shopping in a market, attend social parties, or visit movies. This kept her a virtual prisoner in her home. On free association, her phobia was traced to her early childhood. As a child she had been granted permission to watch the circus parade go by her house but was strictly warned not to follow it into town. On account of the excitement, she forgot this and followed the parade into the center of the town where she soon found herself crowded on all sides. She became frightened and began to cry. A kind gentleman helped her out of the crowd to the front row. After a time her fear subsided and she returned home. Due to fear, she could not discuss her terrifying experiences with her parents. The entire experience was repressed into the unconscious, giving rise to an irrational fear of crowds. Due to its free association, the early experience was recalled and the knowledge of the source of fear gradually helped her to get rid of her phobia (adapted from Page, 1976:142).

Case 2: A young woman 30 years of age had *agoraphobia—the fear of open places*. The phobia became so serious that she had to give up her job and remained home at all times. Psychological investigation revealed that in her early teens she had been sexually promiscuous with several boys in the neighborhood. In her later life she experienced intense guilt feeling about her behavior and repressed all memories of it. The phobia which developed later in her life was based on the fear that she might go astray and be led into a life of prostitution. These repressed memories were revived by the sight of a group photograph and the knowledge of the source of her phobia made her treatment quite possible (adapted from Kisker, 1977:200).

Case 3: A young man had a *phobia of being grasped from behind*. In social gatherings he arranged to have his chair against the wall. It was impossible for him to enter crowded places or go to a movie. When walking on the road, he would look back over his shoulder at intervals to see if he was closely followed. Psychological investigation revealed that as a young boy, he used to steal peanuts from a grocery store. The owner, determined to know who was stealing his peanuts, hid behind a barrel. Just as the boy put his hand in the pile of peanuts, the owner jumped out and grabbed him from behind. The boy screamed and fell fainting on the sidewalk. The terrifying experience was repressed into his subconscious and the present phobia was the result of that earlier repressed experience (adapted from Davison and Neale, 1978:138).

Causes of Phobias

As may be evident from the above three cases, the real cause of a phobia is either unknown to the patient or forgotten on account of being repressed into his unconscious. In general, there are three main causes of phobia:

1. *A forgotten terrifying fear experience at an early age:* In case one above, the young woman had a phobia concerning crowds on account of her terrifying childhood experience. Similarly, an individual frightened by an accident involving a dog, horse or an insect in his childhood may develop zoophobia.
2. *Neurotic defense against anxiety generated by unconscious conflict:* According to psychoanalysts, phobias are merely defense reactions against the anxiety generated by unconscious conflicts related to sexual and aggressive feelings and impulses. In case two above, the young woman was using her phobia of open places as a defense to save her from the situation of being led into a life of prostitution. Similarly, a housewife may develop aichmophobia, fear of sharp and pointed objects, and refuse to keep kitchen knives and scissors in the house on account of her repressed impulses to cut her husband's throat. A husband may develop hydrophobia so that he may keep himself away from rivers because of his repressed feelings of drowning his wife.
3. *Learned pattern of maladaptive behavior:* Phobias, to a great extent, represent a learned pattern of maladaptive behavior either on account of conditioning or social learning. A conditioned response to a fear-producing situation (usually experienced during early childhood) may result in a peculiar phobia. In case three, the young man may be seen to have developed a phobia of being grasped from behind on account of his childhood experience. Similarly, a child with a fearful reaction to an unpleasant experience associated with a cat may learn to be afraid of cats. He may develop an irrational fear of cats, which may include the word cat as well as the sight of it or other animals resembling it. A number of phobias (phobic behaviors) may be an outcome of one's leaning explained through operant conditioning. A phobic symptomized behavior of the child (initially occuring with no substantial reason) when gets reinfoced through positive reinforcers such as sympathy,attention, assistance from others, or excuse of the failure may turn into a habitual pattern of behaving in the same situations. Besides this, fearful parents, family members, and teachers may serve as models for social learning of phobias. A mother who becomes terror-stricken on account of lightning and thunder may communicate her fears to her children, who later on, after being reinforced in the later years of their lives, may develop astraphobia—fear of thunder and lightning.

To Sum Up

Phobic disorders represent the type of psychological disorders in which people are found to experience persistent intense irrational fear of a specific situation or object (such as water, fire, height, darkness, etc.), which interferes with their normal activities and affects their mental health and welfare in an adverse way. They are generally caused by early terrifying experiences and unconscious conflicts or learned on account of conditioning or social learning.

Trauma-and Stressor-Related Disorders

Trauma and stressor-related disorders represent the type of disorders resulting from difficulty coping with or adjusting to a recent stressor (stress-producing stimuli) or trauma.

In its simple meaning, the term stressor stands for all that causes stress to an individual. However, in a technical sense, the term stressor refers to a "type of stimulus that occurs in sufficient amount to cause stress" (Malot and Whaley, 1983). This stimulus can involve any event significant enough to pose a threat, whether real or imagined, to the individual.

The term trauma, on the other hand, stands for a lasting adverse effect on an individual caused by an event that involves threat or danger. According to the DSM-5, trauma can result when an individual directly experiences an adverse event, witnesses that event, or learns about it from others.

If we take into consideration the latest classification systems of disorders of the DSM-5 and DSM-5-TR, the types of disorders included in the category of trauma and Stressor-Related Disorders consist of (i) Posttraumatic Stress Disorder (PTSD), (ii) Acute Stress Disorder, (iii) Adjustment disorder, and (iv) Prolonged Grief Disorder. Let us look into them in brief.

Posttraumatic Stress Disorder (PTSD)

Posttraumatic Stress Disorder represents the type of psychological disorder that results when an individual directly or indirectly experiences an adverse stress- and trauma-related event. People may experience such events when they are caught in a natural catastrophe, like floods, fires, violent storms (tsunamis), rock slides, accidents, and searthquake, as well as manmade catastrophes such as a terror attacks, mass shootings, molestation and rape, robberies, and warfare.

The symptoms visible among those affected with Posttraumatic Stress Disorder (PTSD) are listed in the DSM-5 in four clusters, shown as shown in Table 9.1.

Acute Stress Disorder (ASD)

A person who has experienced or witnessed a life-threatening, terrifying, or otherwise deeply traumatic event may, in some cases, may fall victim to a mental disorder known as acute stress disorder (ASD). While showing several symptoms similar to those exhibited in the previously

Table 9.1 Diagnostic Criteria for PTSD

1. Recurrent experiences of the event, as in memories, dreams, or flashbacks
2. Amplified arousal, including sleep disturbances and reckless behavior
3. Avoiding thoughts, places, and memories about the event
4. Negative thoughts, moods, or feelings
(APA, 2013)

discussed posttraumatic disorder, this differs in the ways as indicated by the DSM-5 and DSM-5-TR in the following manner.

- Acute stress disorder is very similar to PTSD except for the fact that symptoms must be present from three days to one month following exposure to one or more traumatic events.
- Any symptoms manifesting immediately following the trauma that are resolved within three days do not meet the criteria for ASD.
- ASD is a short-term condition. Here the duration of symptoms is at least three days, but no longer than four weeks.
- If the symptoms persist past four weeks, the individual may be then diagnosed with PTSD if the criteria are met. Approximately 50% of individuals with ASD may later develop PTSD. However, an individual may be diagnosed with PTSD without having been previously diagnosed with ASD.
- Symptoms of acute stress disorder follow that of PTSD with a few exceptions. PTSD requires symptoms within each of the four categories discussed in Table 9.1; however, acute stress disorder requires that the individual experience nine symptoms across the five different categories shown in the diagnostic criteria in Table 9.2.

Table 9.2 Diagnostic Criteria for Acute Stress Disorder (ASD)

Presence of nine (or more) of the following symptoms from any of the five following categories beginning or worsening after the traumatic event(s) occurred:

Intrusion Symptoms
1. Recurrent, involuntary, and intrusive distressing memories of the traumatic event(s).
2. Recurrent distressing dreams in which the content and/or affect of the dream are related to the event(s).
3. Dissociative reactions (e.g., flashbacks) in which the individual feels or acts as if the traumatic event(s) were recurring.
4. Intense or prolonged psychological distress or marked physiological reactions in response to internal or external cues that symbolize or resemble an aspect of the traumatic event(s).

Negative Mood
5. Persistent inability to experience positive emotions (e.g., inability to experience happiness, satisfaction, or loving feelings).

Dissociative Symptoms
6. An altered sense of the reality of one's surroundings or oneself (e.g., seeing oneself from another's perspective, being in a daze, time slowing).
7. Inability to remember an important aspect of the traumatic event(s) (typically due to dissociative amnesia and not to other factors such as head injury, alcohol, or drugs).

Avoidance Symptoms
8. Efforts to avoid distressing memories, thoughts, or feelings about or closely associated with the traumatic event(s).
9. Efforts to avoid external reminders (people, places, conversations, activities, objects, situations) that arouse distressing memories, thoughts, or feelings about or closely associated with the traumatic event(s).

Arousal Symptoms
10. Sleep disturbance (e.g., difficulty falling or staying asleep, restless sleep).
11. Irritable behavior and angry outbursts (with little or no provocation), typically expressed as verbal or physical aggression toward people or objects.
12. Hyper-vigilance.
13. Problems with concentration.
14. Exaggerated startle response.

APA (2013, 2022)

Adjustment Disorder

Adjustment disorders represent a simple response to some type of life stress, which may or may not be traumatic (Grohol, 2013). An adjustment disorder, thus, is the least intense of all the four disorders discussed in this chapter in the category of Trauma and Stressor-Related Disorders. The persons suffering from adjustment disorder experience difficulty in getting adjusted to their self and the environment as a consequential outcome of some stressful events happening in their life. Typically, individuals who experience this type of disorder following an identifiable stressor that happened within the past three months and its diagnosis as such need reevaluation if the symptoms persist for more than six months following the termination of the stressor. Regarding the symptoms for its diagnosis, we may find that the people suffering from this disorder may exhibit a number of emotional and behavioral symptoms. However, like PTSD and ASD, we do not have a set of specific symptoms for laying down the diagnostic criteria for adjustment disorder. On this account, here we must see that whatever symptoms the individual is experiencing must be related to the stressor and must be significant enough to impair social, occupational, or other important areas of functioning, as well as causing the individual marked distress that is out of proportion to the severity or intensity of the stressor (APA, 2022).

Prolonged Grief Disorder

Prolonged grief disorder included in both the DSM-5 and DSM-5-TR has been defined as an intense yearning/longing and/or preoccupation with thoughts or memories of the deceased who died at least 12 months ago in the case of adults, and at least 6 months ago for children and adolescents. Individuals suffering from this disorder may experience significant distress or problems regarding their daily functioning, social interaction, and work activities.

Symptoms of prolonged grief disorder (APA, 2022) include:

- Identity disruption (such as feeling as though part of oneself has died).
- Marked sense of disbelief about the death.
- Avoidance of reminders that the person is dead.
- Intense emotional pain (such as anger, bitterness, and sorrow) related to the death.
- Difficulty with reintegration (such as problems engaging with friends, pursuing interests, planning for the future).
- Emotional numbness (absence or marked reduction of emotional experience).
- Feeling that life is meaningless.
- Intense loneliness (feeling alone or detached from others).
- Holding maladaptive cognitions about the self, feeling guilt about the death, and holding negative views about life goals and expectancy.
- Demonstrating harmful health behaviors due to decreased self-care and concern.
- Experiencing hallucinations about the deceased, feeling bitter, angry, and restless, blaming others for the death, and seeing a reduction in the quantity and quality of sleep.

To Sum Up

Trauma and stressor-related disorders represent the type of disorders resulting from the difficulty coping with or adjusting to a recent stressor (stress-producing stimuli) or trauma (lasting adverse effect caused by an event that involves threat or danger). Among these disorders, Posttraumatic Stress Disorder (PTSD) represents the type of disorder that results when an individual directly or indirectly experiences an adverse stress and trauma-related event. Acute stress disorder (ASD) is very similar to PTSD except for the fact that symptoms must be present from day three to one month following exposure to one or more stressful or traumatic events. It is a relatively short-term condition lasting no more than one month. Adjustment disorders represent a simple response to life stressors, which may or may not be traumatic. An adjustment disorder, thus, is the least intense among these four disorders. The persons experiencing adjustment disorder have difficulty getting adjusted to their self and the environment to the extent of impairing their social, occupational, or other important areas of functioning, causing marked distress to them. Prolonged grief disorder is an intense yearning/longing and/or preoccupation with thoughts or memories of the deceased who died at least 12 months ago in the case of adults, and at least 6 months ago for children and adolescents. It causes significant distress or problems regarding the daily functioning, social interaction, and work activities of the afflicted.

Obsessive-Compulsive and Related Disorders

Obsessive behavior represents maladaptive behavior in which an individual is haunted by the persistent recurrence of unwelcome, absurd, and disturbing ideas or thoughts. For example, a wife may have an obsessive idea of stabbing or poisoning her husband, a mother of hurting her little girl, a son of wishing for his mother's death, a husband of pushing his wife down a flight of stairs. Although the patient realizes the absurdity and irrelevance of such thoughts, still he is unable to get rid of them. The more desperately he tries to rid himself of them, the more they persist.

Obsessive behavior, when taken further, becomes compulsive behavior. Compulsion is in fact an overt manifestation of an obsessive thought or an idea. In other words compulsions are obsessions translated into action. Compulsive behavior, in this way, may be defined as maladaptive behavior in which a person is seen to perform repeated acts of unreasonable and irrelevant nature such as washing his hands again and again, checking the alarm clock several times to ensure it has been wound, returning to his house again and again to be certain that the door has been locked, or following an elaborate ritualistic sequence in detail before going to sleep. Such patterns of behavior are maladaptive in the sense that they are unnecessary and irrational. Even the person realizes the absurdity of his compulsive acts, but he feels uncomfortable unless he performs the compulsive act.

While obsessive behavior may exist without compulsion, compulsive behavior cannot even originate without obsession. It is true that thoughts or ideas must compulsorily precede action. But as far as obsessive-compulsive neurosis is concerned, the symptoms of both obsessive and compulsive behavior are present in such neuroses as may be evident from the following definition given in the DSM-II (1968):

> *In this reaction the anxiety is associated with the persistence of unwanted ideas and of repetitive impulses to perform acts which may be considered morbid by the patient. The patient himself may regard his ideas and behavior as unreasonable but nevertheless is compelled to carry out his rituals.*

Some Examples of Obsessive-Compulsive Behavior

1. An adolescent boy was found to have a unique obsessive-compulsive behavior concerning fire, technically known as *pyromania*. He was preoccupied with the idea of fire and possessed

an overwhelming urge to set fires without caring about the consequences. He admitted setting innumerable fires causing damage to properties and lives but could not give any reason for his strange criminal behavior.

2. A pretty young woman of a rich family was found to be suffering from an obsessive-compulsive behavior, *kleptomania* (uncontrollable urge to steal). Whenever she attended dinner parties she could not resist putting selected spoons in her handbag. She had a record of 300 stolen spoons. At one time when she was seen taking the spoons by a friend and asked why she did it, she felt humiliated but replied, "I don't know why it happens but something compels me to do it."

3. Samuel Johnson suffered from an obsessive-compulsive behavior, *coprolalia*. He had a strong urge to utter obscene words for which he was often humiliated. He had no explanation for his strange conduct.

4. A principal of a girls' college was found to suffer from an obsessive-compulsive behavior related to contamination and cleanliness. She used to wash her hands and take baths several times a day. After going outside it was necessary for her to change her clothes. Whenever a visitor came to her drawing room, she had the room cleaned and sprayed with disinfectant.

5. As reported by Freud, an eleven-year-old boy was found to be engaged in a typical obsessive-compulsive ceremony every night before going to bed. He did not sleep until he had told his mother in the minutest detail all the events of the day, there could be no scraps of paper or other rubbish on the carpet of the bedroom, the bed must be pushed right to the wall, three chairs must stand by it, and the pillows must lay in a particular way. In order to get to sleep, he first kicked about a certain number of times with both legs and then lay on his side. When asked why he did these things, he was unable to give a satisfactory reason.

6. A middle-aged man was found to suffer with an obsessive-compulsive behavior related to the drinking of tea. He could not drink his tea for fear that a pin might have been dropped into it. He was forced to pour his tea back and forth several times to make certain that it did not contain a pin.

7. A schoolboy, thirteen years of age, was brought in for help on account of his obsessive-compulsive rituals. When he urinated, he had to wash four times; if he had to put on his socks, he washed seven times; and if he touched something with one hand, he had to touch it with the other. He could give no reason for observing such methodical rituals.

A Few New Varieties of Obsessive-Compulsive Behavior Brought to Light in DSM-5

In the classification of mental disorders, the DSM-5 provided by the American Psychiatric Association in 2013 contains a significant development regarding Obsessive-Compulsive-Related Disorders, i.e., particular patterns of repetitive and excessive behavior that greatly disrupt people's lives in a variety of ways. The DSM-5 has assigned four of these patterns to that group of disorders, namely (i) hoarding disorder, (ii) trichotillomania (hair-pulling disorder), (iii) excoriation (skin picking) disorder, and (iv) body dysmorphic disorder. Let us know about them.

Hoarding Disorder

Individuals suffering from the obsessive-compulsive disorder known as Hoarding disorder are found to feel that they must save items, and they become very distressed if they try to discard them (APA, 2013). Hoarding or making collections of objects or things is an inborn instinctive phenomenon distinctly visible in the behavior of small children. It can be a hobby as well.

However, it may turn into a big problem or mental disorder when it becomes an obsession as well as a compulsion to acquire and hoard things not at all needed. In brief, a person suffering from hoarding disorder may be characterized as follows:

- They have an inherent craving for collecting and accumulating a host of things, and as a result, it is common for them to wind up with numerous useless and valueless items, from junk mail to broken objects and unusual clothes.
- They are extremely unaware of the severity of their behavior. People with hoarding disorders are extremely attached to their possessions, and they are very resistant to efforts to get rid of them (Kring et al., 2012:207).
- The compulsion for afflicted people to resist giving up their possessions results in an extraordinary accumulation of items that clutters their lives and living areas.
- This pattern causes individuals significant distress and may greatly impair their personal, social, or occupational functioning. Parts of their homes may become inaccessible because of the clutter. In addition, it often results in fire hazards, unhealthy sanitation conditions, or other dangers.

Trichotillomania (Hair-Pulling Disorder)

The term *trichotillomania* is derived from the Greek for "frenzied hair-pulling." Accordingly, people suffering from trichotillomania are found to demonstrate the behavioral characteristics summarized as below.

- They are in the habit of repeatedly pulling out hair from their scalp, eyebrows, eyelashes, or other parts of the body (APA, 2013).
- Typically, those with the disorder pull one hair at a time.
- Some sufferers follow specific rituals as they pull their hair, including pulling until the hair feels "just right," and selecting certain types of hairs for pulling.
- There lies a strong emotional element in the shape of sizable anxiety or stress responsible for triggering or accompanying the hair-pulling behavior.
- The demonstration of such undesirable behavior causes much distress, impairment, or embarrassment to the affected individual.
- Despite making resolutions not to engage in such behavior and trying to reduce or stop the hair-pulling for the time being, the sufferers may find themselves helpless in overcoming this habit.

Excoriation (Skin-Picking) Disorder

Individuals suffering from Excoriation (skin-picking) disorder are found to demonstrate behavior characterized as follows:

- Much like the practice of hair pulling from a particular body part, people suffering from skin picking disorder are engaged in using their fingers to pick on one area of their body, most often the face.
- Most of the time the preferred area or body part chosen for skin picking remains one's face. However, the other common areas of the body used for this practice may include the arms, legs, lips, scalp, chest, and extremities such as fingernails and cuticles.

- Repeated picking of skin on one area of the body results in significant sores or wounds (APA, 2013).
- Like hair-pulling, skin-picking behavior is also typically triggered or accompanied by anxiety or stress.
- It is designated as an obsessive-compulsive behavior in the sense that the affected person is habituated to doing it again and again despite the agonies, impairment, and embarrassment suffered, and resolutions made to quit this bad practice are difficult to follow through with.

Body Dysmorphic Disorder

Individuals suffering from the obsessive-compulsive disorder known as body dysmorphic disorder are found to engage in behavior characterized as follows:

- They become preoccupied with the belief that they have a particular defect or flaw in their physical appearance. The perceived defect or flaw is imagined or greatly exaggerated in the person's mind (APA, 2013).
- The perception or belief that there is definitely something wrong with their body part or appearance, drives afflicted individuals to engage in obsessive-compulsive acts such as repeatedly checking themselves in the mirror, grooming themselves, picking at the perceived flaw, comparing themselves with others, seeking reassurance, or performing other similar behavioral activities.
- Of course, it is quite common in our society for teenagers and young adults to worry about their appearance and body makeup. The concerns of people with body dysmorphic disorder, however, are extreme. Sufferers may severely limit contact with other people, be unable to look others in the eye, or go to great lengths to conceal their "defects"—for instance, always wearing sunglasses—to cover their supposedly misshapen eyes. As many as half of people with this disorder seek plastic surgery or dermatology treatment, and often feel worse rather than better afterward. A large number are housebound, and more than 10% may attempt suicide (Comer, 2015:171).
- It is also quite common to witness people suffering from body dysmorphic disorder to experience difficulties, distress, impairment, and embarrassment on account of their repetitive undesirable behavior.
- The people affected by body dysmorphic disorder, according to researchers in this area, are generally found to focus on specifics such as wrinkles on the face; spots on the skin; excessive facial hair; swelling of the face; a misshapen nose, mouth, jaw, or eyebrow; the appearance of their feet, hands, breasts, penis, or other body parts; or even concerned about bad odors coming from sweat, breath, genitals, or the rectum, as witnessed in the case history depicted below.
  A woman of 35 had for 16 years been worried that she smelled terrible. Due to this fear, for five years she had not gone out anywhere except when accompanied by her husband or mother. She had not spoken to her neighbors for three years. She avoided cinemas, dances, shops, cafes, and private homes. Her husband was not allowed to invite friends to their home; she constantly sought reassurance from him about her smell. Her husband bought all her new clothes as she was afraid to try on clothes in front of shop assistants. She used vast quantities of deodorant and always bathed and changed her clothes before going out, up to four times daily (Marks, 1987:371, Quoted by Comer, 2015:171).

The Causation of Obsessive-Compulsive Neurosis

What causes such maladaptive behavior is a matter of concern. Hereditary or other biological factors are not observed to contribute anything to the development of obsessive-compulsive neurosis. This maladaptive behavior is predominantly a learned reaction pattern. Conditioned learning, in a variety of environmental learning situations, provides opportunities for the origin and development of many obsessive-compulsive rituals. The source of such maladaptive behavior patterns may be the result of any one of the following possibilities.

1. An obsessive-compulsive act may be a direct expression of an undesirable motive or impulse. What is not accepted by the ego and thus repressed in the unconscious may become conscious, but the individual is not aware that it represents the fulfillment of his own desire. For example, pyromania (compulsion to set fire) and homicidal mania (compulsion to kill) may be interpreted behaviorally as a revenge reaction arising out of basic frustrations and conflicts. These reactions provide opportunities for the satisfaction of hostile thoughts, outlets for aggressive feelings, and achievement of some kind of power and a sense of satisfaction.

2. The feelings of guilt and self-condemnation associated with past, or sometimes with present, misdeeds may also give rise to an obsessive-compulsive behavior. As a result, an individual may be forced to counteract or cleanse himself of guilt by means of compulsive rituals, for example, the compulsive handwashing ritual. It may be taken as a symbolic attempt to wash away a feeling of guilt relating to sexual or other undesirable behavior. In literature, the compulsive handwashing behavior of Lady Macbeth, a key character in Shakespeare's *Macbeth*, illustrates the dynamics of such behavior. She had an excessive guilt feeling on account of her participation in the murder of the King Duncan and her compulsive handwashing was nothing but an attempt to cleanse her hands of the imaginary blood.

3. Obsessive-compulsive reactions are often generated as defense reactions based on the reaction-formation mechanism. In such situations, the individual behaves in ways which are directly contradictory to his unsocial or otherwise dangerous thoughts or impulses. As a consequence, one may defend himself from abnormal sexual desire by developing a strong attitude of condemnation toward such behavior. Similarly, one may defend himself against his hostile impulses toward his wife or son by obsessively thinking and compulsively doing acts demonstrating concern for their safety.

4. Indecisiveness coupled with the feeling of inadequacy may be the reason for certain obsessive-compulsive behavior. It may breed compulsive doubts and one may be forced to engage in such rituals such as returning again and again to check the lock on the door or cleaning plates again and again before eating. The compensatory behavior for this feeling of inadequacy or helplessness may also force an individual to resort to such compulsive behavior as compulsory stealing, killing, or protecting himself from unknown enemies and dangers.

5. The basic element in obsessive-compulsive behavior is the personal satisfaction which an individual derives in performing such acts. In doing so he relieves himself of the immediate anxiety tension or pressure. He feels satisfied with a sense of achievement in the form of fulfillment of his desires, which, in turn, further reinforces his compulsive behavior, and gradually a reaction pattern involving obsessive-compulsive neurosis is developed and the person becomes fixed to behave in a peculiar way despite being aware that his behavior is irrational.

To Sum Up

Obsessive-compulsive neurotic behavior represents maladaptive behavior in which an obsession (haunting on the part of a person by the recurrence of an absurd thought or idea) is necessarily followed by a compulsion to act upon the felt idea or thought. Such patterns of behavior are maladaptive in the sense that they are unnecessary and irrational. Even the person realizes the absurdity of his compulsive acts, but he feels uncomfortable unless he performs the compulsive act. Certain new varieties of obsessive-compulsive-related disorders have been pointed out in the DSM-5. Among these, *hoarding disorder* is the disorder in which people are compelled to save items and become very distressed if they try to discard them, resulting in an excessive accumulation of items. *Trichotillomania* (also called hair-pulling disorder) is a type of disorder in which people repeatedly pull hair out from their scalp, eyebrows, eyelashes, or other parts of the body. Excoriation disorder (also called skin-picking disorder) is a disorder in which people repeatedly pick at their skin resulting in significant sores or wounds. *Body dysmorphic disorder* is a disorder in which people become preoccupied with an imagined or greatly exaggerated belief that they have certain defects or flaws in their physical appearance.

In the causation of such maladaptive behavior, it can be safely inferred that it is predominantly a learned reaction pattern. The beginning in this direction may be the result of: (i) a direct expression of an undesirable motive or impulse, (ii) feelings of guilt and self-condemnation associated with past or present misdeeds, (iii) defense reactions based on the reaction-formation mechanism, (iv) one's indecisiveness coupled with the feeling of inadequacy, and (v) the personal satisfaction felt in performing such acts.

Depressive Disorders

Depressive disorders are characterized by disproportionate reactions to distressing situations like the death of a loved one, an occupational failure, or a financial setback. In such a distressing situation, it is not abnormal to have feelings of grief and despair in a reasonable amount. It is when these feelings become exaggerated in intensity and duration and begin to interfere with an individual's personal or social adjustment that they turn into a depressive behavioral disorder.

Moreover, time is found to be a great healing factor in normal depressive reactions. The memories of normal stress situations become hazy with the passage of time, coupled with the creation of new interests. Life becomes worth living once more. However, when this reaction turns into a depressive disorder, the depressed mood does not return

A Case of Depressive Disorder

A young woman was found to be suffering from depressive disorder. She had hardly been married for one year when her husband died of poisoning by drinking milk he had taken at night before going to bed. A lizard was found in the milk pot, and this convinced the young woman that she was to blame for the death of her husband. She often thought that she had murdered her husband since she had not covered the milk pot while boiling the milk. Thus, instead of experiencing normal grief or sadness, she developed depressive disorder.

to normal even after a reasonable period of time, as it ordinarily does in normal depressive reactions. Here the symptoms concerning depression of mood are also severe. The patient may have intense feelings of dejection, discouragement, and sadness. There is a high level of anxiety and apprehensiveness and extreme feelings of self-condemnation. The person is unable to concentrate, and his level of activity and initiative is lowered. In its more severe form, the anxiety and desperation are heightened to such an extent that the person is unable to work, sits in despair viewing the dark side of life alone, and sometimes thinks of committing suicide.

Depression may be viewed as hostility or anger directed against the self instead of being turned outward. Instead of blaming others, the person blames himself for the loss and the distressing situation. This guilt raises his level of anxiety and apprehensiveness, and forces him to relieve his tension through the mechanism of self-criticism and a relatively continued mood of depression. Thus, the formula for becoming affected with depressive disorders is self-condemnation plus an external loss precipitated in the case of predisposing personality traits as an inability to express hostility and aggression directly and outwardly, submissiveness, dependence, sensitivity to criticism, and self-criticism. Here, the person may be viewed as punishing himself by feeling responsible for the loss or the distressing situations.

Next, consider a case of depressive disorder described below in the box.

The dynamics of neurotic depressive behavior in the above case study reveal that the process starts when there is a considerable emotional loss for which the person thinks his self responsible. He begins to condemn himself and is overwhelmed with feelings of intense guilt. The depression then employed is a defense that satisfies the person when he inflicts punishment on himself through a continued period of depression. In some cases, it turns out to be the last resort and is adopted as an illness, especially when the person sees no silver lining among the dark clouds of despair and frustration in his life. The seriousness of this illness increases with the intensification of despair when many patients attempt suicide.

To Sum Up

Depressive disorders represent psychological disorders in which people are found to show *disproportionate* reactions to distressing stress situations (like the death of a loved one, an occupational failure, or a financial setback) strong enough to interfere with their personal or social adjustment. There is a high level of anxiety and apprehensiveness and extreme feelings of self-condemnation. In its more severe form, the anxiety and desperation are heightened to such an extent that the person is unable to work, sits in despair viewing the dark side of life alone, and sometimes thinks of committing suicide.

Conversion Disorders

This type of mental disorder represents a behavior disorder in which a person's anxiety or psychological conflict is converted into a physical symptom like paralysis of the legs or an inability to hear. It is a sort of learned reaction to frustration in which the individual tries to seek a neurotic defense by a psychogenic impairment of bodily sensation or action. Here a distinction needs to be made between conversion hysteria and psycho-physiological disorders discussed in the previous chapter. In the words of Kisker (1977:206), it may be summarized as follows:

> *When the symptom is expressed through the sensory or motor pathways of the central nervous system, the condition is called a conversion neurosis. However, when neurotic Symptoms involve the autonomic nervous system, the maladaptive behavior is called psycho-physiological disorder.*

Symptoms: Conversion symptoms appear mainly in two areas, namely sensory and motor.

Sensory symptoms: Conversion symptoms may involve any of the senses. Anesthesia (lack of skin sensation) is one of the most common conversion reactions. As a result, the person no longer feels pain even when sharp objects are pressed in the affected parts. Contrary to anesthesia, a person may feel painful sensations that are difficult for him to describe into some areas of the body, especially when the area is stimulated. In the conversion reactions involving visual and auditory senses, the person may become blind or deaf, in a sense—unable to see or hear things that he actually does not like to see or listen to. It is natural for a soldier to develop conversion blindness (even though the eyes and optic nerves are normal) after seeing a very close friend blown apart by an exploding shell. Similarly, a traumatic experience may give such a shock to an individual that he may not dare to use his ears for fear of what he may hear and, consequently, he develops conversion deafness.

Motor symptoms: Conversion hysteria frequently involves motor symptoms of voluntarily controlled muscles like tremors or shaking, tick-like movements, minor cramps, contraction of muscles, disorders of speech, paralyzed limbs, convulsive seizures, and so on.

In conversion paralysis, a limb becomes useless and so makes it possible for the individual to escape from what is to him an impossible situation. Thus, in many cases, conversion paralysis becomes a preferred way of reacting to stress. As an example, we may cite the case of a soldier who became paralyzed when the order was given to attack the enemy, or a person whose arms got paralyzed when he could not protect his wife from the clutches of violence.

The interesting thing to note with conversion paralysis is that it usually amounts to a functional disorder. Here too, the loss of the function may be selective. Similar is the case with another conversion disorder known as writer's cramp. Persons suffering from writer's cramp cannot write but are able to use the same muscles for other activities, for example, to shuffle a pack of cards or to play a harmonium.

Disorders of speech constitute one of the most common motor manifestations of conversion hysteria. In *aphonia*, the person is able to speak only in whispers. Stuttering, in the majority of cases, is known to result from psychological reasons. In such cases, the individual, afraid of saying the wrong thing, sets up inhibitions that interfere with the normal functioning of the speech organs.

A convulsive seizure, in many respects, resembles epilepsy. The individual falls and may become unconscious. This usually happens when others are present. Although he may throw himself around, his papillary reflex to light remains unaffected, he does not bite his tongue as usually happens in epilepsy, and he is nearly always careful not to injure himself.

In addition to these two types of conversion symptoms, some psychology professionals include visceral symptoms as a third type. But it is proper to classify symptoms like headaches, choking sensations, coughing spells, difficulty breathing, belching, and nausea as psycho-physiological disorders rather than neurotic disorders, as these symptoms also involve the autonomic nervous system along with involuntary muscles of the body.

In some cases of conversion disorders, there exists an exaggeration of actual organic symptoms. Thus, an individual who has a minor organic disorder may build a hysterical superstructure on this foundation. Therefore, in an actual sense, all hysteric individuals attempt to convert their psychological disturbances into physical disorders or diseases, and thus seem to resort to an escape mechanism for justifying their otherwise unjustified behavior. The following example illustrates the mechanism of the conversion reactions.

A successful fifty-year-old businessman, married to an attractive and considerably young wife, suddenly developed paralysis of his arm. Upon medical examination, no organic cause was found for his disorder. The psychological evaluation of the patient revealed that while he seemed anxious to be cured of his disorder, he displayed his arm with some satisfaction, demonstrating the lack of sensation by touching his lit cigarette to the affected part. With the possibility of a conversion reaction, psychotherapy was recommended. It resulted in the removal of the symptom but it returned a few days later. However, the psychological nature of the disorder had been proved and psychotherapy was continued. It became clear to the therapist that the patient had been using his neurotic symptoms to solve his problems. His young and attractive wife was fond of nightclubs, while the patient merely wanted to come home at night, have dinner, read his paper, and go to bed. The difference in age and interests resulted in serious conflict. Finally, the wife began to go out without her husband, and it was at this point that the symptom appeared. The therapist concluded that his paralysis was serving a number of purposes such as (i) a good excuse for staying home at night, (ii) forcing the wife to spend more time with him at home in the evenings, (iii) seeking sympathy and attention of friends and relatives, and (iv) a good excuse for coming home from his office at any hour of the day, as he was jealous of his wife and suspected infidelity. Interestingly, the eventual cure in this case was brought about by the sudden disappearance of his wife with a police officer. When he was convinced that his wife would never return to him, his symptom disappeared spontaneously, as he had no problem of living with his wife now (adapted from Kisker, 1977:208).

To Sum Up

Conversion Disorders stands for the type of disorders in which an individual's anxiety or psychological conflict is converted into a physical symptom like paralysis of legs or inability to hear in order as a matter of seeking a sort of neurotic defense by a psychogenic impairment of bodily sensation or action. The persons affected with these disorders are thus found to exhibit two types of symptoms, (i) sensory (involving any of one's senses such as skin sensation, hearing, vision, touch, or smell) resulting in the loss or unusual response from such sensation, and (ii) motor (involving the impaired ability to control voluntary muscles) resulting in the possibilities such as paralysis of limbs, disorders of speech, and so on.

Dissociative Disorders

Dissociation may be known as a disconnection between a person's thoughts, memories, feelings, actions, or sense of who he or she is. In a normal course of functioning it may happen with us in a mild form at one or the other times, such as daydreaming, getting lost in a book, watching a movie, or sightseeing, all resulting in cutting connection with what is happening around us. It becomes a problem and abnormality turning into a type of disorder when it gets intensified in its severity and consequences.

In this sense, the term dissociative disorders stands for the form or type of disorders in which individuals are found to show a greater degree of severity in cutting the connection between their self and present reality. In dissociative disorders, the affected individuals, thus, may experience a variety of problems concerning their memory, identity, emotion, perception, behavior, and sense of self—strong enough to disrupt every area of their mental functioning.

With regard to their causation, it has been observed these disorders are often the result of trauma experienced in the form of rape, natural or manmade catastrophes, incidents, or accidents.

There are three types of dissociative disorders, known as (i) Dissociative identity disorder, (ii) Dissociative amnesia, and (iii) Depersonalization/Derealization disorder. Let us look into them.

Dissociative identity disorder, known as multi-personality disorder, refers to a type of dissociative disorder in which affected people are found to live in two personalities and shift from one to another, dissociating them from their own real identity without their awareness.

Accordingly, they feel as if they have within them two or more entities, each with its own way of thinking and remembering about them and their life. Their ways of thinking, including attitudes and preferences for one or the other things, may suddenly shift and then shift back. Criteria for diagnosis of Dissociate identity disorder, according to the APA (2013) include:

- The existence of two or more distinct identities or personality states.
- The distinct identities are accompanied by changes in behavior, memory, and thinking. The signs and symptoms may be observed by others or reported by the individual.
- Ongoing gaps in memory about everyday events, personal information, and/or past traumatic events.
- The symptoms cause significant distress or problems in social, occupational, or other areas of functioning.

Dissociative amnesia refers to a type of dissociative disorder in which the person suffers from abnormal forgetting by not being able to recall information or happenings about oneself. This loss of one's memory does not result from physical causes, such as head injury or the consequence of some neurological dysfunction. Such memory loss may be witnessed occurring among affected individuals in various forms, such as: (i) Localized (unable to remember an event or period of time), (ii) Selective (unable to remember a specific aspect of an event or some events within a period of time), (iii) Generalized (complete loss of identity and life history), and (iv) The state of Fugue in which people are found to travel a distance from home and workplace, or do certain acts by assuming another identity, and are later unable to recall what they have done.

Regarding its causation, cases of dissociative amnesia are often linked with past experiences in the form of childhood trauma, and are particularly related to emotional neglect, abuse, and sexual assault, as well as the enormous stresses felt in their present.

Depersonalization/derealization disorder is the type of dissociative disorder in which people are found to be affected by one or the other types of abnormalities in their behavior, referred to as (i) Depersonalization and (ii) De-realization.

Depersonalization here refers to a type of disorder in which affected individuals are found to experience a dreamlike state, causing them to feel separation or detachment from their mind, self, or body. It alters their perception of the self and consequently, they may feel as if they are outside their bodies, watching events that are happening to them as an observer.

The term *derealization*, on the other hand, refers to a type of disorder in which the affected individuals are found to experience detachment or separation from the reality lying before them. In fact, here their sense of reality is temporarily lost or changed; their sense of perception feels unrealistic. Accordingly, they may feel as if things and people in the world around them are not real.

To Sum Up

Dissociative Disorders are the type of disorders in which individuals are found to show a great degree of severity in cutting the connection between their self and the reality existing at present, or experienced by them in their past, causing them to experience a variety of problems concerning their memory, identity, emotion, perception, behavior, and sense of self—strong enough to disrupt every area of their mental functioning. There are three types of dissociative disorders, known as (i) Dissociative identity disorder (people living in two personalities and shifting from one to another for dissociating them from their own real identity without their awareness), (ii) Dissociative amnesia (people suffering from abnormal perception by not being able to recall information or happenings about themselves), and (iii) Depersonalization/Derealization disorder (individuals who experience a dreamlike state, making feel as if they are outside their bodies and watching events as an observer, and experiencing a distorted perception of things in an unrealistic or unusual way).

Causes and Treatment of Psycho-Neurotic Disorders

The most important causative factors of all neuroses are psychological. We see that psychoneurotic reactions often represent learned maladaptive behavior patterns. Factors such as a difficult upbringing, improper childhood experiences, uncongenial home and school environment, and the stresses and strains suffered in later life provide sufficient predisposing and precipitating causes for learning neurotic reactions. An individual feels satisfied in behaving neurotically as it helps him to fulfill his otherwise unsatisfied needs. He derives pleasure in seeking sympathy, attention, and care from his well-wishers or even strangers for his limitations on account of his illness or disease. Thus his neurotic symptoms are reinforced and make his disorder more severe in intensity and duration.

The psycho-neurotic disorders vary in respect to their nature (characteristics and symptoms) and causation. Therefore, no common treatment may be prescribed for all such disorders. However, in general, neurotic patients are curable. They respond more favorably to behavior therapy and psychotherapy than patients suffering from conduct disorders or functional psychoses. The treatment adopted for major types of psychoneurotic disorders is summarized ahead. For more detail about the use of these therapies, readers may go to Chapter 19 of this text.

Anxiety disorders: Neurotic anxiety patients may be helped by chemical therapy, sedatives, or mild tranquillizers. In chronic cases, insulin therapy may be given. They may also be given psychological treatment through (i) supportive psychotherapy; (ii) insight therapy; (iii) group psychotherapy; and (iv) finding other outlets for the patient's drives.

Phobic disorders: The following therapeutic measures may be adopted for the treatment of these disorders:

a. Insight therapy
b. Relaxation and desensitization (de-conditioning)—The patient is relaxed sometimes with the help of drugs, and then gradually introduced to the phobic situation, starting with the least terrifying kind.
c. Implosion (or flooded) therapy—The patient is immediately immersed in the most frightening phobic situation until he no longer experiences fear.
d. Adaptation therapy—The patient observes (in real life or film) someone else handling his phobic situation.

Obsessive-compulsive disorder: "Thought-stopping" is a technique of help in such disorders. In using this technique, the patient is asked to say stop inside their mind for the unwanted thoughts, use attention diverting, relaxation and meditation techniques for taking them away from the unwanted thoughts and then try for replacing the unwanted thoughts with the desirable ones. Even lobotomy, a brain operation, in which the nerve pathways between the frontal lobes of the brain and the thalamus and hypothalamus are cut, has shown to be helpful for this neurosis. Psychotherapy measures are the preferential alternative.

Depressive disorders: The following methods, often in combination, are useful in the treatment of neurotic depression:

- Drug therapy
- Psychotherapies like supportive psychotherapy and insight psychotherapy.
- Modifying the stressful environmental situation.

- In extreme cases of depression, electroconvulsive therapy (ECT) is used.

Conversion and dissociative disorders: The symptoms of these psychoneurotic disorders may be alleviated by hypnosis. The release of an individual from an emotionally stressful situation and intensive psychotherapy, such as supportive psychotherapy, group therapy and re-educative therapy, are the measures needed for better results.

- Phobic neurosis represents disorders in which a person experiences persistent intense irrational fear of a specific situation or object that interferes with his normal activities and affects his mental health. They are generally caused by early terrifying experiences and unconscious conflicts or learned on account of conditioning or social learning.

To Sum Up

The most important *causative factors* of all psychoneurotic disorders are psychological. The early unhappy experiences, repressed wishes, and unresolved conflicts initiate the process. Later, the unfavorable circumstances, stresses, and strains provide sufficient cause for learning neurotic reactions. In many cases, psychoneurotic reactions often represent learned maladaptive behavior patterns.

The *treatment* of psychoneurotic disorders varies in relation to their nature and causation. No common treatment can therefore be prescribed for all these disorders. However, neurotic patients are curable. They respond more favorably to behavior therapy and other psychotherapies than patients suffering from conduct disorders or functional psychoses.

Review Questions

1. What do you understand by the term neuroses or psychoneurotic disorders? Provide its definition and throw light on the underlying characteristics of psychoneurotic behavior.
2. Describe the characteristic features of neurotic behavior and differentiate it from psychotic behavior.
3. Name the specific forms or types of neuroses or psychoneurotic disorders, and describe any one of them in detail.
4. What are anxiety disorders? What types of symptoms are usually visible among individuals suffering from anxiety disorders?

5. Discuss in brief the meaning, nature, and impact of the anxiety disorders known as generalized anxiety disorder, panic disorder, separation anxiety disorder, and social anxiety disorder.
6. What are phobias? Describe the different types of phobias and discuss the how and why of their causation.
7. What is meant by the term trauma- and stressor-related disorders? Discuss the occurrence of the disorders known as posttraumatic stress disorder (PTSD), acute disorder (AD), adjustment disorder, and prolonged grief disorder, along with their accompanying symptoms.
8. What is an obsessive-compulsive behavior? Explain and illustrate with examples and throw light on its causation.
9. Throw light on the nature and impact of the new varieties of obsessive-compulsive behavior known as hoarding disorder, trichotillomania (hair-pulling disorder), excoriation (skin-picking disorder), and body dysmorphic disorder.
10. What are the depression disorders? Throw light on their meaning, nature, and impact on affected individuals.
11. What are conversion disorders? What types of symptoms (sensory and motor) are usually visible among persons suffering from conversion disorders?
12. What are dissociative disorders? Throw light on the nature and impact of the dissociative disorders known as (i) dissociative identity disorder, (ii) dissociative amnesia, and (iii) depersonalization/derealization disorder.
13. What is a dissociative identity disorder/dissociative amnesia/depersonalization/derealization disorder? Explain with the help of an example.
14. What are psychoneurotic disorders? How are they caused and treated? Discuss in detail.

References

American Psychiatric Association (1968), *Diagnostic and statistical manual of mental disorders, DSM-II* (2nd ed.), Washington, DC: American Psychiatric Association.

American Psychiatric Association (2013), *Diagnostic and statistical manual of mental disorders* (5th ed.), Washington, DC: American Psychiatric Association.

American Psychiatric Association (2022), *Diagnostic and statistical manual of mental disorders: DSM-5-TR*, Washington, DC: American Psychiatric Association.

Comer, R. J. (2015), *Abnormal psychology* (9th ed.), New York, NY: Worth Publishers (A Macmillan Education Imprint).

Davison, G. C., & Neale, J. M. (1978), *Abnormal psychology* (2nd ed.), New York, NY: John Wiley & Sons.

Grohol, J. (2013), DSM-5 changes: PTSD, trauma & stress-related disorders, retrieved from https://pro.psychcentral.com/dsm-5-changes-ptsd-trauma-stress-related-disorders/004406.html

Kisker, G. W. (1977), *The disorganized personality* (3rd ed.), New York, NY: McGraw-Hill.

Kring, A. M., Johnson, S. L., Davison, G. C., & Neale, J. M. (2012), *Abnormal psychology* (12th ed.), New York, NY: John Wiley & Sons.

Malot, R. W., & Whaley, D. L. (1983), *Psychology*, Holmes Beach, FL: Learning Publications.

Marks, I. M. (1987), *Fears, phobias and rituals: Panic, anxiety, and their disorders*. Oxford: Oxford University Press.

Page, J. D. (1976), *Abnormal psychology*, New Delhi: Tata McGraw-Hill.

Price, J. H. (1972), *Psychiatric investigations*, London: Butterworths.

Chapter 10

Psychoses or Psychotic Disorders

Learning Objectives

After going through this chapter, you will be able to:

- Discuss the meaning and characteristic features of the psychoses or psychotic disorders.
- Describe the meaning, nature, causation, and treatment of schizophrenia.
- Throw light on the nature and impacts of Simple, Hebephrenic, Catatonic, and Paranoid schizophrenia.
- Elucidate the meaning and nature of bipolar and related disorders (Mood or affective disorders).
- Differentiate between schizophrenic and affective disorders.
- Know about the meaning and nature of the different types of affective disorders known as Manic, Depressive, and Manic-depressive disorders.
- Throw light on the nature of manic behavior occurring in the shape of hypomania, acute mania, and hyper-acute or delirious mania.
- Discuss the depressive disorder occurring in the shape of mild or simple depression, acute depression, and depressive stupor.
- Describe the meaning and nature of manic-depressive disorder along with its classic behavioral signs or symptoms.
- Throw light on the nature and impact of the manic-depressive disorders classified as Bipolar I disorder, Bipolar II disorder, and Cyclothymic disorder.
- Discuss the causes and treatments of affective disorders.

What are Psychoses or Psychotic Disorders?

Psychoses or Psychotic disorders are more "serious disorders" of the mind and in this sense represent a major illness in comparison with the minor illnesses of neurotic disorders. A psychotic behavior is characterized by a serious form of personality disturbance in which the patient shows periodic or prolonged loss of contact with the world of reality. The legal and social term "insanity" is frequently used for the psychotic disorders. A person who is judged insane is considered unable to act consciously, and therefore, lawyers often plead the insanity of their clients for saving them from being punished for crimes committed by them.

DOI: 10.4324/9781003398325-10

The general characteristics of psychosis as summarized by Thorpe and Katz (1948:449) are as follows:

> **Psychoses or Psychotic Disorders**
>
> The more serious disorders of the mind than the neuroses are characterized by a serious form of personality disturbance in which the patient shows periodic or prolonged loss of contact with the world of reality in his behavioral functioning, proving injurious to himself, to society, or both.

- The individual's mental functions are usually so disturbed that he is incapable of carrying out his daily activities.
- The individual manifests symptoms of a severe nature, often in the form of delusions, hallucinations, stupor, incoherence, or violent reactions.
- The individual is more or less out of contact with reality.
- The individual usually lacks insight; that is, he does not appreciate or realize the psychological nature of his symptoms and disabilities.
- The individual's behavior may be injurious to himself or to society, or both; he usually must be placed under guardianship or in confinement, as in a mental hospital.

The Major Mental Disorders Falling in the Category of Psychoses or Psychotic Disorders

Looking into the latest classification system available in the form of the DSM-5 (APA, 2013), DSM-5-TR (APA, 2022), ICD-10 (WHO, 2010) and ICD-11 (WHO, 2022), we see that the major mental disorders falling in the category of psychoses or psychotic disorders are the following:

1. Schizophrenia Spectrum and other Related Disorders
2. Bipolar and Related Disorders (Mood or Affective disorders)

Let us examine these two types or forms of Psychoneurotic disorders.

Schizophrenia Spectrum and Other Related Disorders

In frequency, schizophrenic disorder leads all psychoses, in terms of severity or seriousness. Consequently, the hospitalization of schizophrenic patients is longer (10 to 45 years) than that of any other group.

The term schizophrenia means splitting of the mind. Here, splitting of the mind does not mean a split personality as in amnesia and multiple personalities, but a marked separation of the self from reality. "The term schizophrenia," according to Coleman (1970:275), "is now used to include a group of psychotic reactions in which there are fundamental disturbances in reality relationships and in emotional and intellectual processes."

Schizophrenics, as a rule, manifest a number of symptoms, the significant ones of which are:

1. Lack of coherence in the thought process
2. Disorganized patterns of thinking and feeling
3. Apathy, absence of feeling
4. Disorganised patterns of speech
5. Peculiarities of movements or bizarre actions

6. Preoccupation with private fantasy
7. Withdrawal from reality or seclusiveness
8. Neglect of conduct and personal habits
9. Delusions and hallucinations

Types of schizophrenia: For the purpose of diagnosis as well as treatment, schizophrenic disorders may be sub-divided into the following four major types:

• Simple schizophrenia
• Hebephrenic schizophrenia
• Catatonic schizophrenia
• Paranoid schizophrenia

Simple schizophrenia: Simple schizophrenia is characterized by an attitude of indifference, or in advanced stages, by extreme apathy. The disorder usually begins with a decreased interest in the normal activities of life during adolescence or early adult life, and then gradually develops into a loss of ambition, emotional indifference, and withdrawal from social relations. The individual becomes increasingly indifferent and seclusive, begins to obtain his satisfaction through daydreaming, and eventually sinks into an apathetic state. At this stage, he does not care at all. There is nothing to wish for, nothing to fight for. He has no connection with reality to assume responsibility and is content to lead a simple, irresponsible, indifferent, and dependent life.

Simple schizophrenic disorder may be distinguished from other types of schizophrenia on the ground that it rarely shows the more dramatic symptoms such as disorientation, delusions, hallucinations, or disturbances of language or action. Simple schizophrenics are sometimes mistaken for being intellectually disabled on account of their apathy, indifference, lack of concentration, and low levels of motivation. Psychological tests, however, may reveal that they are not mentally disabled. Another difficulty occurs in differentiating simple schizophrenia from inadequate personality. The difference between the two is that those with inadequate personalities may appear to try to function effectively, while schizophrenics do not try at all.

Hebephrenic schizophrenia: The onset of this disease usually occurs in adolescence and develops gradually. In this disorder, the affected person retreats from the stresses of life by regressing to a silly, childish level of behavior, and by withdrawing into a fantasy world of his own, with accompanying emotional disintegration of the personality, as well as dramatic psychotic symptoms like symbolic language disturbances and symbolic actions hallucinations, particularly auditory, and delusions of a sexual, religious, hypochondriacal, and persecutory nature.

Hebephrenic schizophrenia represents withdrawal in an extreme form. The patient no longer remains interested in the world around him. His silly and inappropriate giggling, weeping, or laughing behavior does not result from external stimuli but from stimuli from within the imaginary world in which he lives. In severe cases, the withdrawal and regression is so extreme that the person behaves in many ways like an infant. It is an incurable stage and the patient continues to exist on the level of his choice in the strange world of his own creation.

Catatonic schizophrenia: Catatonic schizophrenia is diagnosed mainly by the patient's behavior fluctuating between stuporous depression and wild excitement. Consequently, his motor behavior may be inhibited (stupor), or alternately, he may break out into an inexplicable burst of overactivity (catatonic excitement). During his periods of stupor, the patient may remain for hours in a bizarre posture. For example, he may sit, stand, or keep his limb in a particular position for hours on end, or he may manifest symptoms like muscular rigidity (rigidity of the muscles and a general resistance to movement), waxy flexibility (remaining in any position in which he is put), echopraxia (mimicry or imitation of what others do), echolalia (automatic repetition of words said by another), and negativism (resisting even the simplest request). He may repeatedly carry out complicated stereotyped movements such as banging the parts of his chair in a certain sequence symmetrically with both hands or walking endlessly up and down the ward; some steps in one direction and an equal number of steps in the other.

In the excited phase of catatonia, the patient becomes extremely overactive, agitated, aggressive, and destructive. During such periods he may shout, throw himself around, tear his clothes, assault others, or injure and mutilate himself. The violence of the catatonic patient is unbridled. In addition to the motor symptoms, the catatonic patients display typical schizophrenic thinking and affect. They may frequently experience fears, hallucinations, and delusions involving ideas of grandeur and of persecution.

The genesis of catatonia may be examined on a psychological basis. The meaningless behavior, the stereotyped physical activity, the stupor or violence are rarely senseless in light of the patient's inner conflicts and repressions. Any psychological trouble arising out of conflicts and frustrations (for example, sex frustrations and feelings of guilt concerning sex behavior) may become a potent source for catatonic functional psychosis.

Paranoid schizophrenia: The term paranoid means "beside oneself." Consequently, a paranoid person is said to be a person who believes himself to have a special relationship with other people. The paranoid patient is intensely preoccupied by his relationship with other people, bad though this relationship may be. As a result, paranoid schizophrenia is diagnosed mainly by disorders of thought content involving systematic delusions and hallucinations, frequently of a persecutory nature, resulting in loss of critical judgment and unpredictable behavior. The term "delusions" stands for the "fixed beliefs, that are not amenable to change in light of conflicting evidence" (APA, 2022:101). This means that despite evidence contradicting their thoughts, people are unable to distinguish their thoughts from reality. A wide range of delusions are seen in the schizophrenia-related disorders of paranoid patients, known as (i) Delusions of grandeur (the belief they are God or have exceptional abilities, wealth and fame), (ii) Delusions of control (the belief that others control their thoughts/feelings/actions), (iii) Delusions of persecution (the belief they are going to be harmed, harassed, or plotted against by somebody), and (iv) Delusions of reference (the belief that specific gestures, comments, or environmental cues are directed directly to them). On the other hand, hallucinations are "perception-like experiences that occur without an external stimulus" (APA, 2022:102). They can occur in any of the five senses: hearing (auditory hallucinations), seeing (visual hallucinations), smelling (olfactory hallucinations), touching (tactile hallucinations), and tasting (gustatory hallucinations).

In the beginning, the individual who develops paranoid schizophrenia feels unworthy and suffers from feelings of inferiority. He resorts to the defense mechanism of blaming others for his failure to achieve. He carries this defense to extremes by distrusting everyone to the extent that he feels certain that they have designs against him. Suspicions of others gradually grow into ideas of reference, and ideas of reference, in turn, become delusions of persecution.

Hallucinations and delusions of persecution of the paranoid schizophrenic may take many forms, sometimes of a very peculiar nature. The patient may falsely believe that an event has a particular significance for him individually. He may believe that the events described by the news reader on the television are oblique references to his own life; the newspapers say things about him in code; there is a special meaning for him in the nods and glances exchanged by others on the train.

The persecutory beliefs and the element of mystery combine to produce a preoccupation with plots to kill or injure the patient. A businessman was sure that his partner was trying to get rid of him and take over the company. Another patient used to wear a rubber suit at home to protect himself from the rays of an "influenced machine" that a spiteful neighbor was directing against him. A laborer declared that some people were going to lower him into hot acid and make hot iron out of him. Another interesting case involved a woman patient who remarked that "one of the doctors has stolen my mind out of my head and he is going to use it to make a lot of money."

The paranoid schizophrenic is inclined to be very verbal about his or her ideas and beliefs. Such patients are generally alert, agitated, talkative, and aggressive, but also confused and afraid. At times when they believe that someone wants to destroy them, they destroy them first in order to save themselves. The hostile attitude and aggression shown by some paranoid patients reflect such trends. However, as their personality deteriorates with time, paranoid schizophrenics tend to become withdrawn and apathetic rather than aggressive.

Etiology of Schizophrenia (Causation)

Genetic factors (heredity): There have been many studies to support the claim that schizophrenia is inherited. These studies may be grouped into three major types: family-risk studies, twin studies, and studies of adopted children.

It has been observed in family-risk studies that the families of schizophrenics had a disproportionately large number of schizophrenic cases. The fact that the disorder runs in families has led to the conclusion that schizophrenia is inherited.

In twin studies, where one of the twins has schizophrenia, then the chances of the other twin having schizophrenia are higher when he is identical than when he is non-identical. Since identical twins are genetically the same in comparison with non-identical ones, the findings suggest that hereditary influences play a part in the inheritance of schizophrenia.

The studies carried out with the children of schizophrenic parents adopted by normal parents and children of normal parents adopted by schizophrenic parents also suggest that there are genetic influences in schizophrenia. It was noticed that when the child of schizophrenic parents was separated from his family soon after birth and nurtured in a proper environment by normal parents, he was still found to be affected by this disorder.

In spite of the evidence put forward by hereditarians, hereditary influences provide only the necessary explanation of causes, but not sufficient ones. Genetic influences are not the sole cause of schizophrenia. Children belonging to schizophrenic parents of families are not bound to become schizophrenics. There are instances of one of the identical twins not being schizophrenic, though both parents or one of them was schizophrenic. If schizophrenia itself is inherited, then its emergence in one identical twin should always be accompanied by its emergence in the other identical twin. We may conclude that schizophrenia is not exclusively the product of hereditary influences. On the other hand, there are some psychiatrists who would deny that the genes and chromosomes may be loaded for schizophrenia in the children of schizophrenics. Therefore, the controversy lies not in the existence of hereditary influences in schizophrenia, but in the extent of this influence.

We may conclude that genetic influences provide some genetic predisposition to schizophrenia. This explains why the disorder seems to be hereditary, and also why it is not essential for identical twins to both be schizophrenics. Genetic influences, thus, may be the first step in the process of making of a schizophrenic by providing a relatively weak constitution that may not be able to resist the many stresses of life.

In summary, heredity influences appear to be relatively unimportant in the development of schizophrenia. Whether a child predisposed to schizophrenia through his genetic influences will become schizophrenic or not depends upon the environmental influences to which he shall be exposed in his future.

Environmental factors: Besides genetic influences, researchers have tried to link schizophrenia with biochemical disturbances and metabolic errors in the body. But this possibility has not made much headway. The accepted causal theory of schizophrenia in recent years speaks of the psychosocial causes inherent in one's environment. It asserts that schizophrenic reactions are learned patterns of behavior and are acquired in the same way in which normal behavior is acquired. These patterns are the results of defective upbringing, faulty environment, improper models of imitation, and emotionally traumatic experiences of life.

A schizophrenic seeking to escape reality may learn to withdraw into a private world of fantasy and social isolation; he feels safer in his private world or in his state of regression. Schizophrenic withdrawal often represents an avoidance of threatening interpersonal relationships, criticism, and failure. Family environment plays an important role in the development of schizophrenic behavior. The improper relationships prevailing in familial situations, particularly between the mother and father, on one hand, and between parents and the child, on the other, may provide sufficient ground for the development of schizophrenia.

In many cases, the behavior of mothers toward their children may be considered a sufficient cause. One such factor occurs when the mother's nonverbal behavior does not match her verbal behavior. She may appear to be rejecting, stressing the child's independence, and at the same time, may show affection, overprotection, and a self-sacrificing attitude. This "double bind" dilemma, coupled with discord between parents, may result in an irrational and maladaptive behavior of the offspring. Consequently, a child may learn:

- To avoid close interpersonal relationships
- Improper emotional behavior
- Indecisiveness and suspicious nature
- Thought disorders

All such learning patterns in early life may gradually develop into schizophrenic behavior.

Stress situations at any stage, in early or later life, may be considered important precipitating factors for causing schizophrenia. In a genetically predisposed brain and nervous system, stress events trigger biochemical and metabolic changes that result in schizophrenic symptoms. The stresses (the miseries of one's life in their sociocultural context) cause abnormality in the patterns of interpersonal relationships. They also cause feelings of inferiority, frustration, tension, anxiety, and fearful attitude in the individual, who may lose confidence in his abilities, isolate himself, and become suspicious of everything in his environment, and may learn to attack others in imaginary self-defense.

In conclusion, it can be said that genetic influences are a necessary, but not sufficient cause, for the development of schizophrenia. What is acquired as a predisposition to the disorder in the form of genes and biological structure is further subjected to environmental influences. Difficult early childhood experiences and family situations coupled with the stress events of later life may act as causative and precipitating factors in the development of schizophrenic behavior. The likelihood of an individual becoming schizophrenic depends upon the magnitude or degree of the genetic predisposition (heredity) and stress (environment).

Treatment of Schizophrenia

Schizophrenic reactions, besides being a learned behavior, have a hereditary and biological base. The treatment of this disorder, therefore, involves physical as well as psychological methods. No time should be lost in commencing treatment, as delay may leave the patient schizophrenic forever.

Physical methods involve the use of insulin coma therapy, electric shock, psychosurgery, and chemical therapy—that is, the use of tranquilizers, energizers, and anti-anxiety drugs. In view of the risks involved, insulin coma therapy is rarely used. Psychosurgery is also rarely performed on schizophrenics unless all other available forms of treatment have failed. Physical treatment is usually performed through medication (use of drugs). It is often supplemented by electroconvulsive therapy (ECT) for better results. However, ECT is reserved for cases where drugs are not successful, or for patients who are particularly agitated or distressed. Since schizophrenia is a disorder of arousal, drug therapy works well, as most of the drugs such as phenothiazines, butyrophenones, raw-wolffian alkaloids, trifluoperazine (stelazine), diazepam (valium), and other tranquilizers decrease arousal.

It is to be remembered that the principal characteristic of schizophrenic behavior is withdrawal. It follows that the principal ingredient in its psychological treatment should therefore be relationship. The classical form of psychoanalytically oriented psychotherapy should not be used. The removal of defenses and use of uncovering techniques involve great risk of precipitating overt schizophrenia in previously borderline or latent cases. Individual and group psychotherapy may work well with schizophrenics if the personal relationships between the patients and the therapist are properly established. The therapist has to win the confidence of his patient and should try to remove the suspicion and distrust amidst the patient's interpersonal relations. The patient must trust and like the therapist and not fear him. At times the schizophrenic may attempt to hurt the therapist merely on the assumption that he wishes to destroy him (as he has been hurt in other relationships). In such a delicate situation, a good therapist must exercise patience and tolerate the hostility of the patient without fear or counter-hostility. Persons who care for the treatment of schizophrenics should always remember that schizophrenics are, after all, human beings. Like normal persons, they respond negatively to punitive treatment and positively to warmth and understanding. They should be sympathetically understood and, as far as possible, their ideas and beliefs should never be challenged, but they should be gradually made to come to terms with reality.

To Sum Up

Schizophrenia Spectrum and other Related Disorders lead all psychoses, in terms of their severity and potential to become injurious to the self and others. The term schizophrenia means splitting of the mind. Accordingly, schizophrenia spectrum and other psychotic disorders represent the group of psychotic disorders in which people experience fundamental disturbances in relationships and in emotional and intellectual processes. For the purpose of diagnosis as well as treatment, the schizophrenic disorders may be sub-divided into four major types: (i) *Simple schizophrenia* (characterized by an attitude of indifference, or in advanced stages by extreme apathy), (ii) *Hebephrenic schizophrenia* (representing withdrawal in an extreme form), (iii) *Catatonic schizophrenia* (diagnosed mainly by the patient's behavior fluctuating between stuporous depression and wild excitement), and (iv) *Paranoid schizophrenia* (diagnosed mainly by the disorders of thought content involving systematic delusions and hallucinations, frequently of a persecutory nature).

The likelihood of an individual becoming schizophrenic depends upon the magnitude or degree of their genetic predisposition (heredity) and their stress (environment). The treatment of schizophrenics involves the use of physical means (drugs and ECT) as well as psychological methods (psychotherapies based on building relationships).

Bipolar and Related Disorders (Mood or Affective Disorders)

Affective disorders of psychotic origin are characterized by severe disturbances of mood (or affect, as the emotional state is known technically). The patient is either excessively elated and high in spirits (manic state) or excessively depressed and low in spirits (depressive state). Sometimes he may show a combination of ups and downs in mood, resulting in a manic-depressive state. Disturbances in emotional state—that is, the mood—are accompanied by changes in the patient's thought processes. Consequently, the patient may be preoccupied with unpleasant thoughts concerning disease, poverty, unworthiness, or guilt, or may develop ideas of grandeur. He may suffer from misrepresentation of reality, delusions, or hallucinations. Changes in mood and thought contents lead to changes in the patient's behavior. He may show signs of abnormal overactivity, sometimes harming others or himself.

Schizophrenic and Affective Disorders

In spite of much overlapping of symptoms, the differences between schizophrenic and affective disorders are:

(i) In schizophrenia, there is a complete retreat from reality. The patient adopts it as a means for his adjustment. On the other hand, in affective disorders, the individual appears to be desperately trying to do something about the situation. The reaction is that of fighting, as seen in manic states. Even in depression, there may be an element of aggression.

(ii) Schizophrenic disorders are more frequent than affective disorders. The percentage of schizophrenic patients entering mental hospitals is three to four times more than patients with affective disorders.

(iii) Patients with affective disorders are more extroverted and less withdrawn than schizophrenics.

(iv) A large percentage of affective disorder patients are married. In contrast, most schizophrenics never marry.

(v) In comparison to affective disorder patients, schizophrenics remain hospitalized for a long period of time. The possibility of their improvement is much less certain than for manic-depressives.

(vi) Affective disorders are more common in women than in men, while most schizophrenics are found to be men.

Classification of Affective Disorders

According to the DSM-II (APA, 1968), affective disorders may be classified into three categories:

- Manic disorder
- Depressive disorder
- Bipolar affective disorder (Manic-depressive disorder)

1. Manic disorder: Manic disorder or mania is associated with the elation of mood and excessive excitement. The patient is high in spirits, overactive, and bursting with energy. Manic behavior is of three degrees: hypomania, acute mania, and hyper-acute or delirious mania. *Hypomania* is a relatively mild form of excitement that manifests itself through a state of apparent happiness coupled with unusual restlessness or nervousness. An individual suffering from hypomania is found doing something at high speed. For example, in conversation,

he speaks rapidly or engages himself in drumming with his fingers, or keeps moving his feet while others are talking. The patient appears quite friendly, self-confident, and energetic. His thoughts are usually on pleasant topics or wish-fulfilling fantasies. While the depressed patient has ideas of unworthiness, the patient with hypomania has ideas of grandeur. Instead of worrying about illness, he denies the fact that he is currently ill. Similarly, instead of remaining within his means, he is liable to spend lavishly. All seems to be going well with such individuals. But overactivity, excitement, high spirits, and ideas of grandeur may compel this individual to behave foolishly and impulsively. This is so because the patient is out of touch with reality. He must therefore be saved from the stage when he starts cursing himself for his behavior and being frustrated by excessive irritations, leading to acute stages of this disease.

Acute mania is a more severe degree of manic disorder. While hospitalization is rarely needed for persons suffering from hypomania, the acute manic may be a case for hospital care when restlessness or excitement is more marked and elation more extreme. There is a quickening of thought process, speech, and motor excitement. The patient is extremely gay and confident. As a result of his overconfidence and excitement, he loses the little self-control that he has and becomes unfriendly, uncooperative, insensitive, careless (even of his appearance and surroundings), irritable, vulgar, aggressive, and even assaultive to others. He resents any form of restraint or criticism and wants to have his own way. He frequently has delusions and hallucinations, usually of the grandeur type for maintaining his feeling of self-importance.

Hyperacute or delirious mania is the most extreme form of manic disorder. The patient becomes very restless and excited. He experiences hallucinations and delusions of both persecution and grandeur and loses all contact with reality. In his wild excitement, the patient may shout and laugh constantly, tear his clothes, and is likely to become dangerous both to himself and others. He, then, must be kept isolated in a room.

2. *Depressive disorder:* Depression is the polar opposite of mania. The patient remains in low spirits, and feels discouraged and sad. He loses his interest in things around him and may even neglect his appearance and bodily care. The patient's movements become slow. He may either sit doing nothing or even remain in bed in a form of stupor ignoring his surroundings and need for food and hygiene. There is a marked retardation of thought processes, and he has difficulty summoning enough energy to think. He talks slowly and hesitantly or not at all. By contrast, some patients with severe depression may also show signs of agitation. They pace up and down restlessly wringing their hands in despair. Agitation and retardation have some common elements also. The element of anger (rage) is likely to be present in both as the depressed individual may express hostility inwardly and outwardly. The other common feature exhibited through retarded or agitated behavior is a severe lack of useful energy. Loss of appetite, loss of weight, and constipation are common. Sexual desire tends to diminish and the patient is likely to become frigid or impotent. The patient suffers from insomnia. Early morning wakefulness is a characteristic found in severe forms of depressive disorder.

Depressive disorder also involves delusions and hallucinations usually associated with feelings of guilt. The patient may hear voices accusing him of sins that he has committed. Ideas related to disease, unworthiness, and poverty are also found. The patient may be preoccupied with disease and retains his convictions despite medical examination. Feelings of depersonalization are colored by the mood in depressive illness. Declarations like "my mind is dead," "my legs have been turned to lead," "my liver has been taken away," often reflect the state of affective disorder in individuals. Another common feature of depressive disorder is a loss of confidence and a pessimistic outlook. The world looks gloomy for the patients and nothing gives delight. The profound helplessness and ideas of unworthiness may lead to suicidal attempts or the passive contemplation of suicide.

Subtypes of depressive disorder: Based on the degree of severity of the symptoms, depressive disorder may be classified under three subheads: (i) mild (simple), (ii) acute, and (iii) depressive stupor.

Mild or simple depression characterizes the initial stage of the disorder. In *acute depression,* the symptoms characterizing depression are more marked and reach their peak in depressive stupor. *Depressive stupor* is the most extreme form of depressive reaction, where the patient is unresponsive, lies motionless, and usually requires forced feeding. While a mild depressive requires no hospitalization and is often treated as an outpatient, an acute depressive needs hospitalization and supervision for guarding against suicide attempts. In the stupor stage, the need for looking after the patient becomes pronounced and the treatment becomes most difficult.

BIPOLAR AFFECTIVE DISORDER (MANIC-DEPRESSIVE DISORDER): This category of affective disorder involves reactions that are neither manic nor depressive, but a blend of the two, with the mood of elation (excitement and overactivity) accompanying morbid ideas and despair. The classic signs of manic-depressive illness as suggested by J.H. Price (1972:57) are listed as follows:

(i)   Sudden, unexplained, often profound changes in mood to either sadness or elation, with no degree-by-degree shift.
(ii)   The illness occurs without any appropriate external stimulus.
(iii)   Depression is at its worst in the early morning.
(iv)   When ill, the patient is out of touch with reality. At such times one cannot reason with him.
(v)   The manic phase has the appropriate characteristics—ecstasy, euphoria, flight of ideas, overactivity, and expansiveness.
(vi)   In a depressive episode, patients often resign from their jobs or may give up all their possessions.
(vii)   The illness is known to respond to electroconvulsive therapy.
(viii) Manic-depressive psychosis is classically a genetic illness, and inheritance follows the dominant single autosomal gene.
(ix)   The additional clinical features are somatic delusions and vague hypochondriacal complaints such as, "My bowels are blocked, I have not defecated for years."
(x)   The major risk of the illness is suicide, particularly in the early morning when the patient has no one with whom he may share his problems.

In their behavioral functioning, people with bipolar disorders experience extreme states of mania and depression typically occurring during distinct periods of days to weeks, called mood episodes, proving quite damaging to them and others in their interactions.

For their diagnosis and treatment, bipolar and related disorders are further categorized as: bipolar I, bipolar II, and cyclothymic disorder.

Bipolar I Disorder represents that form or type of bipolar and related disorders in which the state of manic behavior in the form of acute and hyperacute mania dominates the scene. People with bipolar I disorder thus experience extremely excited and erratic behavior with manic "up" periods that last at least a week and may be so severe that one needs medical care. It may be followed by a neutral mood or, more commonly, with extreme "down" periods of depressive moods lasting at least two weeks.

Bipolar II Disorder represents that form or type of bipolar and related disorders in which the afflicted individual is diagnosed with having at least one major depressive episode and also at least one hypomanic episode. People may return to their usual functioning between these episodes. In this way, in this disorder one also has erratic highs and lows, but it not as extreme as in bipolar I.

Cyclothymic Disorder represents a milder form of bipolar disorder in people. They may experience many mood swings with hypomania and depressive (ups and down) symptoms that occur frequently but with less severe symptoms than are found in bipolar I and II disorders.

Causes and treatment of affective disorders: A number of studies have established that mania and depression, either separately or combined, are more frequently encountered in families than schizophrenia. But this is not sufficient reason for providing a genetic basis for affective disorders. The possibility of learning this type of behavior as a consequence of environmental influences from early childhood cannot be eliminated. However, recent researches in this field have helped in establishing the genetic and biochemical factors responsible for affective disorders.

Apart from genetic and biochemical conditions, psychological factors appear to be by far the most significant in the development of affective disorders. Affective reactions are the learned reaction patterns that an individual adopts to cope with his adjustment and the satisfaction of his basic needs. For example, when a child learns that his depressed state catches attention and brings sympathy and support from friends and relatives, he adopts depression as a preferred pattern of behavior. Early life experiences and stressful events of the later years often trigger incidences of the affective disorder. Guilty feelings, lack of love and affection, frustrations, and situations giving rise to conflicts, tensions, and stresses all produce hostility which may compel an individual either to seek its outward expression or inward sufferings, as found in most affective psychoses.

The treatment of affective psychosis involves both physical as well as psychological methods. Electroconvulsive therapy and medication constitute the physical methods of treatment. In depressive disorder, antidepressant drugs (mostly tricyclic antidepressants) are widely used, while the use of tranquilizers is recommended for manic disorder. In the agitated type of depression, a combination of tranquilizing and antidepressant drugs is sometimes useful.

In psychological methods of treatment of depressive disorders, psychotherapies like supportive therapy, insight-oriented therapy, and listening therapy may be effectively used.

In the case of mania, neither supportive nor insight-oriented therapy works well. Hospitalization is the first need for such patients. A well-organized psychological approach known as management of the interpersonal relationship between the therapist and the patient has been found useful in the treatment of manic patients.

To Sum Up

Bipolar and Related Disorders (Affective or mood disorders) represent those psychological disorders in which people are found to experience changes in their mood and ability to function to a great degree, in a bipolar way—traveling from one extreme to another extreme, from a positive state (known as mania) to a negative state (known as depression). While in the state of mania, they experience elation of mood and excessive excitement, the state of depression, on the other hand, is marked with feelings of discouragement and sadness. The bipolar and related disorders for their diagnosis and treatment are further categorized as: bipolar I, bipolar II, and cyclothymic disorders.

In view of the latest researches, the genetic and biochemical factors contribute significantly to causing affective or mood disorders. However, in this concern, psychological factors appear to be by far the most significant in the development of affective disorders. Somehow the affective reactions are the learned reaction patterns that an individual adopts to cope with his adjustment and satisfaction of his basic needs. The treatment of patients suffering from affective disorders usually involves physical as well as psychological methods.

Review Questions

1. What do you understand by the term psychoses or psychotic disorders? Discuss and point out the characteristic features of such disorders.
2. What are Schizophrenia spectrum and other related disorders? Discuss their nature, causation, and methods of treatment.
3. Throw light on the nature and impact of various types of schizophrenia, known as Simple, Hebephrenic, Catatonic, and Paranoid schizophrenia.
4. What are bipolar and related disorders (Mood or affective disorders)? Throw light on their meaning and nature.
5. What are schizophrenic and affective disorders? Differentiate between them.
6. Discuss the meaning and nature of the different types of affective disorders, known as manic, depressive, and manic-depressive disorders.
7. Throw light on the nature of manic behavior occurring in the shape of hypomania, acute mania, and hyper-acute or delirious mania.
8. Discuss depressive disorder occurring in the shape of mild or simple depression, acute depression, and depressive stupor.
9. Describe the meaning and nature of manic-depressive disorder along with its classic behavioral signs or symptoms.
10. Throw light on the nature and impact of the manic-depressive disorders classified as Bipolar I disorder, Bipolar II disorder, and Cyclothymic disorder.
11. Discuss in detail the causes and treatment of affective disorders.

References

American Psychiatric Association (1968), *Diagnostic and statistical manual of mental disorders, DSM-II* (2nd ed.), Washington, DC: American Psychiatric Association.

American Psychiatric Association (2013), *Diagnostic and statistical manual of mental disorders* (5th ed.), Washington, DC: American Psychiatric Association.

American Psychiatric Association (2022), *Diagnostic and statistical manual of mental disorders: DSM-5-TR*, Washington, DC: American Psychiatric Association.

Coleman, J. C. (1970), *Abnormal psychology and modern life*, Bombay: D.B. Taraporewala & Sons.

Price, J. H. (1972), *Psychiatric investigations*, London: Butterworths.

Thorpe, L. P., & Katz, B. (1948), *The psychology of abnormal behaviour*, New York, NY: The Ronald Press Company.

World Health Organization (WHO) (2010), *The ICD-10 classification of mental and behavioural disorders: Clinical descriptions and diagnostic guidelines* (10th ed.), Geneva: World Health Organization.

World Health Organization (WHO) (2022), *ICD-11 for mortality and morbidity statistics* (version: 02/2022), https://icd.who.int/browse11/l-m/en

Chapter 11

Neurodevelopmental Disorders

Learning Objectives

After going through this chapter, you will be able to:

- Understand the meaning and nature of Neurodevelopmental disorders
- Define the term mental retardation and throw light on its meaning, nature, and characteristics.
- Discuss mental retardation or deficiency in its various forms—mild, moderate, severe, and profound.
- Throw light on the common clinical types of mental retardation known as Down syndrome, cretinism, microcephaly, hydrocephaly, phenylketonuria (PKU), and amaurotic idiocy.
- Discuss the causes of mental retardation and treatment measures taken for it.
- Define the term ADHD.
- Know about the diagnosis of ADHD based on the criteria laid down by the APA.
- Discuss the causes of ADHD and throw light on its treatment measures.
- Define the term autism.
- Discuss how autistics behave in their environmental situations.
- Tell about the diagnosis and identification of autism in light of the criteria laid down by the APA.
- Throw light on the underlying causes and treatment measures for autism.
- Define the term learning disabilities, and throw light on its meaning and concept.
- Discuss dyslexia along with its various forms and types.
- Discuss dyscalculia and its various forms and types.
- Throw light on the measures taken for the treatment of dyslexia and dyscalculia.

What are Neurodevelopmental Disorders?

The term neurodevelopmental disorders is used for the type of mental disorders affected individuals experience mental malfunctioning that is essentially developmental—developed among them during the developmental period of their early childhood years.

DOI: 10.4324/9781003398325-11

The DSM-5 provided by the APA (2013) has named Neurodevelopmental disorders as one of the prevalent categories of mental disorders. It also lists the types of mental disorders falling into this category. In this chapter, we would like to throw light on some of the important ones known as Mental

> **Neurodevelopmental Disorders**
>
> The type of mental disorders in which one experiences mental malfunctioning that developed in him during the developmental period.

retardation, ADHD, Autism, and Learning disabilities. Let us engage in discussion about these one by one.

Mental Retardation

Meaning and Definition

This disorder is also referred to as mental deficiency or mental subnormality. Although it is not associated with any specific illness yet, it certainly affects the development and functioning of the mind and behavior of the affected person. It is, in fact, an arrested or incomplete development of the brain beginning usually at birth and leading to a diminution of intellectual powers

> **Mental Retardation**
>
> A condition or state of retarded or deficient development of one's mind or brain coming to light through his subnormal intellectual functioning or inadequate adaptation to the environment.

relative to one's chronological age. Some of the definitions explaining the meaning of the term mental retardation or mental deficiency are reproduced ahead.

Page (1976:354): Mental deficiency is a condition of subnormal mental development, present at birth or early childhood and characterized mainly by limited intelligence and social inadequacy.

Rosen et al. (1972:356): Mental retardation refers to a chronic condition present from birth or early childhood which is characterized by both impaired intellectual functioning as measured by standardized tests and impaired adaptation to the daily demands of the individual's social environment.

American Association on Mental Retardation (1983): Mental retardation refers to significantly sub-average intellectual functioning existing concurrently with deficits in adaptive behavior and manifested during the developmental period (Grossman, 1983, p. 11).

British Mental Deficiency Act (1929): Mental retardation is a condition of arrested or incomplete development of mind existing before the age of 18 years whether arising from inherent causes or induced by disease on injury (cited by Shanmugam, 1981:197–198)

All these definitions reveal that:

(i)   Mental retardation is a condition or state of mind.
(ii) It is not a disease or illness of the mind.

(iii) It is related to the subnormal development of the mind or brain.

(iv) It is also related to one's inadequate adjustment or adaptation with the environment.

(v) The deficiency may be observed at birth or in early childhood.

(vi) Both inherent and external factors may cause mental retardation.

In this way, mental retardation or deficiency may be considered a retarded or deficient growth and development of one's mind or brain, exhibiting subnormal intellectual capacities or inadequate adaptation to one's environment on account of inherent or external factors.

Classification of Mental Retardation or Mental Deficiency

From the very beginning, right from early childhood, developing children may be found to be inflicted with one or the other types of mental deficiency and subnormality. On the basis of intelligence tests, individuals suffering from such deficiency or subnormality were previously classified as dull, morons, imbeciles, or idiots. However, the criteria for classifying the mentally retarded or deficient on the basis of their IQ has been replaced by the criterion of Adaptive behavior.

This criterion describes one's adaptive behavior expected of his age and cultural group, in two ways for the required assessment, namely (i) the degree to which the individual is able to function and maintain himself independently, and (ii) the degree to which he meets satisfactorily the culturally imposed demands of personal and social responsibility. Attempts have been made to devise measures for the assessment of deficiency in adaptive behavior through the Vineland Social Maturity Scale, the Adaptive Behavior Scale (AAMD), and the Maxfield Buckholz Social Maturity Scale.

The consideration of deficiency in adaptive behavior along with very low scores on an intelligence test has resulted in the development of an altogether new classification of subnormality. The terms moron, imbecile, and idiot are now completely avoided for determining one's level of retardation. The new terminology in terms of obtained IQ on different test scales is represented in Table 11.1.

In view of typical subnormal intelligence and deficient adaptive behavior, these categories are described below.

Mild retardation: A majority of approximately 85% of retarded people belong to this category. In adult life, these individuals attain intellectual levels comparable to that of the average 10-year-old child. Their social adjustment may be compared with that of an adolescent. Here, too, they lack the innovative and vigorous nature of normal adolescents. They show signs of delayed development early in life, and learn to walk, talk, feed, and

Table 11.1 Level of Retardation

Level of retardation	IQ Standford Binet	Wechsler scales
Profound	Under 20	Under 25
Severe	20–35	25–39
Moderate	36–51	40–54
Mild	52–67	55–69

toilet themselves a year later than the average. They may be identified in schools as slow learners and are frequently required to repeat early grades. Speech disturbances are common among them.

In comparison with normal individuals, the mildly retarded exhibit immature behavior, have poor control over their impulses, lack judgment, and fail to anticipate the consequence of their actions. Their sexual behavior and adjustment, despite normal sexual development and fertility, is unpredictable, and may lead to a variety of problems and difficulties.

Mildly retarded individuals generally do not show any organic pathology and require little supervision. They are considered to be educable. With early diagnosis, parental assistance, and aid of special classes, they can be expected to reach a reasonable degree of educational achievement and to make an adequate social and economic adjustment in the community.

Moderate mental retardation: Approximately 10% of mentally retarded people belong to this category. In adult life, these individuals attain intellectual levels similar to that of the average six-year-old child. Physically they appear clumsy, suffer from motor incoordination, and present an affable, dull, and somewhat vacuous personality. As a result of their inadequate development and deficient capacities and abilities, they are regarded as "trainable" instead of being "educable," like the mildly retarded. From early infancy or childhood, they show signs of retardation in almost all areas of development, and though they manage to speak, their rate of learning is slow. They are unable to do work that requires initiative, originality, abstract thinking, memory, or consistent attention, and cannot be expected to acquire the basic skills of reading and writing.

However, with early diagnosis, parental help, and adequate training and support, most moderately retarded people can achieve considerable independence in all spheres of life. Nevertheless, they require constant supervision and support and may need institutionalization depending on their general level of adaptive behavior.

Severe mental retardation: Nearly 3.5% of all retarded individuals—mostly children and adolescents—belong to this category. They never attain an intellectual level greater than that of the average four-year-old child. The mortality rate due to high susceptibility to disease is quite high among these individuals. They are severely retarded in development from birth or infancy onward and show severe motor and speech retardation. Sensory defects and motor handicaps are common. The majority of them display relatively little interest in their surroundings and many of them never master even the necessary skills and functions like feeding and dressing themselves, or bladder and bowel control.

People with severe mental retardation are neither "educable" nor "trainable," and the majority of them remain dependent on others throughout their lives. They need the care and supervision of others, with a great need for institutionalization. They may benefit from proper care, timely treatment, and specialized training and management of their own physical well-being, as well as doing manual labor.

Profound mental retardation: This group makes up 1.5% of the total mentally retarded population. It is characterized by the most severe symptoms of mental retardation. The individuals belonging to this category never attain in adult life an intellectual level greater than that of the average two-year-old child. They are severely deficient both in their intellectual capacities and adaptive behavior. The symptoms associated with them are retarded growth, physical deformities, pathology of the central nervous system, mutism, severe speech disturbances, motor incoordination, deafness, and convulsive seizures. They are unable to protect themselves against common dangers and are unable to manage their own affairs nor satisfy their physical needs. Their life span, as a result of their low resistance, is short. Such individuals are completely dependent on others and need the care and supervision given to an infant. Essentially, they need to be institutionalized as their condition may deteriorate on account of the biased attitudes of the parents and the stressful demands of their environment.

Common Clinical Types of Mental Retardation

Knowledge of the well-known categories of mental deficiency or retardation based on a number of clinical symptoms and syndromes is useful in the identification, treatment, and care of the retardates.

Mongolism: The mental deficient whose facial characteristics bear a superficial resemblance to members of the mongolian race are classified as mongols. The retardation in them ranges from moderate to severe (IQ approximately 20–50).

Mongoloids tend to be short in stature with small round heads, an abnormally short neck, thumbs and fingers, with slanting almond-shaped eyes, and short flat noses. They usually have a small mouth and fissured, dry lips and tongue. Their hands and feet are broad and clumsy, and they have a deep voice. Motor coordination is awkward. They are handicapped in any learning or training but most of them can learn self-help skills, acceptable social behavior, and routine manual skills.

The causes of mongolism are faulty heredity (possible chromosomal anomalies), and metabolic factors (glandular imbalance often involving pituitary glands). But once it occurs, it is irreversible. There is no effective treatment or workable preventive measures.

Cretinism: This mental deficiency (also known as congenital hypothyroidism) ranging from moderate to severe retardation results from thyroid deficiency. The severity of the disorder depends on the age at which the deficiency occurs as well as the degree and duration of the deficiency.

The physical symptoms in the case of persons suffering from cretinism consist of a dwarf-like, thick-set body, coarse and thick skin, short and stubby extremities, abundant hair of wiry consistency, and thick eyelids that give a sleepy appearance. Other pronounced symptoms include a broad, flat nose, large and flabby ears, a protruding abdomen, and failure to mature sexually. Early timely treatment in the form of injection of thyroid gland extract produces favorable results in all cases except those of long standing where the damage to the nervous system and to general physical development is beyond repair.

Microcephaly: It refers to the mental deficiency associated with failure of the cranium to attain normal size on account of the impaired development of the brain. The microcephalic person has an unusually small head that rarely exceeds a circumference of 17 inches, as compared with the normal of approximately 22 inches. In addition, he is short-statured with a cone-shaped skull and receding chin and forehead. Depending upon the degree of severity of mental retardation, microcephalics fall into the profound, severe, and moderate categories of mental retardation. Both genetic as well as non-genetic factors impair the development of the brain and thus cause microcephaly. There is no proper medical treatment available for microcephaly if there has been impaired brain development.

Hydrocephaly: This mental deficiency results from the accumulation of an unusually large amount of cerebrospinal fluid within the cranium, causing damage to the brain and enlargement of the skull. The degree of mental retardation in this disorder varies from moderate to profound depending upon the extent of neural damage, which, in turn, depends upon the age of onset, the duration, and the size of the skull. The chief symptom of hydrocephaly consists of the gradual increase in the size of the skull. The causes seem to be genetic as well as non-genetic. In some cases, the disorder is present at birth, or the head begins to enlarge soon after birth on account of prenatal disturbances. More often, the disorder develops during infancy or early childhood on account of intracranial neoplasm or acute inflammatory brain disease. An early diagnosis and proper surgical treatment show favorable results in checking further damage to the brain tissue. However, the advanced acute stage does not respond to any treatment and eventually results in death.

Phenylketonuria (PKU): This disorder has a genetic base and is assumed to be transmitted through a recessive gene carrying a metabolic disturbance. As a result, the child at birth lacks an enzyme needed to break down phenylalanine, an amino acid found in protein foods. Consequently, there is an abnormal accumulation of phenylalanine in the blood, causing damage to the brain tissue.

The symptoms such as vomiting, a peculiar musty odor, infantile eczema and seizures, motor incoordination, signs of mental retardation, and neurological manifestations relating to severe brain damage are found to be common with this disorder. However, the diagnosis of the disorder is primarily made on the basis of the presence of phenyl pyruvic acid in the urine. The treatment of PKU depends on early detection. A special diet, low in phenylalanine, is recommended for affected infants. Timely treatment helps in restraining or preventing brain damage.

Amaurotic idiocy: It is a rare hereditary disorder of fat metabolism transmitted as a simple recessive characteristic. It is never transmitted directly from patient to offspring because death generally occurs before puberty. The only mode of transmission is through the mating of persons who, although free of overt symptoms, are carriers of the defective genes. This disorder has been described to occur in two different forms—infantile and juvenile—depending on the age at which it occurs. The major symptoms of this disorder include muscular weakness, inability to maintain normal posture, loss in the ability to grasp objects, visual difficulties leading to progressive blindness, seizures, and neurological manifestations.

Infantile amaurotic idiocy, also known as Tay-Sachs disease, is common among infants. This disorder appears at about six months of age and death occurs between the ages of two and three years. Juvenile amaurotic idiocy occurs at five or six years of age and the patient may live up to thirteen years.

Causes of Mental Retardation

It is difficult to postulate standard causes for mental retardation applicable to every case. A number of factors are believed to cause mental retardation, which may be divided into two broad categories:

A. Organic or biological factors
B. Socio-psychological factors

A. Organic or Biological Factors

Causes listed in this broad category are described as follows.

1. Genetic factors: Mental deficiency may be established by genetic factors operative at the time of conception in two ways—either through transmission of some defective genes in the chromosomes of one or both parents, or on account of chromosomal aberrations.

The transmission of defective genes gives rise to many disorders causing mental deficiency. Mental retardation or deficiency attributable to a dominant gene is very rare because the persons affected are generally incapable of reproduction. It is often the result of the pairing of two defective recessive genes. When defective recessive genes are paired, as in PKU, the production of an enzyme, necessary for an important metabolic process, is usually disturbed. This, in turn, affects the development of the embryo and causes mental deficiency. In some cases, like Tay-Sachs disease, mental deficiency may also be transmitted by the pairing of single recessive genes.

Several chromosomal anomalies determine mental retardation at the time of conception. Down syndrome or mongolism is one such disorder that is said to be caused by chromosomal aberrations. The majority of mongoloid children are found to have 47 chromosomes instead of the usual 46. The number of chromosomes increases as a result of the tripling of chromosomes 21 (during the fertilization of the egg, the chromosomes of pair 21 become three instead of two). Another example of chromosomal abnormality is Klinefelter's syndrome in which an extra X chromosome is usually at fault. This disorder occurs only in males and symptoms are usually noticed at puberty when the testes remain small and the boy develops feminine secondary sex characteristics such as enlarged breasts and round hips.

2. Infection: Mental retardation can also be the result of infectious diseases, such as syphilis, rubella (German measles), toxoplasmosis, or encephalitis, which can damage brain tissue and the nervous system, resulting in severe mental deficiency or retardation. If the mother suffers from one or the other of these infectious diseases, she may transmit the infection to the developing fetus. A child at birth or afterward may be infected with diseases that cause lifelong mental subnormality. Encephalitis and meningococcal meningitis cause irreversible brain damage and even death if contracted in infancy or early childhood. Besides directly damaging brain tissues, such infectious diseases may indirectly lead to mental abnormality by causing congenital physical defects such as blindness, deafness, paralysis, and epilepsy.

3. Intoxication: Mental retardation may be caused by intoxication. A number of toxic agents like carbon monoxide, mercury, lead, and various immunological agents like anti-tetanus serum or the use of the smallpox, rabies, and typhoid vaccines may result in brain damage during development after birth. Similarly, large doses of X-rays in radiotherapy in the abdominal region of the pregnant mother, drugs administered to the mother during pregnancy, incompatibility in blood types between mother and fetus, and an overdose of drugs administered to the infant may also lead to toxicity and brain damage.

4. Trauma: Mental retardation may be caused on account of physical damage to the brain in the form of injuries prior to birth, at the time of delivery, or following birth, in the manner as follows.

- Prenatal injuries adversely affect the brain and the nervous system of the fetus. One of the main causes of such damage is asphyxia, which results from oxygen deprivation and consequently causes suffocation of the tissues. It is accounted for by the compression of the umbilical cord which supplies the fetus with blood carrying oxygen and nutrition from the mother. Another example of prenatal injury is the damaging effects of irradiation on the uterus of the pregnant mother.

- Abnormal delivery and birth injuries make for another cause of mental retardation. Difficulties during labor result in damage to the infant's brain. Any abnormal delivery also involves the risk of brain injuries. An abnormal position of the fetus, breech extraction, the use of forceps, and other obstetrical procedures may cause hemorrhage of the brain and thus lead to mental retardation.
- Premature birth exposes the child to an increased risk of brain damage from mechanical trauma and anoxia (the condition associated with changes in the oxygen supply, discussed next). Similarly, post-mature birth also results in an increased risk of anoxia for the child, during the later weeks of pregnancy and childbirth.
- Another birth trauma in the form of anoxia results from delayed breathing of the newborn infant or as a result of anesthetic accidents that may also damage the brain. Anoxia may also occur after birth as a result of cardiac arrest associated with operations, heart attacks, gas poisoning, or near drowning.
- Accidental brain injuries received in infancy, childhood, or later in life, may cause damage to the brain leading to serious mental retardation.

5. *Metabolic and endocrine disorders:* Mental retardation may be caused by various disturbances in the metabolism by which body cells are built up and broken down, and by which energy is made available for their functioning. The chemical errors involving the metabolism of fat may cause Tay-Sachs disease, while disturbed protein metabolism causes PKU. Both these disorders lead to severe mental retardation. Similarly, metabolic disorders like galactosemia, involving an inability to metabolize galactose, and maple syrupurine disease, involving chain amino acids, lead to mental retardation. Several metabolic disorders involving endocrine imbalances may also result in various degrees of mental retardation. Hypothyroidism (usually referred to as cretinism) is one such metabolic disorder.

6. *Tumors:* Mental retardation may be caused by brain damage associated with brain tumors and other new growths. Tuberous sclerosis or epiloia is characterized by numerous nodules and tumors throughout the brain and other parts of the body. A butterfly shaped rash, initially appearing on the face, spreads over a wider area. It may lead to convulsions and mental retardation. Similarly, macrocephaly (large headedness), microcephaly (small headedness), and hydrocephalus (accumulation of an abnormal amount of cerebrospinal fluid in the cranium) are some of the other conditions resulting in mental subnormality that may be caused by tumors.

B. Socio-Psychological Factors

Psychological factors coupled with an adverse sociocultural environment play a leading role in the causation as well as the perpetuation of mental retardation. Children who are denied the satisfaction of their psychological and social needs become oversensitive to psychological stress in the same way as a patient with a vitamin deficiency is susceptible to infection. Deprivation during early childhood, such as lack of adequate mothering and parental care. results in a retarded rate of development.

In an inadequate sociocultural environment, children are deprived of the basic necessities of life for their proper physical, intellectual, emotional, and social development. A poverty-ridden, deprived, crowded, and uncongenial family environment provides sufficient as well as necessary grounds for the germination and perpetuation of mental subnormality. The deprived members tend to marry spouses like themselves and their poverty compels them to suffer. The severe environmental deprivation in the form of physical, cultural, emotional, and intellectual poverty, especially during infancy and childhood, results in the retardation of the child's intellectual development, even when his potential at birth is normal. The child may have difficulty in developing verbal abilities on account of such an unfavorable environment, or may suffer from a lack of emotional and social maturity, and thus may not be able to adapt to the needs of his environment.

In some cases, the failure of the school system has adverse effects. School maladjustment tends to retard the development rate of the child who, once labeled as a slow learner or retarded on the basis of speech, IQ scores, achievement test scores, and observable behavior, becomes subnormal on account of the perpetuation of inferiority feelings and complexes.

Treatment Measures for Mental Retardation

Whatever preventive measures we may adopt, it is neither possible nor feasible to eliminate the possibility of the occurrence of mental retardation. We can neither exercise much control over hereditary influences nor can we avoid accidental hazards and traumas. Moreover, we also feel handicapped in controlling the evil influences of defective sociocultural environments, and are unable to overcome the deficiency of psychological deprivations. Therefore, cases of mental retardation are bound to exist and hence, we have to think and plan the treatment and remedial measures for mental retardates.

One thing that should be made clear while seeking treatment of mental retardation is the fact that there is no cure for mental deficiency. Mental retardates are essentially incurable in the sense that they cannot be given more intelligence and made normal. No amount of training or medical care can transform a mental retardate into a normal individual. Mental subnormality should never be confused with the persons who are mentally ill or suffer from a mental disease. In this connection, the observation of Wechsler (1935) is worth quoting:

> Mental deficiency unlike typhoid fever or paralysis is not a disease. A mentally deficient is not a person who suffers from a specific disease process but one who by reasons of intellectual arrest or impairment is unable to cope with his environment to the extent that he needs special care, education and institutionalization.

It will be appropriate to consider the treatment or remedial measures for the adjustment, rehabilitation, and education of the mentally retarded in light of the above observations.

1. *Medical or physical measures:* Mental retardation, to some extent, is said to be a medical problem. The following medical measures may prove helpful in some cases:

    (i) *Cretinism:* This mental retardation resulting from a deficiency in thyroid secretion, if recognized at birth or in its early manifestations, may be corrected or controlled by the institution of thyroid therapy.
    (ii) *Congenital syphilis:* Children infected with congenital syphilis are usually found to be suffering from severe mental subnormality. Early detection and prompt penicillin therapy are found to be helpful in the prevention as well as control of many of the effects of congenital syphilis.

   (iii) *Phenylketonuria (PKU):* On early detection with the help of a simple urine test, PKU, a metabolic disorder causing mental retardation, may be checked or controlled, to a great extent, by placing the infant on a special diet relatively free of phenylalanine found in most protein foods.

   (iv) *Hydrocephalus:* Hydrocephalus, resulting from the accumulation of an abnormal amount of cerebrospinal fluid within the cranium, results in mental retardation. Surgical treatment is found to be very effective in the treatment of this disorder. It is aimed at the reduction of the normal production of cerebrospinal fluid, or the channeling of the fluid by removing obstruction resulting from congenital malformations or post-natal infections.

   (v) *Epileptic seizures:* In the case of patients suffering from epileptic seizures, the administration of anti-convulsant medication may prove helpful in controlling and minimizing intellectual deterioration.

   (vi) *Controlling disturbed behavior:* The administration of tranquilizers proves useful in controlling hyperactive and disturbed behavior among mental retardates.

2. *Psychological treatment;* Often on account of the link between mental subnormality and psychological factors, psychological treatment in the form of individual or group psychotherapy is found to be useful in providing remedial measures for mental retardation. Children can be helped in solving problems of their emotional and social maladjustment and resolving their mental conflicts through psychological measures.

3. *Educating the parents:* Parents can also help in the welfare, care, as well as treatment of the mental retardate. For this purpose, there is a need for proper counseling services for them. Moreover, on account of their emotional involvement, the parents may not realize the shortcomings and deficiencies of their children and waste a lot of time and money in the hope that some magic cure will be found, or the deficiency will be automatically eliminated with the lapse of time. Sometimes, they become disturbed by the responsibilities of looking after their mentally retarded child. Such disappointed, insecure, and guilt-ridden parents begin to demand behavior and intellectual achievement beyond the abilities of the child, who is often abused, snubbed, and punished for no fault of their own. Some parents adopt an overprotective approach in their effort to shield the child from challenging situations and thus make him completely dependent by interfering with the development of whatever abilities or capacities he may have. It is therefore essential that:

   (i) Parents should first realize the truth about their child. They should accept the child's limitations and mental deficiency in the sense that the child cannot be given more intelligence and made normal.

   (ii) Secondly, they should be educated to behave normally with their mentally subnormal child without being overprotective or rejecting the child.

   (iii) Thirdly, the parents should be given training and education for handling the emotional and social adjustment problems of their children. They should never compare their achievements and abilities with their normal siblings or other children in the home and neighborhood. It should be understood that the child should not be unnecessarily criticized or ridiculed by others.

   (iv) Fourthly, they should be educated to provide essential training at home to their mentally retarded child; training the child on how to manage his affairs independently, and encouraging the child to seek his maximum potential are some of the areas where useful education and support can be provided by the parents.

(v)   Finally, the parents should be made to realize that, if needed, there is no harm in sending their children to special schools meant for mental retardates. They are the best place for their education and training.

4. *Provision of special education and training:* It is a cardinal educational as well as psychological error to educate or train mental retardates with normal children. The involved attitude of the parents at home may also interfere with the development of the retarded child. The remedy lies in the provision of special education or training for them. The institutes or boarding schools meant for subnormal children serve a useful purpose in this direction. For better results, special institutes or schools must be managed in view of the following considerations:

(i)   There should be proper grouping and classification of mentally retarded children on the basis of the degree of the severity of their retardation.

(ii)   The "educable" should be educated and the "trainable" should be trained. Those who are neither easily educable nor trainable should be cared for and efforts should be made to train them for managing their essential day-to-day affairs.

(iii) The schools should provide the essential environment for the maximum development of the abilities and capacities of all mental retardates. Curriculum, methods of teaching, and tools for evaluation should be adjusted according to individual needs.

(iv)   There should be a provision for specially trained teachers able to utilize new materials and techniques for their education or training. They should be able to deal with the special problems of these children, understand them sympathetically, and help them to grow with their deficiencies.

(v)   In these schools, greater emphasis should be placed on co-curricular experiences and the children should be provided opportunities for learning the ways of their emotional and social adjustment, imbibing moral virtues, and desirable personal habits.

(vi)   These institutions should have the provision for vocational education and training. The mental retardates should be trained for manual work, crafts, and specialized vocations according to their abilities. The general attitude toward the mentally handicapped needs to be changed. They are not to be pitied, protected, and ridiculed, but to be helped in growing and developing within their strengths and limitations. Their education or training should begin at home. Thereafter special schools or institutions may be involved in their education and training. The society and the state, then, should take responsibility for their rehabilitation and adjustment.

To Sum Up

The term mental retardation stands for a retarded or deficient growth and development of one's mind or brain exhibiting subnormal intellectual capacities or inadequate adaptation to the environment on account of inherent or external factors. On the basis of intelligence tests, the mentally retarded were previously classified on a spectrum of dull, moron, imbecile, and idiot. However, based on the consideration of deficiency in adaptive behavior along with considerably low scores on an intelligence test, they are now classified as individuals with mild, moderate, severe, and profound retardation. We can also classify the mentally retarded on the basis of a number of distinguishable clinical symptoms and syndromes into categories such as mongolism, cretinism, microcephaly, phenylketonuria (PKU), and amaurotic idiocy.

Mental retardation may be the result of organic causes such as factors operative at the time of conception, infection, intoxication, trauma, metabolic and endocrine disorders, and tumors. Besides this, psychological factors coupled with an adverse sociocultural environment are said to play a significant role in the causation as well as the perpetuation of mental retardation.

Treatment regarding mental deficiency involves (i) medical or physical measures, (ii) psychological treatment, (iii) educating the parents, and (iv) provision of special education and training.

Attention-Deficit Hyperactivity Disorder (ADHD)

What is Attention-Deficit Hyperactivity Disorder (ADHD)?

In its simple meaning, as suggested through its naming, Attention-Deficit Hyperactivity Disorder, briefly referred to as ADHD, stands for a type of behavioral disorder characterized by significant deficiencies in one's attention behavior devoid of necessary self-restraint. Various authors and researchers have provided their own conceptions and definitions for the term ADHD. We can take considerable help from their points of view for understanding what ADHD means.

> **Attention-Deficit/ Hyperactivity disorder (ADHD)**
>
> A type of neurodevelopmental disorder or serious behavioral problem of developing children often visible among them in early years of the schooling characterized by lack of attention, hyperactivity, and impulsivity chronic enough for causing a lot of adjustment problems to them in their life functioning.

1. **Barkley (2000:9):** ADHD is a development disorder of self-control. It consists of problem with attention span, impulse control, and activity level. . . . It is not just a temporary state that will be outgrown, a trying but normal phase of childhood. It is not caused by parental failure to discipline or control the child, ant it is not a sign of some sort of inherent "badness" in the child. ADHD is real—a real disorder, a real problem, and often a real obstacle. It can be heartbreaking and nerve-wracking.
2. **Cooper and Bilton (2002:9):** Attention-Deficit/Hyperactivity Disorder (AD/HD) is a medical diagnosis that is applied to children and adults who are experiencing significant behavioral and cognitive difficulties in important aspects of their lives (e.g., in their familial and personal relationships; at school or work). These difficulties can be attributed to problems of impulse control, hyperactivity and inattention. It is believed that these problems are caused primarily by dysfunctions in the frontal lobes of the brain.
3. **Goldstein (1999):** ADHD is characterized by a constellation of problems with inattention, hyperactivity and impulsivity. These problems are developmentally inappropriate and cause difficulty in daily life.

The definitions and views cited above may help us to draw the following conclusions about the meaning and nature of Attention-Deficit Hyperactivity Disorder (ADHD).

- It is a quite chronic behavior or psychological disorder of childhood (usually beginning in the early school years) that may follow them to their adult years, if not diagnosed and treated properly earlier.
- It may cause them to experience significant behavioral and cognitive difficulties in their day-to-day life, schooling, and work situations at the different stages of their life.
- Parents and teachers cannot be blamed for the upsurge of this disorder in children. It is not caused by parental or school failure to discipline or control the child.
- Although what causes ADHD exactly is not known, the researchers believe that it results from deficiencies or dysfunctions of the brain (caused through genetic inheritance or injury to the brain).
- Deficiencies like deficits in certain chemicals called neurotransmitters and dysfunctions of certain lobes of the brain bring impairment to the controlling functions of the brain. This is responsible for making the affected child disabled in terms of self-control.
- Inability in exercising self-control may give birth to three major problems particularly related to inattention, hyperactivity (exhibiting excessive acting out behaviors), and impulsivity (acting without thinking), the very hallmarks or symptoms of ADHD.
- The symptoms of ADHD provide red signals that should be noticed as earliest possible. Its presence in children provides a big challenge to parents and teachers in terms of its control and treatment. If not cared for properly, it may cause unimaginable damage, not only to the affected child, but it also may prove a source of danger to society.

Known in this way, we can draw the following summarized conclusion about the nature and concept of ADHD.

Attention Deficit Hyperactivity disorder (ADHD) refers to a type of behavioral or psychological disorder of childhood often visible in the early years of schooling. It has been found to be caused by biological reasons mainly associated with deficiencies and dysfunctions of the brain, generating a lack of ability to exercise self-control, and causing three major problems—namely inattention, hyperactivity, and impulsivity chronic enough to cause serious difficulties in one or more major life areas—home, school, work or social relationships.

The next example, of an ADHD child named "Danny," may portray exactly what ADHD is.

Danny, a handsome 9-year-old boy, was referred to us because of his difficulties at school and at home. Danny had a great deal of energy and loved playing most sports, especially baseball. Academically, his work was adequate, although his teacher reported that his performance was diminishing and she believed he would do better if he paid more attention in class. Danny rarely spent more than a few minutes on a task without some interruption: he would go up out of his seat, rifle through his desk, and constantly ask questions. His peers were frustrated with him because he was equally impulsive during their interactions: he never finished a game, and in sports he tried to play all positions simultaneously.

At home, Danny was considered a handful. His room was in a constant mess because he became engaged in a game or activity only to drop it and initiate something else. Danny's parents reported that they often scolded him for not carrying out some task, although the reason seemed to be that he forgot what he was doing rather than that he deliberately tried to defy them. They also said that, out of their own frustration, they sometimes grabbed him by the shoulders and yelled "Slow down!" because his hyperactivity drove them crazy.

Adapted from Durand and Barlow (2013:486)

The behavior demonstrated by the child in this example may be helpful in highlighting the important symptoms and characteristics of children suffering from ADHD, such as:

- Having great difficulty attending to tasks, or behaving overactively and impulsively, or both. ADHD often appears very early in life, before the child starts school.
- The symptoms of ADHD often feed into one another. Children who have trouble focusing attention may keep turning from task to task until they end up trying to run in several directions at once. Similarly, children who move constantly may find it hard to attend to tasks or show good judgment.
- In many cases, one of these symptoms stands out much more than the other. About half of the children with ADHD also have learning or communication problems; many perform poorly in school; a number have difficulty interacting with other children, and about 80% misbehave, often quite seriously.
- It is also common for these children to have anxiety or mood problems (Comer, 2015:583).

Diagnosis of ADHD

The diagnosis of ADHD among children is not a simple task. However, for helping us on this account, we may study these objective criteria available in the DSM-5. Let us review them.

Table 11.2 Diagnostic Criteria Prescribed for ADHD by the American Psychiatric Association (APA)

1. Individual presents one or both of the following patterns:
   (a) For six months or more, the individual frequently displays at least six of the following symptoms of inattention, to a degree that is maladaptive and beyond that shown by most similarly aged persons:
   - Unable to properly attend to details, or frequently makes careless errors
   - Finds it hard to maintain attention
   - Fails to listen when spoken to by others
   - Fails to carry out instructions and finish work
   - Disorganized
   - Dislikes or avoids mentally effortful work
   - Loses items that are needed for successful work
   - Easily distracted by irrelevant stimuli
   - Forgets to do many everyday activities

(Continued)

Table 11.2 (Continued)

(b) For six months or more, the individual frequently displays at least six of the following symptoms of hyperactivity and impulsivity, to a degree that is maladaptive and beyond that shown by most similar aged persons:
  • Fidgets, taps hands or feet, or squirms
  • Inappropriately wanders from seat
  • Inappropriately runs or climbs
  • Unable to play quietly
  • In constant motion
  • Talks excessively
  • Interrupts questioners during discussion
  • Unable to wait for turn
  • Barges in on others' activities or conversations.
2. Individual displayed some of the symptoms before 12 years of age
  (i) Individual shows symptoms in more than one setting
  (ii) Individual experiences impaired functioning

Source: American Psychotic Association (2013), *Diagnostic and Statistical Manual of Mental Disorders (5th ed.),* American Psychiatric Association: Washington DC.

Causes of ADHD

ADHD is usually attributed to three types of factors: (i) Neurological or Biological Factors, (ii) Genetic or Hereditary Influences, and (iii) Environmental or Sociocultural factors.

For the neurological or biological factors responsible for causing ADHD, the researchers often name (i) abnormality or dysfunction of the brain (particularly pre-frontal and frontal lobes of the cerebrum, basal ganglia, and cerebellum) and (ii) impairments in neurological functioning (particularly related to the impairment in the functioning of the two transmitters known as Dopamine and Norepinephrine).

Regarding the role of genetic or hereditary influences in causing ADHD, Barkley (1988) on the basis of research evidence, has claimed that heredity accounts for about 80% of children with ADHD.

Besides the genetic and neurological factors causing ADHD, environmental factors—the negative and damaging happenings in one's physical and sociocultural environment—may be seen to work as germinators as well nourishing or inflaming agents of developing ADHD among children.

Treatment of ADHD

The more commonly used approaches adopted currently for treating ADHD consist of the use of Medical or Drug therapy, Behavioral therapy, and/or a combination of both.

Medical or Drug Therapy: The medications that seem to be most effective in the treatment of people with ADHD are a class of drugs known as stimulants (stimulating or activating neurological functioning). The most common type of stimulant used for ADHD is *methylphenidate* (trade name Ritalin). The other useful stimulants are Adderall, Concerta, Dexedrine, Dextrostat, Metadate, Cylert, and Focalin.

In addition to the aforementioned stimulant medications, non-stimulation medications can also be used for normalizing the executive functions of the brain. A widely used medication is called Strattera, or atomoxetine. Administered once per day, this medication is proving quite helpful in controlling the levels of norepinephrine (a type of neurotransmitter other than Dopamine believed to play a role in ADHD). The combination of the stimulants (primarily working on dopamine) and non-stimulant (mainly working on norepinephrine) may thus be a better formula often prescribed by physicians for children. However, medication as a treatment of ADHD should not be used at the first sign of a behavioral problem, and if needed (after the proper recommendation of a physician/neurologist), these should be always used in combination with other behavioral management techniques.

Behavior Therapy: The techniques involving behavior therapy are aimed to decrease or reduce the occurrence of inappropriate behavior with an equal emphasis on increasing the probability of the child's appropriate or desirable behavior. For this purpose a number of behavior management strategies may be followed, such as the following.

1. In one such strategy (known as token money or point receiving strategy), the desired behaviors that a child needs to exhibit on his part are brought into his awareness by noting them in his diary or putting them on a chart. He is to earn points (say five) or a token (say a card) for each of his good/desired behaviors, but also has the risk of losing the same (the five points or token) if he behaves otherwise. After a fixed interval of say a day or week, the points or tokens left with the child may be exchanged for rewards (things that have value to the child).
2. In another strategy, the phenomenon of "shaping of behavior" (a technique of behavior modification through operant conditioning) may be utilized for producing appropriate behaviors and reducing or eliminating inappropriate ones. In this technique, one behavior or its component is chosen as the target behavior. The child is told clearly about the type of behavior or behavioral elements expected from him (as an acceptable or desirable behavior). Whenever the child demonstrates the desired behavior or provides a clue for stepping up to the desired behavior, a suitable reinforcement in terms of earning points or any reward (valuable for him) is given and the process (emitting good behavior and responding to it through reinforcement/reward) is continued until the desired behavior *in toto* is learned by the child. In between, the undesirable responses are ignored. In doing so, the principle "Don't mind the small errors but don't ignore the right step no matter how insignificant it looks" should always be followed.

As a third approach for treating ADHD, a combination of behavioral and drug therapies is also desirable because, according to research, children who receive both treatments require lower levels of medication, meaning, of course, that they are less subject to the medication's undesired effects.

To Sum Up

Attention-Deficit/Hyperactivity Disorder (ADHD) refers to a neuro-behavioral disorder of childhood often visible before the age of six or seven through the symptoms of excessive inattentiveness, hyperactivity, and impulsivity (often also accompanied by problems of deficient and aggressive behavior).

The children themselves are not responsible for learning or developing these symptoms in their behavior. The disorder is caused by some dysfunction in their brain and neurological functioning. In turn, it makes them lose control over their ability for inhibition or self-regulation, resulting in ADHD behavioral problems chronic enough for causing major difficulties in one's life areas like home, school, work, or social situations.

The diagnostic criteria prescribed by the American Psychiatric Association through its publication of the DSM-5 prove quite useful in the proper diagnosis of ADHD.

ADHD is attributed to a multiplicity of factors classified as neurological, genetic, and environmental. However, most substantial causes of ADHD fall in the neurobiological realm, indicating some or the other impairments in the structure and functioning of the brain contributed through genetic inheritance and environmental factors like brain injuries, brain diseases, and fatal exposures to alcohol, drug abuse, and high levels of lead at both the pre- and post-natal stages. Besides causing dysfunctions and impairments in the brain, environmental factors may also work as a nourisher for problems related to ADHD among children.

The treatment of ADHD involves a combination of approaches including medication (using stimulant as well as non-stimulant drugs), as well as the use of behavior modification or management techniques.

Autism

Meaning and Definitions of the Term "Autism"

It is quite natural that most children follow a normal course of development in terms of their speaking, language acquisition, and interactions with their peers and family members. As social creatures, children are often smiling, cuddling, laughing, interacting, and responding eagerly to games

> **Autism**
>
> A type of neurodevelopmental disorder taking root among developing children from early ages causing serious impairments in their mental and behavioral functioning, exhibited through social aloofness and bizarre activities like repetitive and unusual responses to sensory experiences, and affecting adversely their educational performance and adjustment in life.

like "peek-a-boo" or "hide-and-seek." However, in some cases, we have a different story to tell. Some children, instead of needing and desiring contact with others, isolate themselves in a world of their own, a place characterized by repetitive routines, odd and peculiar behavior, problems in communication, and a lack of social and emotional awareness and bonds with others. Children characterized by such deviancy and sub-normality in their normal development are often referred to as having a specific developmental disorder called autism. Let us look into the meaning and nature of this disorder from some of its available definitions.

1. **Cohen et al. (1987):** Autism, a poorly understood condition, is now considered a pervasive developmental disorder because children who are autistic are challenged by a range of impairments in the normal development of communication, social and cognitive capacities (p. xvi).
2. **Autism Society of America:** The essential features of the condition (named as autism) typically appear prior to 30 months of age and consist of disturbances of (i) developmental rates and/or sequences, (ii) responses to sensory stimuli, (iii) speech, language and cognitive capacities, and (iv) capacities to relate to people, events and objects (Sturmey and Servin, 1994).
3. **Advani and Chadha (2003):** Autism is a brain disorder that typically affects a child's ability to communicate, form relationships with others and respond appropriately to the

environment. Some children with autism are relatively high functioning, with speech and intelligence intact. Others are mentally retarded mute, or have serious language delays. For some, autism makes them seem closed off and shut down, and there are others who seem locked into repetitive behaviors and rigid pattern of thinking (p. 211).

4. **Individuals with Disabilities Education Act, (IDEA) USA (1994):** Autism is a "developmental disability, affecting verbal and nonverbal communication and social interaction generally evident before age 3, that affects a child's performance. Other characteristics often associated with autism are engagement in repetitive activities and stereotyped movements, resistance to environmental change or change in daily routines, and unusual responses to sensory experiences" (34 CFR, part 300, 300.7[b][1]).

The definitions cited above may lead us to derive the following conclusions about the meaning and nature of the term autism.

i) Autism, as indicated in the first definition, is a pervasive development disorder. That is why in the diagnostic manual used to classify disabilities, the DSM-IV (American Psychiatric Association, 1994), "autistic disorder" is listed as a category under the heading of "Pervasive Developmental Disorders," and in the DSM-5, it has been accepted as within the category of Neurodevelopmental disorders and has been a given a new name, "Autism spectrum disorder."

ii) Children affected with autism display limitations and defects in terms of their communication, social and cognitive behaviors, and performances as early as 30 months or 3 years of their age. In addition to their developmental deficiencies or performance deficits in three major areas—communication, social and cognitive behaviors—children with autism may also be seen to demonstrate the following types of abnormalities in their behavior.

- Engagement in repetitive activities and stereotypical movements.
- Resistance to environmental change or change in daily routine.
- Unusual responses to sensory experiences.

iii) Autism, defined as a neurological or brain disorder by Advani & Chadha, is mainly caused by impairments in one's neurological functioning or brain damage.

iv) A child with autism is adversely affected in terms of educational performance and day-to-day adjustment in his life.

Understood in this way, the term autism may be functionally defined as:

Usually evident before age three and mainly caused by brain dysfunction, autism refers to a pervasive developmental disorder that may bring serious impairments and disabilities in the communication, social, emotional and cognitive behaviors of affected children, demonstrated often in terms of social aloofness and bizarre activities like repetitive and unusual responses to sensory experiences and affecting adversely their educational performance and adjustment in life.

How do Autistics Behave in Their Environment?

For identifying how an autistic child may behave in his environment, consider the following examples of autistic children.

Example 1: A parental description of autistic behavior

We start with an image—a tiny, golden child on hands and knees, circling round and round a spot on the floor in mysterious, self-absorbed delight. She does not look up, though she is smiling and laughing, she does not call our attention to the mysterious object of her pleasure. She does not see us at all. She and the spot are all there is, and though she is eighteen months old, an age for touching, tasting, pointing, pushing, exploring, she is doing none of these things. She does not walk, or crawl upstairs, or pull herself to her feet to reach the objects. She does not want any objects, instead she circles her spot, or she sits, a long chain in her hand, snaking it up and down, watching it coil and uncoil for twenty minutes, half an hour, longer.

Source—Park, 1998b:30 quoted in Hunt Nancy and Marshall Kathleen (2002)

Example 2: Bizzare behavior of an autistic child

Consider the case of George, an eight-year-old. He is difficult to understand because he makes up and uses his own words. He often sits in the backyard holding a branch in his hand, rocking back and forth and talking gibberish to it. He drags a moth-eaten stuffed animal—he calls it "Toe Bunny"—around the house, and will not go to bed without it. Yet he scored above the retarded range on intelligence tests not requiring verbal responses.

Source—Kirk et al. (1993:468)

Example 3: Autistic child Amy roaming in her own world

Amy, three years old, spends much of her day picking up pieces of lint. She drops the lint in the air and then watches intently as it falls to the floor. She also licks the back of her hands and stares at the saliva. She hasn't spoken yet and can't feed or dress herself. Several times a day she screams so loudly that the neighbors at first thought she was being abused. She doesn't seem to be interested in her mother's love and affection but will take her mother's hand to lead her to the refrigerator: Amy likes to eat butter—whole pats of it, several at a time. Her mother uses the pats of butter that you get at some restaurants to help Amy learn and to keep her well behaved. If Amy helps with dressing herself, or if she sits quietly for several minutes, her mother gives her some butter. Amy's mother knows that the butter isn't good for her, but it is the only thing that seems to get through to the child. The family's pediatrician has been concerned about Amy's developmental delays for some time and has recently suggested that she be evaluated by specialists. The pediatrician thinks Amy may have autism and the child and her family will probably need extensive support.

Source: Durand and Barlow (2013:496)

Criterion for the Diagnosis and Identification of Autism

The satisfactory and reliable psychological diagnostic criteria have been given by agencies such as the American Psychiatric Association (APA) from time to time in its published documents— the DSMs (Diagnostic and Statistical Manuals of Mental Disorders). Table 11.3 provides extracts regarding the diagnosis of autism from the current manuals of the DSM-5.

Table 11 3 APA Criteria for the Diagnosis of Autism Spectrum Disorder

Autism Spectrum Disorder (APA, 2013)
1. Individual displays continual deficiencies in various areas of communication and social interaction, including the following:
   (i) Social-emotional reciprocity, (ii) Nonverbal communication, (iii) Development and maintenance of relationships.
2. Individual displays significant restriction and repetition in behaviors, interests or activities including two or more of the following:
   (i) Exaggerated and repeated speech patterns, movements, or object use, (ii) Inflexible demands for same routines, statements, and behaviors, (iii) Highly restricted, fixated, and overly intense interests, (iv) Over or under reactions to sensory input from the environment.
3. Individual develops symptoms by early childhood.
4. Individual experiences significant impairment.

Causes of Autism

What causes autism has been a subject of wide research and controversy over a long period of time. At one time, autism was considered an emotional or psychological disorder caused by sociocultural factors such as an uncongenial environment at home and other unfavorable, stress-related factors present in one's sociocultural environment. However, recent work in the psychological and biological spheres has persuaded clinical theorists that cognitive limitations and brain abnormalities are the primary causes of this disorder. This is why autism (in the name of Autism spectrum disorder) has been placed in the category of neurodevelopmental disorders.

It is a known fact that what we do, think, and feel is almost entirely decided and executed through our brain and neurological apparatus. If one's brain is not found to function in a normal way and there is some sort of brain dysfunction or neurological impairment, then it is natural for affected individuals to experience disturbances and abnormalities in their communication, social and emotional behavior—the known hallmarks of an autism disorder. It is what happens with autistics.

It has been established through contemporary researches that the brain of an autistic child shows marked deficits and deficiencies in terms of its structure and functioning in comparison to his non-disabled peers. Let us cite a few examples.

(i) A portion of the brain called the Amygdala (responsible for directing our emotional responses) has been found impaired in most severely affected autistic children.
(ii) The parietal areas of the brain (responsible for the control of hearing, speech, and language) and corpus callosum (a portion of the brain responsible for passing information from one side of the brain to the other) of autistic children have been found less active than their normally abled peers.
(iii) The frontal lobes of the cerebrum (the portion of the brain responsible for problem-solving, planning ahead, restraining impulses, and understanding the behavior of others) of autistic children have been found quite less active and energized than in their peers without autism.

In this way, at present, we may claim to have significant research evidence in favor of declaring brain dysfunction or neurological impairments as a strong causative factor for autism disorder.

The question may now arise: What is behind these brain dysfunctions or neurological impairments? All the elements and factors like the transmission of defective genes, improper happenings with the child in the womb of the mother during pregnancy, accidents at the time of delivery, as well as maladjustments suffered by them after birth in their sociocultural environment may be potential causative factors for germinating as well as perpetuating the dysfunction or impairment in the brain.

On the basis of such findings it is proper to conclude that autism may have multiple neurodevelopmental or biological causes (genetic, prenatal, birth, and postnatal). Each of them on its own and in combination may lead growing children to a common problem in the brain—a *final common pathway*, such as neurotransmitter abnormalities or dysfunction in the brain resulting in the distinguishable features of autism.

Treatment Measures for Autism

Treatment measures for any ailment, disturbance, or disorder are very much based on the findings of what causes that ailment or disorder. Since autism, as discussed earlier, may be caused by a host of factors in one's heredity and environment, there is no single method or measure that can be termed as a sure shot for the cure and treatment of autism. A number of treatment measures are listed as follows.

1. *Use of Medication and Biochemical treatment:* The following medication and biochemical measures have been found to be useful in the treatment of autism:

   (i) Eliminating or decreasing foods in the diets to which these children show sensitivity or food allergy.
   (ii) Administering doses of vitamins B6, B12, and magnesium, or giving an injection of gamma globulin for decreasing negative behavior associated with autism.
   (iii) Providing drug therapy to disturbed and agitated autistic children.

2. *Use of Sensory integration Treatment:* In providing sensory integration therapy to autistic children, they are provided with structured experiences and activities that may challenge their ability to respond properly to sensory stimuli, and in this way, it may help them in getting rid of their improper behavior regarding sensory stimulation and its integration.

3. *Providing Communication treatment or training:* This treatment measure is meant for bringing improvement to the deficits and disorders of autistic children in their communication skills. The services of a person called a facilitator may provide physical assistance to the autistic child in spelling words using a keyboard of a typewriter, computer, communication board, or other letter display. The facilitator plays the role of an active assistant and offers physical support to the disabled child. The support provided by him may range from hand-over-hand support to a simple touch on the shoulder.

4. *Treatment involving Applied Behavior Analysis:* The technique of applied behavior analysis, as a behavior therapy, rests on the basic principles of classical and operant conditioning, schedules of proper reinforcement, and shaping of the appropriate behavior. It adopts a systematic approach in its application:

   i) The first step in the treatment is the analysis of the behavior of the affected child in the context of his environmental setup. It is aimed to determine the role or function of his inappropriate behavior in his environment.

ii) The second step consists in identifying some alternative behaviors that can serve the same function that is being served by the present inappropriate behavior of the child.

iii) The third step now consists of arranging the environment and providing consequences for increasing the desired new alternative behaviors and decreasing the inappropriate ones.

To adopt applied behavior analysis as a technique of behavior modification, several methods and approaches have been invented for the treatment of autism. For this purpose, a popular and widely used method has been invented by the psychologist Ivar Lovaas and his colleagues at the University of California at Los Angeles. Known as the Lovaas method, it can be understood and applied as described ahead:

The Lovaas method consists of an intensive intervention program originally designed for preschool-aged children with autism. It begins when the child is two to three years of age and involves intensive training of teachers or parents. It makes use of behavior modification techniques—molding and rewarding desired behavior, and ignoring or discouraging undesirable ones—to achieve its goals. The trained interventionists—parents or teachers—then provide intensive, discrete trial training to the affected children on a one-on-one basis in the child's home and the natural settings of the child's behavior. As an intensive and persistent effort approach, this therapy usually consists of four to six hours per day, five to seven days a week. In this way, it generally aims to provide essential training to the affected child on a one-on-one basis (in areas like basic communication skills), for up to 30 to 40 hours per week, continued for a minimum of three years (Lovaas, 1994).

To Sum Up

Usually evident before age three and mainly caused by brain dysfunction, autism refers to a pervasive developmental disorder that may bring serious impairments and disabilities in the communication, social, emotional, and cognitive behaviors of affected children. It is usually demonstrated by them in terms of their social aloofness and bizarre activities, such as repetitive and unusual responses to sensory experiences, and it adversely affects their educational performance and adjustment in life. For the diagnosis and identification of autism, the Diagnostic Criteria provided by the American Psychiatric Association in the DSM-5 may serve a useful purpose.

Autism is the outcome of dysfunction or impairment of the brain and neurological transmission. These abnormalities of the brain and neurological functioning may be caused by a single factor or a combination of factors, such as the transmission of defective genes, pregnancy complications, accidents at the time of delivery, as well as maladjustments they experience after birth in their sociocultural environment.

The treatment applied to cases of autism may consist of a number of measures in the shape of Medication and biochemical treatment (involving drug and vitamin therapy); Sensory integration treatment (aimed to rectify the deficiencies related to sensory integration ability); and Communication training or treatment (concentrating on improving communication skills); as well as treatment involving applied behavior analysis or behavior therapy.

Learning Disorders or Disabilities

Meaning and Concept of Learning Disorders or Disabilities

Children suffering from serious learning difficulties or disabilities are labeled as learning-disabled children. The question may arise as to what these learning difficulties or disabilities are. A learning difficulty or disability is nothing but a sort of handicap or helplessness that can be felt by the sufferer in terms of his academic performance (learning or understanding something), much in the same way as experienced by a physically handicapped person in terms of his physical functioning, or by a mentally handicapped in terms of his mental

---

Learning disability

A type of neurodevelopmental disorder, evident from school-going age, causing severely impaired learning inefficiency or handicapping conditions among affected children in one or the other cognitive areas (e.g., use of language or doing mathematical work), leading to a distinctive gap between one's potential and actual educational achievement to the extent of requiring special care, attention, and remedial measures.

---

functioning. Interpreted in this way, a learning-disabled child suffers from inconveniences and problems in learning areas, much like those experienced by people who are mentally retarded or handicapped in mental or cognitive areas, or by a physically handicapped in the physical and motor areas, or even by a socially or emotionally handicapped in the social and emotional areas.

Let us try to know more about the terms learning-disabled and learning disabilities with the help of some well-known definitions:

USA National Advisory Committee to the Education for the Handicapped, 1969: A specific "learning disability" means a disorder in one or more of the basic psychological processes involved in understanding or in using language, spoken or written, that may manifest itself in an imperfect ability to listen, think, speak, read, write, spell or to do mathematical calculations. The term includes such conditions as perceptual disabilities, brain injury, minimal brain dysfunction, dyslexia and developmental aphasia. The term does not apply to children who have learning problems that are primarily the result of visual, hearing, or motor disabilities, of mental retardation, of emotional disturbance, or of environmental, cultural, or economic disadvantages.

(*Federal Register*, 1977)

Kirk and Kirk (1971): The term learning disability is not meant to be used for children with minor or temporary difficulties in learning but with a severe discrepancy between ability and achievement in educational performance and such severed discrepancy described as learning disabilities with significant learning problems that cannot be explained by mental retardation, sensory impairment, emotional disturbance or lack of opportunity to learn.

Kavale and Forness (1985): People with learning disabilities belong to a group of very diverse individuals but they do share one common problem: They do not learn in the same way or as efficiently as their nondisabled peers. Although most possess normal intelligence, their academic performance is significantly behind their classmates. Some have great difficulty learning mathematics, but most find the mastery of reading and writing to be their most difficult challenge.

A close analysis of all these definitions may reveal the following things concerning meaning and concepts of the term learning disabilities and learning-disabled.

1. Learning disabilities refer to certain kinds of disorders in the basic psychological processes of an individual.
2. These disorders are mainly caused by intrinsic factors (the things lying within the individual), such as central nervous system dysfunction (brain or neurological damage impeding one's motor or learning abilities), and specific deficits in information processing or the ability to learn.
3. Although learning problems may be caused by extrinsic factors like mental retardation, sensory impairment, emotional disturbance, cultural differences, lack of educational opportunities, and poverty, the learning disability is not the direct result of such external factors or conditions.
4. Disorders associated with learning disabilities are usually manifested in specific severe learning problems confined to one or two cognitive areas, such as the inability to grasp or understand things, difficulties in language-related areas such as communication, written language, or reading, or handicap in terms of acquiring mathematical or social skills.
5. Individuals with minor or temporary difficulties in learning are not termed as learning-disabled. Only those who have severely impaired learning inefficiency and serious learning problems are included in this category.
6. The learning disability may allow an individual to have intelligence scores within the normal range, but it essentially makes them substantially delayed in academic achievement. He always lags behind in terms of his educational progress in comparison to the peers of his age and class.
7. The impaired learning inefficiency coupled with serious learning problems in one or the other cognitive areas leads to a distinctive gap between an individual's potential and actual educational achievement, and as a result, he becomes disabled or handicapped in one or the other learning areas so much so that he needs special care, attention, and educational services for his adjustment and welfare.

In this way, learning disabilities may provide a lot of obstacles and difficulties in the path of learning. Gradually the learning problems may become so acute as to cause severely impaired learning inefficiency in one or the other cognitive areas. It leads to a distinctive gap between one's potential and actual educational achievement requiring special care, attention, and remedial measures; when this happens, the learner is labeled as learning-disabled.

The Common Learning Disabilities Found In Children

It is quite common to find the prevailing learning disabilities among individuals in their two popular distinctive forms, known as (i) Dyslexia and (ii) Dyscalculia. Let us examine these two types of learning disabilities.

DYSLEXIA

Meaning and Definition of the Term Dyslexia

Etymologically, the word dyslexia is composed of dys and lexia, where "dys" stands for a type of disorder or disturbance, and the Greek word "lexia" stands for "pertaining to words." In this sense, the world "dyslexia" in its word meaning stands for a type of disorder or disturbance related to words or language, written or spoken (Webster's Seventh New Collegiate Dictionary, 1969:259).

Dyslexia

A type of learning disability or disorder experienced by developing children making them handicapped in the acquisition and use of necessary language skills.

In this way, Dyslexia represents a particular type of learning difficulty or disability that may create a big problem for a developing child in making use of the words or language in his study or day-to-day communication and adjustment.

In its broader aspect, Dyslexia causes difficulty in the acquisition of necessary language skills pertaining to reading, writing, listening, and speaking on the part of a developing child. Taking note of such outcomes of the disorder Dyslexia, the World Federation of Neurologists has termed dyslexia as "a disorder in children who, despite conventional classroom experience, fail to attain the language skills of reading, writing and spelling commensurate with their intellectual abilities."

The nature of this particular type of learning disability may become clear through the description of some experiences and concerns of persons with Dyslexia and their parents.

Case I

My son has always had difficulties in reading and writing since Pre-K, and I had taken him to his doctor for possibly having ADD (Attention-Deficit Disorder). She determined that my son did not have any problems. As the years went by, my son still struggles with reading/comprehension and writing. My son is now in the third grade, and after speaking with his teacher, my son is again struggling in writing his thoughts on paper. When reading, he adds words that are not there or makes up his own words. He still has problems with writing "b" and "d"; as well as, "p" and "q." He changes the words "the" to "and," and "from" or "for" to "of." I have my son enrolled in Tutoring for reading and writing but still he is performing below grade level. His teacher is also going to help tutor him before school. I do not want to overwhelm my son but I want to help him improve.

Case II

With my dyslexia, I often say words I did not intend to say. For example, I'll mentally mean to have said "I went walking yesterday" when I meant today. Or I'll say, "Have you fed the cat?" when I meant to say "dog." This has been happening for more than 10 years (I am 45). The numerical confusion has been with me for longer, dating back to childhood. Needless to say, I was no good with arithmetic as a youngster, and although my numerical skills have improved, I live in fear of making mathematical errors in my calculations.

The study of cases such as these may help us to conclude a number of things about the meaning and nature of the learning disability known as dyslexia.

1. Dyslexia is essentially a language- or communication-based learning difficulty or disability that is experienced by an individual from a young age of their schooling.
2. It is reflected through inability shown, difficulty experienced, and acute deficiency demonstrated by the developing child in terms of his acquisition and use of essential language skills—reading, writing, listening, and speaking—and thus results in his failure to comprehend and convey ideas in a way commensurate with his age and intellectual level.
3. Beginning in the early years of one's childhood, it may persist throughout one's life. However, if detected early and treated with suitable remedial measures, it may be managed in an effective way.
4. In case it goes undetected with no care for the suffering child's difficulties and problems, it can cause a number of academic as well as behavioral problems for the developing child. The child may show signs of utter frustration, depression, and low self-esteem. He may become truant, aggressive, delinquent, or may retreat into solace.
5. The learning disability experienced by the suffering child is not caused by hearing, vision, or speech problems. The disorder is a specific information processing problem; it occurs when there is a problem in areas of the brain that help in the interpretation of language—auditory sensation or visual symbols to convey information.
6. It may appear simply as a reading problem or may be accompanied by other language problems, such as (i) difficulty in writing (script or numeral), (ii) difficulty in understanding what has been said, or (iii) difficulty in saying what is to be conveyed.
7. Dyslexia as a learning disability or disorder is a language-based disorder. It results from the failure of a portion of the brain to properly recognize and process certain symbols (script or numerals). Other portions of the brain may thus remain functioning in a normal, or in some cases, above normal and exceptional ways. This is why it is no surprise to find individuals who have achieved much in spite of their dyslexia; we may cite the names of the famous dyslexics Albert Einstein, Walt Disney, Tom Cruise, and Magic Johnson.
8. Dyslexia (the learning disability related to language) and Dyscalculia (the learning disability related to mathematics) may or may not go side by side. These are two different types of disabilities, as may be seen through the discussion carried out ahead.

In conclusion, we can define dyslexia as *a type of disability or disorder causing problems to the individual in the acquisition and application of language, related to one or the other language skills, such as reading, writing, listening, and speaking, causing considerable harm to his educational progress and adjustment in life.*

Various Forms and Types of Dyslexia

Dyslexia can be found in individuals in a variety of forms and ways, as described ahead.

A. Classification Based on the Degree of Severity

The World Federation of Neurologists has classified Dyslexia into the following three types:

1. **Primary or Hereditary Dyslexia:** It is hereditary—passed down family lines through transmitted genes—and is found more often in boys than in girls. There is a dysfunction of the left

side of the brain (cerebral cortex) that may cause problems in the interpretation of language. It is dangerous in the sense that (i) it does not change with age, (ii) individuals with this type of dyslexia are rarely able to read above a fourth-grade level, and (iii) they may struggle with reading, spelling, and writing as adults.

2. **Secondary or Developmental Dyslexia:** It is not hereditary but acquired in the developmental period either at the early stages of fetal development or in the first few years after birth. It is controllable and may diminish as the child matures. Its frequency is also more common in boys than girls.

3. **Trauma or Accidental dyslexia:** It is neither hereditary, nor does it result from developmental deficiencies. It usually occurs after some form of brain trauma or injury to the area of the brain that controls language functions. It may occur evenly in boys or girls as a matter of accident or incidence. It is quite severe in the sense that it is incurable and uncontrollable; it may impact the communication/linguistic ability of the person for life.

B. Classification Based on the Nature of the Effect on Functioning

Dyslexia may affect the visual, auditory, and kinesthetic functioning of a person with respect to their acquisition and use of a language. Accordingly, we may classify the Dyslexia found in children into three distinct types:

1. **Visual Dyslexia:** It is characterized by number and letter reversals (writing 9 for 7, *p* for *q*, or vice versa) and the inability to write symbols in the correct sequence.

2. **Auditory Dyslexia:** Here, one experiences difficulty in comprehending the sounds of letters or sentences on account of perceiving them as jumbled or not heard correctly.

3. **Dysgraphic or Kinesthetic Dyslexia:** It is concerned with the difficulty faced by the child in holding and controlling a pen or pencil and thus causing his disability in terms of writing something on paper.

Treatment of Dyslexia

Treatment lies in the proper diagnosis. Therefore, for treatment measures of the problems associated with Dyslexia, all attempts should be made to first get acquainted with the exact nature of the difficulties faced by the child in learning and using language. Then, attempts should be made for chalking out the appropriate treatment and remedial plans. The treatment plans chalked out for children with dyslexia may be implemented in the regular classroom or a special education setting. It remains quite beneficial psychologically, socially, and educationally for these children to try for the remedial instruction or treatment plan, in the inclusive setup of regular classroom teaching. The specialized setup or individual private tutoring are best resorted to in severe cases of language learning difficulties. Let us, therefore, discuss the possible remedial measures in the regular classroom setup for children with dyslexia.

In seeking treatment for children with dyslexia, it should be remembered that learning disabilities caused on account of dyslexia vary widely in their nature and occurrence. We cannot prescribe a single remedy for all cases of dyslexia. It is advisable to use many techniques for teaching children with dyslexia, such as the following:

(1) They may be asked to approach reading tasks by tracing over letters, using the sense of touch, showing pictures along with words, and using toys and other concrete materials along with the word.

(2) A direct approach may include a systematic study of phonics.

(3) There may be some well-thought-out attempts involving general language enrichment programs for helping them in solving their language problems.

(4) There must be structured formats or programs and they should receive training in the task of processing information into language or cognitive systems (e.g., asking the child to listen to a taped lecture or watch a video recording of a presentation and then respond to a series of oral or written questions).

(5) In all cases of implementing the needed treatment plan, one should focus on strengthening the child's weaknesses while utilizing their strengths.

(6) Techniques designed to help all the senses work together efficiently can also be used. Specific language learning approaches that require a child to hear, see, say, and do something (multisensory) may also be used.

(7) Mobile and computer technology may suit the requirements of these children by providing valuable opportunities for the learning and use of language skills.

(8) Children with dyslexia should be taught and trained in the acquisition of necessary compensation and coping skills for managing academic and psychological problems.

(9) As far as possible, individual attention should be paid for arranging the optimum learning conditions and alternative avenues for demonstrating their language learning performance in and outside the school.

(10) The work strategy for these children should be planned wisely. Because the academic demands on a child with dyslexia may be great and the child may tire or frustrate easily, work increments should be broken down into appropriate chunks. Frequent breaks should be built into class and drill work or homework time. Reinforcement should be given for efforts as well as achievements in a judicious way as to promote learning and achievement.

(11) Wherever needed, earnest attempts should be made to make use of the behavioral and psychoanalytic approach for the correction and reinforcement of the desired behavior of children with dyslexia.

Dyscalculia

Meaning and Definition

The word "Dyscalculia" has its origin in Greek and Latin, standing for "counting or calculating badly," as its prefix "dys" meaning "badly" has been derived from Greek, and "calculia" derived from the Latin means "to count, calculate or compute." In this way, etymologically the term dyscalculia stands for a state or condition that adversely affects one's ability to perform calculation or computation in Mathematics. Dyscalculia is therefore fundamentally different from dyslexia. Whereas in dyslexia, a learner is found to experience difficulty and disability in dealing with words, in dyscalculia he faces difficulty and disability relating to numbers. Elaborating on this concept, The United Kingdom Department for

> **Dyscalculia**
>
> A type of learning disability or disorder experienced on the part of the developing children making them handicapped in the acquisition and use of necessary mathematical skills.

Education and Skills in its report submitted to the British Parliament in the year 1999 described the term dyscalculia as:

> a condition that affects the ability to acquire arithmetical skills. Dyscalculic learners may have difficulty understanding simple number concepts, lack an intuitive grasp of numbers and have problems learning number facts and procedures. Even if they produce a correct answer or use a correct method, they may do so mechanically and without confidence.

However, further researches in the field of dyscalculia have suggested that there may be several subsets of mathematical difficulties other than number-based difficulties that may be experienced by dyscalculic learners. These may include procedural and sequencing difficulties, as well as difficulties in problem-solving and understanding basic concepts in areas other than arithmetic, such as algebra, geometry, trigonometry, and statistics. In this way, dyscalculia may prove a great handicap and obstacle to dyscalculic learners, not only in terms of numeracy and calculations in arithmetic but also in learning essentials pertaining to all aspects and areas belonging to the subject mathematics. It is responsible for creating disinterest and phobia toward mathematics, instilling a feeling of helplessness and a lack of confidence, and raising their level of anxiety around engaging in any mathematical learning or performing tasks involving mathematical abilities.

As a result of such adverse impact and influences conveyed through the term dyscalculia, it can be properly defined as a particular type of learning disability that is responsible for adversely affecting one's learning and performance in the subject of mathematics, demonstrable through early symptoms such as:

- Inability to write numerals and mathematical symbols correctly
- Difficulty in recalling the meaning of the symbols
- Difficulty in counting and performing mathematical calculations and computation work
- Difficulty in carrying out basic arithmetical operations e.g., addition, subtraction, multiplication, and division
- Difficulty in following the proper steps and reasoning for the solution of mathematical problems—particularly word problems
- Difficulty in acquiring a proper understanding of basic mathematical concepts like place value, directed numbers, directions and dimensions, decimals, fractions and percentages, measuring units and time sense, etc.

Treatment Measures for Dyscalculia

For employing treatment measures for problems associated with dyscalculia, the beginning should be made by getting acquainted with the exact nature of the problems or difficulties faced by the child in learning and using mathematics. Then, the appropriate treatment measures may be taken in the manner given as follows:

1. Keep in mind that remedial measures taken or support provided may differ for each dyscalculic as well as each problem associated with dyscalculia. For illustration, here we can cite some measures as follows:

    - In case the child is suffering from short-term memory difficulty preventing them from remembering instructions, the remedy lies in (i) repeating instructions, probably, in separate chunks rather than in one long string, (ii) ensuring that new vocabulary is explained carefully so that child may grasp the contents of the instruction.

- In cases where the child is suffering from word problems, these can be solved by allowing them to be read aloud to by the teacher or another child (a study buddy).
- In case there is a problem with retrieving basic facts, such as multiplication tables, the remedy lies in giving the child a small tables square.
- In cases of the child feeling difficulty in performing a mathematical task by considering it overdemanding or beyond his capabilities, the remedy may lie in adjusting the content of the task or way of performing the task.
- A child may encounter problems concerning number transpositions, that is, writing 51 for 15. Here, the cause of the problem lies in our saying "fifteen," which sounds like "five-ten," and consequently, the child may fall into the trap of writing it as 51. In this case, correction should come immediately before it becomes a habit for the child.

2. For tackling a variety of problems related to dyscalculia, a teacher may be advised to take into consideration the use of the following practices for helping students:

   - Allow the use of finger counting, circles, pencil marks, etc., if the child feels comfortable doing so.
   - Try to provide clear and concise instructions for the meaningful understanding of the basic concepts and skills related to diagnosed areas of weakness/difficulties.
   - Try to provide examples and non-examples for the clarification of fundamental concepts and principles.
   - Present yourself as a model for learning the right way of doing calculations and solving problems and also use peers as models.
   - Try to provide enough time for explaining mathematical symbols and mathematical language. Repeat this information often and in different manners to ensure that the learners understand it well.
   - Make sure the child understands the process that occurs in a calculation.
   - Create an environment where making mistakes are seen as part of the learning process.
   - Make use of concrete, meaningful examples and materials for the understanding of mathematical concepts, problems, processes, and functions.
   - Allow the use of note-taking technology or a tape recorder for learners whose visual processing speed poses problems in classroom learning so that they can concentrate on the lessons rather than on taking notes.
   - Use real-life situations that make problems functional and applicable to everyday life and provide opportunities to see patterns, rhythm, symmetry, and reasoning in the structure and functioning of mathematics.
   - Always follow the teaching maxim "simple to complex" (teaching easier knowledge and skills before difficult ones) and "concrete to abstract" (use of concrete material visual and auditory examples for understanding abstract concepts and processes).
   - Remember that the acquisition of skills in mathematics needs a lot of practice. Hence, provide enough opportunity to do so through distributed practice (plenty of practice in small doses). Don't forget to have proper supervision for preventing students from practicing misconceptions and "misrules" and help them in their learning through immediate corrective and positive reinforcement.
   - Use visual methods and rhymes to help children learn mathematical facts, and build retention by providing review within a day or two.

- ○ Help students in visualizing math problems by drawing and following systematic problem-solving steps via structural worksheets, video display, and modeling.
- ○ Teach that much of mathematics is interconnected. For example, you can teach that division is the opposite of multiplication and show how this is beneficial in actual work (e.g., 180 divided by 15 can be rephrased as $15 \times ? = 180$ or $12 \times ? = 180$).
- ○ Help students to track their progress—which facts they have mastered and which remain to be learned.
- ○ Make use of well-prepared material, remedial programs, and computer-assisted instructions.
- ○ Allow dyscalculic children to make use of tools, such as an abacus, calculators, and computers, for learning and performing tasks in mathematics.
- ○ For dealing with a dyscalculic student, go back to what he knows and understands. This will almost certainly be further back than you think. It is important to build on a firm base to bring him up to speed on his learning.
- ○ Keep in mind that children should be taught in such a way as not to make mathematics dry and boring, beyond their comprehension and utility. Try to make use of the proper strategies by setting a required level of mastery for inculcating self-confidence in the art of calculation and problem-solving.

To Sum Up

Learning Disorders or Disabilities refer to those psychological disorders in which individuals are found to suffer seriously from impaired learning inefficiency to the extent that they require special attention, care, and remedial programs for the rectification of their learning problems and disabilities. In general, two types of learning disabilities, known as dyslexia and dyscalculia, are more common and require special attention. Dyslexia is a type of learning disability that cause problems to the individual in the acquisition and application of language skills. such as reading, writing, listening, and speaking; dyscalculia, on the other hand, creates problems in the acquisition and application of abilities to calculate or compute in mathematics.

In seeking treatment for individuals with dyslexia and dyscalculia, it should be well remembered that learning disabilities caused on account of dyslexia and dyscalculia may vary widely in their nature and occurrence. We cannot prescribe a single remedy for all cases related to dyslexia or dyscalculia. Therefore, in the treatment of children with dyslexia or dyscalculia, we may witness a number of specialized techniques for their education and adjustment, depending upon the nature of the learning problems they suffered on this account.

Review Questions

1. What are Neurodevelopmental disorders? Name the different neurodevelopmental orders mentioned in DSM-5 provided by the APA.
2. What do you understand by the term mental retardation or mental deficiency? Discuss it in its various forms or kinds: mild, moderate, severe, and profound mental retardation.
3. Define the term mental retardation and throw light on its common clinical types, known as down syndrome, cretinism, microcephaly, hydrocephaly, phenylketonuria (PKU), and amaurotic idiocy.

4. How is mental retardation caused among affected individuals? Discuss the measures taken for possible treatment.
5. What is Attention-Deficit/Hyperactivity Disorder (ADHD)? Explain it with the help of a suitable example.
6. Discuss the diagnosis and identification of ADHD in light of the criteria laid down by the APA.
7. Throw light on the causes behind cases of ADHD and discuss the possible measures taken for their treatment.
8. Define the term autism and throw light on its meaning, nature, and characteristic features.
9. What is autism? How do autistics behave in their environmental situations? Illustrate with the help of examples.
10. Discuss the diagnosis and identification of autism in light of the criteria laid down by the APA.
11. Throw light on the underlying causes behind cases of autism and suggest possible measures for their treatment.
12. Define the term learning disabilities and throw light on their meaning and concept.
13. What is dyslexia? Discuss its various forms and types.
14. What is dyscalculia? Throw light on its various forms and types.
15. Discuss in detail the possible measures taken for the treatment of dyslexia and dyscalculia.

References

Advani, L., & Chadha, A. (2003), *You and your special child*, New Delhi: UBS Publishers, Distributors Pvt. Ltd.

American Psychiatric Association (1994), *Diagnostic and statistical manual of mental disorders, DSM-IV* (4th ed.), Washington, DC: American Psychiatric Association.

American Psychiatric Association (2013), *Diagnostic and statistical manual of mental disorders*, (5th ed., DSM-5), Washington, DC: American Psychiatric Association.

Autism Society of America quoted by Sturmey, P., & Servin, J. A. (1994), Defining and assessing autism, In J. L. Matson (Ed.), *Autism in children and adults: Etiology, assessment and intervention* (pp. 33–36), Pacific Grove, CA: Brooks/Cole.

Barkley, R. A. (1988), *ADHD and the nature of Self-control*, New York: Wiley.

Barkley, R. A. (2000), *Taking charge of ADHD: The complete authoritative guide for parents*, New York, NY: The Guilford Press.

British Mental Deficiency Act (1929), *Quoted in Shanmugam, T.E., Abnormal psychology*, New Delhi: Tata McGraw Hill, 1981.

Cohen, D. J., Donnellian, A. M., & Paul, R. (Eds.) (1987), *Handbook on autism and pervasive developmental disorders*, Silvers Springs, MD: V.H. Winston & Sons.

Comer, R. J. (2015), *Abnormal psychology* (9th ed.), New York, NY: Worth 'Publishers (A Macmillan Education Imprint)

Cooper, P., & Bilton, K. M. (2002), *Attention deficit/hyperactivity disorder: A practical guide for teachers* (2nd ed.), London: David, Fulton Publishers.

Department of Education USA (1994), *Individuals with Disabilities Education Act (IDEP), USA (1994)*, Washington, DC: Department of Education.

Durand, V., & Barlow, D. (2013), *Essentials of abnormal psychology* (6th ed.), Wadsworth: Cengage Learning.

Federal Register (1977), *Report of the USA National Advisory Committee to the Education for the Handicapped, 1969*, Washington, DC: U.S. Government Printing Office.

Goldstein, S. (1999), The facts about ADHD: An overview of attention deficit hyperactivity disorder, retrieved from http://www.samgoldste4in.com/articles/ 9907.html

Grossman, H. G. (Ed.) (1983), *Classification in mental retardation*, Washington, DC: American Association on Mental Retardation.

Kavale, K. A., & Forness, S. R. (1985), *The science of learning disabilities*, San Diego, CA: College Hill.

Kirk, S. A, Gallagher, J. J., & Anastasiow, N. J. (1993), *Educating exceptional children*, Boston, MA: Houghton Mifflin Company.

Kirk, S. A., & Kirk, W. D. (1971), *Psycho-linguistic learning disabilities; Diagnosis and remediation*, Urbana, IL: University of Illinois Press.

Lovaas, I. (1994), *Quoted in Heward, William L. (2000), Exceptional children: An introduction to special education* (6th ed.), Upper Saddle River, NJ: Merrill.

Page, J. D. (1976), *Abnormal psychology*, New Delhi: Tata McGraw-Hill.

Park, C. C. (1998b), *Quoted in Hunt Nancy, and Marshall Kathleen, Exceptional Children and Youth (2002), An Introduction to Special Education*, Boston, MA: Houghton Mifflin Company, 30.

Rosen, E., Fox, R., & Gregory I. (1972), *Abnormal Psychology* (2nd International Student ed.), Philadelphia, PA: Saunders.

Webster's Seventh New Collegiate Dictionary (1969), Springfield, MA: Merriam Webster's Publishers.

Wechsler, D. (1935), The concept of mental deficiency, *Psychiatric Quarterly,* 9: 232–236.

Chapter 12

Disruptive, Impulse-Control, and Conduct Disorders

Learning Objectives

After going through this chapter, you will be able to:

- Know about the meaning of the terms disruptive, impulse-control, and conduct disorders.
- Discuss the meaning and nature of the term oppositional defiant disorder.
- Throw light on the meaning and nature of intermittent explosive disorder.
- Describe the meaning and nature of conduct disorder.
- Know about the meaning and nature of antisocial behavior and antisocial personality.
- Elucidate the meaning and concept of the term delinquency.
- Throw light on the underlying causes, prevention, and treatment of delinquency.
- Tell about the meaning and concept of the term crime.
- Discuss the underlying causes and prevention of criminality.
- Throw light on the methods of treatment and rehabilitation of criminals.

What are Disruptive, Impulse-Control, and Conduct Disorders?

It may be natural for children to act impulsively and violently, to become disruptive and defiant, and act in socially undesirable ways at one or the other times for a while in the form of short-lived episodes. However, when these conducts or behaviors become much more severe and longer lasting affecting their social interaction, and proving harmful to them and others, then they may turn into problematic behavior and behavioral disorders named as Disruptive, impulse-control, and conduct disorders.

In the DSM-5 classification system of mental disorders provided by the American Psychiatric Association (2013), Disruptive, Impulse-control, and conduct disorders have been provided a separate prominent category with the objectives of their proper diagnosis and treatment.

In a formal way, disruptive, impulse-control, and conduct disorders among children are also known as Oppositional

> **Disruptive, impulse-control, and conduct disorders**
>
> A group of mental and behavioral disorders consisting of oppositional defiant, intermittent explosive, and conduct disorders of children, later developed as antisocial behavior and antisocial personality among adults, proving harmful to self and others.

DOI: 10.4324/9781003398325-12

defiant disorder, Intermittent explosive disorder, and Conduct disorders. When found among adults, these behavior patterns are known by a common name: Antisocial personality disorder. Let us look into them one by one.

Oppositional Defiant Disorder

Children with this type of disorder are found to show age-inappropriate opposing and defiant behavior in a hostile way, in the manner as follows:

- They often lose their temper and get angry, irritated, and resentful, often on unreasonable grounds.
- They often argue with authority figures, refuse to comply with requests or rules, and willfully and deliberately try to annoy others.
- They are found to possess an attitude or feelings comprised of vindictiveness.
- They do not realize the inappropriateness of their angry, defiant, and oppositional behavior. Rather, they try to argue and convince others about the appropriateness of their otherwise inappropriate behavior.

Intermittent Explosive Disorder

This type of behavioral disorder is more severe and damaging in its occurrence and consequences than oppositional defiant disorder. The impulsive actions and aggressive reactions or responses here are quite inflammatory and explosive, like an explosion from a bomb blast. This occurs in the behavior of affected individuals frequently and in an untimely manner. The distinguishing features of the behavior demonstrated by people with this type of disorder may be named as (i) quite impulsive in nature, (ii) out of proportion to the event or incident that triggered it, (iii) resulting in loss to the person in question, as well as others to whom reactions or responses are addressed, in the form of causing damage, distress, and serious problems of adjustment and interactions.

Conduct Disorders

It refers to age-inappropriate behaviors that are more serious than oppositional defiant behavior shown by children, involving the frequent and vigorous breakage of social rules and regulations. In this way, antisocial acts or behaviors, when committed in a more severe and deliberate form for inflicting pain, loss, and injury to others, including animals and property, may describe a child afflicted with conduct disorder. We may cite the following as examples of acts or conduct associated with this type of disorder.

- Acting aggressively toward people and animals (such as bullying, physical fights, and use of a weapon to cause harm).
- Destroying public and private property of others wilfully and deliberately.
- Committing unlawful acts such as theft, lying, deceiving, robbery, chain snatching, vehicle lifting, and kidnapping.
- Violating norms and rules enforced in the family, school, playgrounds, or other places of social interaction and activities in a more frequent, deliberate, and severe form, such as frequent truancy from class and school, running away from the home, and so on.

To Sum Up

The term Disruptive, impulse-control, and conduct disorders refer to a group of disorders classified as Oppositional defiant disorder, Intermittent explosive disorder, and Conduct disorders found among children. When found among adults, these behavior patterns are known by a common name—Antisocial personality disorder.

Children suffering from *oppositional defiant disorder* are found to show age-inappropriate oppositional and defiant behavior in a hostile way, without realizing or being convinced of the inappropriateness of their behavior.

Children suffering from *Intermittent Explosive Disorder* are found to exhibit more frequently, untimely, and even more out-of-proportion impulsive and aggressive actions, of a nature similar to a bomb explosion, causing damage and distress to others, and serious problems of adjustment to themselves.

Children suffering from *conduct disorders* are found to engage deliberately in social acts or behaviors involving the breakage of social rules and regulations, frequently and vigorously, for inflicting pain, loss, and injury to others, including animals and property.

Antisocial Behavior and Antisocial Personality

The prevalence of disruptive, impulse-control, and conduct disorders is not limited to children. It may also appear at later stages of their attaining maturity, turning into an antisocial personality, and their conduct into antisocial behavior.

The term antisocial behavior, according to the American Psychiatric Association (1968), stands for "behavior characterized by impulsive, irresponsible actions satisfying only immediate and narcissistic interests without concern for obvious and implicit social consequences." Such behavior is not only harmful to the adequate personality development and well-being of individuals but also affects their social adjustment and proves detrimental to society. In this way, individuals with conduct disorders are likely to be turned into antisocial personalities.

According to the DSM-II (1968:43), antisocial personalities may be defined as

individuals who are basically un-socialized and whose behavior pattern brings them repeatedly into conflict with society. They are incapable of significant loyalty to individuals, groups, or social values. They are grossly selfish, callous, irresponsible, impulsive, and unable to feel guilt or to learn from experience and punishment. Frustration tolerance is low. They tend to blame others or offer plausible rationalizations for their behavior. A mere history of repeated legal or social offenses is not sufficient to justify this diagnosis.

In the subsequent editions of the DSM published by the American Psychiatric Association in the names of the DSM III, DSM IV, DSM IV-TR, antisocial behavior was placed in the category of Personality Disorders. In the DSM-5 published in 2013, it has been placed in the broad category of "Disruptive, Impulse-control and Conduct Disorders," diagnosed and assigned to individuals who habitually and pervasively disregard or violate the rights and considerations of others without remorse. Accordingly, individuals with Antisocial Personality Disorder may be habitual criminals or engage in behavior that are grounds for criminal arrest and prosecution, or they may engage in behaviors that skirt the edge of the law, or manipulate and hurt others in ways that are widely regarded as unethical, immoral, irresponsible, or in violation of social norms and expectations. In general, we may include behavioral acts designated as delinquency and crime in our social world for the designation of antisocial personalities. In the pages ahead, we will be discussing the concepts and implications of the phenomena of delinquency and crime in their essential details.

To Sum Up

The prevalence of disruptive, impulse-control, and conduct disorders is not limited to children. It may accompany them in their adolescence and appear at later stages of their attaining maturity, turning into antisocial personality, and their behavior and conduct becoming antisocial behavior. Such behavior is not only harmful to the adequate personality development and well-being of the individuals, but it also affects their social adjustment and proves detrimental to society. The individuals exhibiting such behavior are known as individuals suffering from antisocial personality disorder, designating them as antisocial personalities engaging in acts of delinquency and crime.

Delinquency

Concept and Meaning

Criminal behavior or the tendency to commit crime in any society or nation is not only found among adults, but minor children and adolescents as well. These individuals are known as juvenile or young delinquents. Juvenile delinquents, therefore, are criminals minors in age legally from 7 to 16, in the case of boys, and 7 to 18 years in the case of girls. On account of their age, delinquents are also referred to as

---

Delinquency

A type of antisocial behavior committed by children or youths (minor in age) deviating seriously from the norms of their culture or society and involving offenses such as murder and robbery or those that are strictly age-related, such as drinking liquor or smoking.

---

minors with major problems. They violate the law and commit offenses like thefts, gambling, cheating, pick-pocketing, murder, robbery, dacoity, destruction of property, violence and assault, intoxication, vagrancy, begging, kidnapping, abduction, and sexual offenses. The term "juvenile delinquents" or "young delinquents" means children or youths (minor in age) who deviate seriously from the norms of their culture or society and commit crimes such as murder and robbery, or offenses that are strictly age-related, such age drinking liquor and sexual activities. Juvenile delinquency should, therefore, be considered a serious challenge to the well-being of society. Young delinquents, if not handled properly, may become a source of concern for society.

Causes of Delinquency

1. *Hereditary factor:* Early researches held heredity responsible for delinquency. The claim of hereditarians such as Henry, Maudsley, Tredgold, and Dugdale that delinquency is inherited was tested by William Healey, Cyril Burt, Conrad and Jones, and Wingfield and Sandiford.

They concluded that delinquency is not inherited and therefore it is unjustified to blame heredity for delinquent behavior.

2. ***Constitutional or physiological factors:*** Defective constitution or glandular systems were also thought to be the cause of delinquent behavior. Udai Shanker (1958:30) observed that "poor health, short or too big stature or some deformity which gives rise to feelings of inferiority, dispose one to more aggression, as a compensatory reaction for his inadequacies." Consequently, this may lead to delinquent behavior. This correlation may seem well founded, but it is not so, as not much scientific evidence has been reported in its support so far. However, in some cases, it may be taken as one of the causes of delinquent behavior.

3. ***Intelligence factor:*** While earlier writers such as Lombroso and Goddard emphasize that the most important cause of delinquency and crime is low-grade mental capacity, Burt, Healey, Bronner, Merrill, and others deny that delinquents are mentally retarded. In fact, a direct causal relationship between intelligence and delinquency is doubtful. High intelligence is no guarantee for good behavior. Often, persons with superior intelligence have been found to be the leaders of notorious gangs and antisocial organizations. Sometimes, it is argued on the basis of statistics that since the majority of delinquents possess low intelligence, defective intelligence therefore causes delinquency. But this conclusion is not well founded. The collected statistics, in such cases, may represent an unreal picture. An intelligent individual may not be caught red-handed, whereas someone with low intelligence may always be taken into custody. Moreover, defective intelligence may lead to delinquency in one situation and may be a barrier to it in another situation. Hence, low intelligence alone cannot be held responsible for delinquent behavior.

4. ***Environmental and social factors:*** It has been proven that delinquent behavior is a learned reaction. Delinquents do not inherit delinquent qualities from their parents or ancestors but are made so by an uncongenial environment and social conditions. Udai Shanker (1958:30) observes that "delinquency is not inherited; it is the product of social and economic conditions and is essentially a coefficient of the friction between the individual and the community. The most important causes of antisocial behavior are environmental and sociological in character." It is therefore the uncongenial environment of the family, school, neighborhood, and society that should be blamed for delinquent behavior of children, since they pick up delinquent traits in such situations. We shall now see how the environment is responsible for delinquent character formation among minors.

(a) Home Environment and Delinquency

A defective and deficient family environment provides fertile ground for the germination of delinquency. As a matter of fact, family life and delinquency are closely related. Findings of various studies indicate that the family environment in which the following relationships or conditions prevail is most susceptible to delinquency:

- Broken home—where the family is incomplete due to death, desertion, separation, or divorce.
- Improper parental control.
- Unusual jealousy and rivalry among siblings and reactions such as, "My parents gave him more love than they gave me"
- The delinquent and criminal behavior of parents or other family members.
- Domestic conflicts.
- Economic difficulties and poverty of the family.

- Dull, monotonous, and uninteresting home environment.
- Denial of reasonable freedom and independence to youngsters.
- Maltreatment and injustice inflicted on youngsters
- Lack of proper physical and emotional security.

In such situations and environmental surroundings, children do not get the opportunity for the satisfaction of their basic needs. They become victim to emotional problems such as feelings of inferiority, insecurity, jealousy, or being thwarted, which make them maladjusted individuals and consequently turn them into hostile, rebellious, and antisocial personalities. Thus, uncongenial home conditions deserve to be blamed for juvenile delinquency, and in all circumstances, the root causes of delinquent behavior must be investigated in the child's family background and home environment.

(b) Uncongenial Environment Outside the Home

Whereas the home provides the roots for delinquent behavior, the social environment outside of the home nourishes it by supplying substitute for the satisfaction of unsatisfied basic needs and urges. For example, the peer group or gang presents itself as a substitute for family love and a sense of belonging. It also satisfies the need for recognition and gives an individual the opportunity for self-dependence and adventurism. Delinquent acts of one's peer group may lead them to delinquent behavior. The neighborhood and the places of social contracts and situations where elder members of society engage in antisocial activities, or the mass media such as newspapers, books, magazines, and cinema that acquaint children with immoral and antisocial acts, provide temptation for youngsters to become delinquents.

(c) Maladjustment in School

In many cases of delinquency, an uncongenial school environment can be a significant contributing factor. It brings about serious maladjustment and consequently increases the probability of delinquent character formation. Such an environment may involve the following elements:

- Defective curriculum
- Improper teaching methods
- Lack of co-curricular activities
- Lack of proper discipline and control
- Slackness in administration and organization
- Antisocial or undesirable behavior of the teachers
- Maltreatment and injustice done to the child
- Failure or backwardness

To conclude, delinquency is an environmental and social disease. Delinquent acts are learned and acquired acts. No child is born delinquent nor is delinquent behavior the product of genes. Thus, delinquents are not a specific type of human being born with innate, physical, mental, or emotional characteristics. They are normal individuals with normal needs and desires. Like normal children, they also want to love, to be loved, and to satisfy their need for security and recognition. The denial of these basic needs leads to maladjustment and makes them hostile and rebellious. Thus, delinquent behavior is a reaction or resentment against the prevailing social and environmental conditions. It is a revolt against parents, teachers, or social organizations that do not provide them the essential environment for the satisfaction of their basic needs and urges.

Prevention and Treatment

Delinquency, besides being a legal problem, is basically a psycho-social problem. All delinquents are essentially maladjusted personalities and the result of faulty upbringing and maltreatment. The solution to the problem requires preventive and curative measures.

Preventive Measures

Initially, these involve improvement of the social or environmental conditions that thwart the satisfaction of an individual's basic needs. Some of the following suggestions may work well in this direction.

Parental education: Parents should be aware of the psychology of delinquency so that they can treat and handle their children with understanding and provide them with an environment for the satisfaction of their basic needs and urges. It requires parental education, which may be provided through guidance services, clinics, and voluntary social services.

The child's company: Parents, family members, and school authorities should keep a close watch on children's activities and social environment, and take care so that they do not fall in bad company. Antisocial elements and criminals often seek out youngsters for their own purposes. Attempts should be made to save children from them, and they should be educated in keeping away from such elements.

Substitute environment: It is difficult to bring a change in a defective family environment or the influences of the neighborhood peer group. In such circumstances, children should be removed from their environment and placed either in foster homes or well-managed reformatories and special schools so that they may be provided with a healthy environment for their emotional and social adjustment.

Rectifying school education and environment: The school environment should be healthy and congenial. The curriculum, methods of teaching, discipline, classroom behavior of the teacher, and the social atmosphere of the school should be rectified so that children do not involve themselves in emotional and social maladjustment problems. The attitudes of teachers who impose their authority on children and do not understand their basic needs should be changed. The headmaster as well as the teachers should be familiar with the psychology of individual differences and delinquency.

Treatment or Curative Measures

The problem of juvenile delinquency should not be regarded as a law and order problem. It is an educational and welfare problem. Juvenile delinquents should not be put behind bars and treated through the panel system. Delinquents require rehabilitation and re-education for which special legal provisions should be made. The legal dealings with juvenile delinquents have changed in the progressive communities of the world.

In our own country, also, we have made a specific legal provision for dealing with delinquents in the name of the Juvenile Justice Act enacted by the parliament of India in 2015 and modified many times in the subsequent years, most recently in 2021 (Ministry of Law and Justice, 2021). The main provisions and features of this act are summarized below.

- A juvenile who has committed an offense can be dealt with only by a juvenile court. A juvenile court differs from other courts in its philosophy, objectives, and functions. The juvenile court is constituted by qualified magistrates and is assisted by honorary social workers. Special knowledge of child psychology and child welfare is an essential qualification for every member of the court. The proceedings in respect of a juvenile are not public and only specified persons are allowed to attend the proceedings. The disclosure of name, address, or other particulars that might lead to the identification of the juvenile is prohibited.
- No delinquent juvenile can be tried in the same way as an adult under the court of criminal procedure. A delinquent juvenile can also not be charged and tried with an adult. Under the Act, a juvenile cannot be sentenced to death or imprisonment. If the court comes to the conclusion that the child has committed the offense they are charged with, then several outcomes might result, ranging from releasing the child on probation of good conduct to placing him under the care of a qualified parent/guardian, institution, or special home.
- Rehabilitation has been made an integral part of such institutional programs. Every neglected and delinquent juvenile must not only be provided accommodation, maintenance, and facilities for education, vocational training, and rehabilitation, but also with facilities for the development of his character and necessary training for protecting himself against exploitation. The importance of aftercare has been recognized as essential for the rehabilitation of the juvenile in the community. The Act provides for the setting up of aftercare organizations for juveniles once they leave juvenile homes or special homes, to help their readjustment, resettlement, and rehabilitation as self-reliant, socially useful citizens. Many state governments have established comprehensive aftercare schemes, the objectives of which are the following:

  a. To extend help, counseling, guidance, support, and protection to all released juveniles whenever necessary;
  b. To help a released juvenile overcome his mental, social, and economic difficulties;
  c. To impress upon the juvenile the need to adjust his habits, attitudes, approaches, and value schemes on a rational appreciation of social responsibilities and obligation and the requirements of community living;
  d. To help the juvenile make a smooth adjustment to his post-release environment;
  e. To encourage the juvenile in making satisfactory readjustment with his family, neighborhood, and community;
  f. To assist the juvenile in functioning as a self-reliant, socially useful citizen;
  g. To assist in the process of the juvenile's physical, mental, vocational, economic, social, and attitudinal post-release readjustment and ultimate rehabilitation;
  h. To complete in all respects the process of the juvenile's final readjustment, resettlement, and rehabilitation.

As a follow-up measure under the Juvenile Justice Act, the Scheme for Prevention and Control of Juvenile Social Maladjustment has been implemented by the Ministry of Welfare since 1986–87 to provide financial support to states/Union territories for setting up or upgrading juvenile homes/special homes/aftercare organizations and for the training of functionaries.

As a result of such legal provisions in our country, and influenced by what is happening in other countries, our attitude toward delinquency is also changing. It has now been realized that children who are called delinquents are ill primarily in their inability to conform to the social milieu. Consequently, in most states, the Juvenile Justice Act has been enforced, and some have gone ahead in the work of rehabilitation and re-education of young offenders. Separate child welfare boards for dealing with the problem of delinquency have been established, and approved schools have come into existence. Some states encourage voluntary organizations to take custody of delinquent children. Provisions for the care of neglected and destitute children are also made so that they do not become delinquents. Some states have started foster care programs in which the court gives custody of a child to a responsible person. There is, however, a need to arouse public consciousness of this problem. No government can solve a social problem without public cooperation. Therefore, there is a need for a change in our attitude toward delinquents so that they may be helped in their readjustment and rehabilitation.

To Sum Up

The violation of the law of the land and committing legal offenses is termed criminal behavior and the person who exhibits such behavior is termed a criminal. However, when such offenses are committed by individuals who are minor in age (in a legal sense, from 7–16 years in the case of boys, and 7–18 years in the case of girls in our country), they are termed delinquents and not criminals, and their criminal behavior is known as delinquency.

Causes of delinquency are traced to a defective and uncongenial home environment, and family and other sociocultural environmental conditions, instead of hereditary or biological factors. While the causes for the delinquent behavior are provided by an uncongenial home and family environment, the social environment outside the home nourishes it by supplying a substitute for the satisfaction of unfulfilled desires and needs.

Preventive measures taken for dealing with the problem of delinquency aim at improving the social or environmental conditions and may involve parental education, protecting the child from bad company and antisocial environment, providing a substitute for the defective environment, and rectifying the school education and environment.

Regarding the employment of curative measures, we should remember that delinquents cannot be cured through legal punishment. The curative measures employed for them, thus, should involve appropriate psychological and rehabilitation attempts on the part of government or voluntary organizations. Moreover, there is a need to bring change in our attitude toward delinquents and delinquency. As a constructive approach toward delinquency, it is a welcome sign to note that appropriate steps in our country in this direction are now taking their roots in the shape of enacting the Juvenile Justice Act and making provision for the reformatories, approved schools, foster-care programs, and remand homes, in the pattern of other developed countries.

Crime

Concept and Meaning: Crime may be defined as an act prohibited by the laws of a country or state, or a failure on the part of an individual to perform an act that is prescribed by that law. In a legal sense, a person of 21 years and above convicted by the court of law for violating the provision of IPC and CPC is labeled a criminal in our country, and the illegal act for which he is convicted is known as a crime. Any behavior like pickpocketing, gambling, burglary, robbery, theft, dacoity, rape, kidnapping, attempts at suicide, murder, riots, destroying another's property, sexual assault, prostitution, cheating, counterfeiting, failure to deposit taxes and revenue, and so on are termed criminal behavior.

> ## Crime
>
> The antisocial behavior and acts committed by persons of 21 years and above that are prohibited by law of the land and convicted by the court of law.

The term criminal needs to be distinguished from other terms used for antisocial personalities, such as delinquents, young offenders, and problem children. We can summarize the meaning of these terms in light of the existing criminal laws prevalent in our country.

Criminals: People 21 years of age and older committing antisocial behavior or acts serious enough for getting them convicted by the court of law in our country for violating the provisions of the Indian Penal Code (IPC) and the Criminal Procedure Code (CPC).

Delinquents: Children or youths (minor in age, i.e., below 16 years of age in the case of boys and 18 years for girls), committing an antisocial behavior of the same nature that would have been termed a crime if committed by an adult of 21 years of age or older.

Young or Youthful Offenders: Individuals between 16–21 among boys and 18–21 among girls committing antisocial acts serious enough to violate the provisions of the Indian Penal Code (IPC) and the Criminal Procedure Code of our country.

Problem children: Children up to seven years committing an antisocial behavior of any nature termed as a crime under the provisions of the IPC and CPC of our country.

Causes Underlying Crime

Although delinquents do not necessarily become criminals, in many cases, adult crime has been found to show a history of juvenile delinquency. Both delinquency and crime have a similar tendency characterized by a unique reaction pattern of aggression against the social setup. The causes underlying crimes are therefore similar to those of delinquency.

Biological factors such as defective heredity and intelligence, poor constitutional makeup, or glandular disturbances, have not been found to play any substantial role in the causation of criminal behavior. The view that a criminal is born has almost been discarded in favor of socio-psychological environmental factors being responsible for the criminal tendency in an individual.

It should be observed that criminal behavior may have a variety of forms and degrees of severity. It may range from an offense that is committed once in a lifetime to a lifestyle of criminal behavior. Hence, the pathology involving socio-psychological causes also varies from crime to crime and criminal to criminal. Criminal behavior is not necessarily generated and developed by a single factor or a few factors.

Criminals are victims of social maladjustment arising out of defective environmental conditions and unfavorable life circumstances. Some of these situations may be summarized as follows.

1. *Learned as a professional art:* Criminal behavior may be learned like any professional act or art like tailoring, woodworking, or haircutting from parents or members of the family and

community. The perpetuation of one or the other specific criminal behaviors such as burglary, prostitution, theft, or bootlegging among certain tribes, castes, or races are some other examples.

2. *The impact of defective family environments:* An uncongenial home environment contributes to criminal character formation. It is often the result of broken homes through desertion, divorce, separation, or the death of one or both parents. Moreover, the defective and deficient environment created by unfavorable intrafamilial tensions and conflicts, lax parental control, poverty, sibling rivalries, and maltreatment is insufficient to fulfill the basic physiological and psychological needs of children. In order to gratify their physical, social, and emotional needs, they are lured and sometimes forced onto a path of crime. Not only young members of the family but also adults may be forced to lead a life of criminals on account of the frustrations caused by deficient family environments and unhealthy interpersonal relationships. For example, sexual frustration may lead one to promiscuity, prostitution, or even causing murder, rape, or other similar offenses.

3. *Economic factors:* Poverty, unemployment, desire for the pleasures of life, competition to earn money by any means, and the evils of industrialization all contribute in pushing an individual toward criminal behavior.

4. *Degradation of moral values:* The crisis of character and degradation of moral values in society also may cause criminal character formation. Crimes such as call-girl rackets in posh colonies and luxury hotels, adulteration of food and drugs, forgery, counterfeiting of money, bank robberies, black money transactions, smuggling, bribery, and selling secrets of one's own country can be attributed to a lack of moral values.

5. *Environment outside the family:* Whereas defective home environments and circumstances provide the basic causes for criminal behavior, the criminal environment outside the home nourishes it by providing a substitute for the gratification of unsatisfied needs and cherished goals. Neighborhoods, communities, and places of social contact where there are opportunities for mixing with criminal characters attract and even push individuals into the world of crime. The unhealthy impact of the mass media, especially cheap literature, obscene pictures, photographs, and films, may encourage individuals toward crime.

6. *Social system and denial of justice:* The defective social system and traditions lead to circumstances where an individual learns criminal behavior. For example, the dowry system, the dominance of men in the social setup, and the status of widows give rise to complications leading to crime. The gulf between the rich and the poor, caste differences, hatred toward other communities, races, linguistic groups, sects and religions, and the exploitation of laborers and landless farmers by landlords often lead to strained relationships and crimes.

7. *Mental illness and abnormal states of mind:* Sometimes crimes are committed by mentally ill persons in an abnormal state of mind. Compulsive behaviors like kleptomania of neurotics and abnormal behavior of sexual deviants may lead to crime. Similarly, psychotic individuals classified as criminally insane may commit a variety of offenses depending upon the situation and their state of mind. Under the influence of liquor and drugs, offenses are committed not only by professional criminals and socially and emotionally maladjusted individuals but also by normal people. Individuals suffering from senile brain degeneration and mental deficiency may also be found responsible for certain offenses committed in an abnormal state of mind without realizing the consequences of their behavior.

Prevention and Treatment

The remedy for criminal behavior demands preventive and curative measures.

Prevention

Preventive measures involve the improvement of the social factors and environmental conditions that are responsible for the germination and perpetuation of criminal behavior. The problem is a gigantic one and needs the cooperation of parents, family members, neighborhood, community, school or college authorities, religious heads, police, and government officials responsible for the improved social and psychological environment of citizens. The following measures may be fruitful in prevention efforts:

- Since today's delinquents are tomorrow's criminals, maximum efforts should, therefore, be made for the prevention, control, and treatment of identified delinquents.
- There is a great need for social reforms and breaking social and caste barriers.
- The task of narrowing the gulf between the rich and the poor, linguistic groups, and religious sects should be given priority.
- The importance of moral values should be inculcated. There should be an end to the crisis of character threatening the existence of the moral basis and legal codes of our society.
- The system of education and national planning needs rethinking and remodification for minimizing the economic difficulties of our youth and adults.
- The problem of unemployment has to be checked, and the professional dissatisfaction and frustration affecting a vast population of the younger generation should be curbed.
- Attempts should be made to minimize undesirable influences of literature, films, and other mass media.
- The parents, elders, government authorities, and social, religious, educational, and political leaders should be such that they become ideals of socially desirable behavior.
- Society should feel the necessity of providing social and legal justice to its citizens. In case of environmental deprivations and hazards of life, the affected individual should be helped, protected, and rehabilitated.

Thus, there is a need for modifying the environmental conditions so that one does not fall victim to social and emotional maladjustment or be lured in by criminals to commit crimes.

Treatment and Rehabilitation

The old notion that criminals are born and nothing can be done for reforming and rehabilitating them still holds its ground. Law enforcement is still largely punitive and vengeful. Even in many civilized societies and developed countries, the treatment provided to criminals is still on the terms of tooth for tooth and eye for eye. Criminals are isolated from society, kept in prisons; punishments such as lashing, severing of hands and legs, and hanging are given in public not only to deter the criminal from further offenses but also to prevent others from indulging in such acts. However, as a result of an increase in the knowledge of human behavior and criminal psychology, there have been changes in the attitude of the general public, police officials, and government authorities toward criminals and crime. It is now understood that for most criminals, their behavior is part of a larger pattern of personality maladjustment. Criminal behavior is nothing but a social disease and criminals are ill primarily in terms of their inability to conform to the social milieu. With serious psychological and psychiatric problems, they need hospitalization, medical and psychological treatment as curative measures for their illness.

The change in attitude has ushered in a new era in the management of jails, which are now called correctional institutions. More progressive prison authorities are now adopting a constructive attitude toward criminals. In addition to custodial care, attempts to resocialize, readjust, and rehabilitate the criminals are employed. The emphasis is on the study of each prisoner as an individual, as a victim of circumstances, and to provide them the medical aid and psychological treatment, training, and help needed for their restoration to society as a self-supporting and law-abiding citizen. The effectiveness of the curative and reformatory measures lies in modifying the behavior of criminals and equipping them with the necessary skills for playing useful roles in society.

Some of the measures used in this new constructive reformatory approach are:

1. The crimes committed by delinquents or young offenders and also by relatively normal adults during periods of acute stress and deprivation have very little chance of being repeated unless they are compelled to do so again. Also, the majority of new criminals are accidental criminals who commit an offense by chance or mishap. The environment of prisons, coupled with their association with hardened criminals, often converts them to a life of criminality. Attempts should be made to keep them out of prison by granting probation and making provisions for their adequate supervision by competent probation officers.
2. The constructive approach calls for change in the environment of the prison and the treatment of prisoners as human beings in need of sympathy and affection in understanding their behavioral problems.
3. Many countries are now experimenting with open prisons, which do not have fences or outer walls, and their dormitories are neither locked nor guarded. They are open fields with situations where prisoners are provided opportunities to work for which they are paid. Their expenses are met out of their earnings, which are partly sent to their families. Occasionally, they too are sent to meet their families. There is an environment of understanding and trust prevailing in such prisons, providing sufficient opportunities for the modification of their behavior. They are made to learn useful social skills and readjustment into society.
4. A humanitarian approach in which prisons are converted into hospitals—the criminals understood as mentally ill, socially maladjusted, and psychologically handicapped individuals—is taking root in the prisons of many countries. Efforts are also being made to study criminal behavior, to investigate its causes, and to find ways of modifying it. The cooperation of the physician, psychiatrist, social worker, and legal authorities is sought by prison authorities for the treatment of abnormal and antisocial behavior of the inmates.
5. In some countries, useful rehabilitation programs are being adopted for the welfare of criminals. In our country, the rehabilitation of the dacoits of the Chambal Valley by Sarvodaya leaders may be cited as a good attempt in providing opportunities for leading a self-supporting and law-abiding life.

To Sum Up

Crime may be defined as an antisocial act prohibited by the law of the land. In a legal sense, people of 21 years and above convicted by the court of Jaw for violating the provision of IPC and CPC are labeled as criminals in our country, and the illegal act for which they are convicted is known as a crime.

Regarding the causes underlying crime, it can be well inferred that criminals are always the victims of social maladjustment arising out of defective environmental conditions and unfavorable circumstances of life. Accordingly, criminal behavior is essentially a learned pattern of maladaptive and antisocial behavior resulting from close interaction of unfavorable social, psychological, and psychiatric factors.

The preventive measures for criminal behavior involve the improvement of social and environmental conditions that are responsible for the germination and perpetuation of criminal behavior. On the other hand, for the treatment and rehabilitation of criminals, the basic requirement demands a change in outlook and attitudes toward criminals and crimes so that criminals may be provided with hospitalization, medical and psychological treatment as curative measures for their serious socio-psychological and psychiatric problems. They should be understood sympathetically, studied individually, treated medically and psychologically, trained and helped educationally as well as vocationally, and finally, rehabilitated to become self-supporting and law-abiding citizens in the interest of their own and that of society.

Review Questions

1. What do you understand by the terms disruptive, impulse-control, and conduct disorders?
2. What is oppositional defiant behavior? Throw light on its meaning and nature.
3. What is intermittent explosive disorder? How does a child suffering from this disorder behave in their environmental situations?
4. What is conduct disorder? Throw light on the behavior exhibited by children inflicted with this disorder.
5. What do you understand by the terms antisocial behavior and antisocial personality? What type of behavior, in general, is expected from an antisocial personality?
6. What is delinquency or delinquent behavior? Throw light on its meaning and concept.
7. While defining the term delinquency, throw light on its causes or factors responsible for its emergence.
8. Discuss in detail the preventive and curative measures taken for dealing with the problem of delinquency.
9. What is crime or criminal behavior? Throw light on its meaning and concept.
10. While defining the term crime, throw light on the probable causes underlying criminal behavior.
11. Discuss in detail the ways and means utilized for the prevention of crimes and treatment as well as the rehabilitation of criminals.

References

American Psychiatric Association (1968), *Diagnostic and statistical manual of mental disorders, DSM-II* (2nd ed.), Washington, DC: American Psychiatric Association.

American Psychiatric Association (2013), *Diagnostic and statistical manual of mental disorders* (5th ed.), Washington, DC: American Psychiatric Association.

Ministry of Law and Justice (2021), *The Juvenile Justice (Care and Protection of Children) Amendment Act, 2021*, New Delhi: Govt. of India Press.

Shanker, U. (1958), *Problem children*, Delhi: Atma Ram & Sons.

Chapter 13

Substance-Related and Addictive Disorders

Learning Objectives

After going through this chapter, you will be able to:

- Know about the meaning and define the term substance-related and addictive disorders
- Name the different disorders classified as substance-related and addictive disorders
- Describe the criteria mentioned in the DSM-5-TR for the diagnosis of substance-induced mental disorders
- Discuss different types of psychoactive substances and their effects
- Discuss the causes underlying alcohol addiction
- Tell about the different stages of turning one a hardened alcoholic
- Evaluate the causes of alcoholism
- Discuss the treatment measures for alcoholism
- Know about the concept and meaning of drug-addiction as an addictive disorder
- Discuss the causes of drug addiction
- Throw light on the prevention and treatment of drug addiction

What are the Substance-Related and Addictive Disorders?

Substance-related and addictive disorders are the outcomes of addiction resulting from substance abuse—the continued use of a psychoactive substance (such as alcohol or a drug) despite significant problems related to its use. Consequently, we may refer to these disorders as a type of mental and behavioral disorders characterized by the symptoms and signs of addictive behavior and the psycho-physiological ill consequences accompanying such behavior.

In fact, an abuse of a psychoactive substance occurs when an individual consumes it for an extended period or ingests large amounts of it to get the same effect it provided previously. It creates an intense *craving* for its consumption more and more on the part of the individual. As individuals consume a substance more and more for getting the desired effects (e.g., relaxation, relief in pain, or a feeling of pleasurable experience), it results in building an increased *tolerance* in them for the consumption of that substance. At this stage, they are fully entrapped and have no way other than taking more and more doses of the substance, despite facing a lot of physiological, psychological, and social problems. It is the stage of

DOI: 10.4324/9781003398325-13

complete dependence and compulsion for the use of the substance. Here, in cases where they intend to reduce or abstain from the use of the substance, they feel a lot of difficulty in doing so on account of the inherent craving for the consumption of that substance, as well as experiencing the resulting *withdrawal* symptoms (such as lack of appetite, loss of weight, constipation, restlessness, nervousness. cramps, anxiety attacks, sweating, nausea, vomiting, tremors, hallucinations, or severe physical and psychological problems like seizures, stroke, or even death).

> ### Substance-related addictive disorders
>
> Substance-related addictive disorders are the type of mental and behavioral disorders visible among people who become addicted to a psychoactive substance such as alcohol or a drug through its abuse and suffer from the physiological and psychological ill consequences arrived at through such addiction.

In this way, the abuse of a psychoactive substance ultimately leads an individual to reach the stage of becoming addicted to the use of a substance with the signs and symptoms of (i) an intense craving for the consumption of the substance regardless of its consequences, (ii) a tendency to increase the doses of the substance with time, (iii) physiological and psychological dependence on the effects of substance consumption, and (iv) manifestation of particular withdrawal symptoms on abrupt discontinuation of the consumption of the substance.

In light of this, we may define the term substance-related addictive disorders, as a type of mental and behavioral disorder found among people who demonstrate the signs and symptoms of addictive behavior (resulting from the abuse of one or the other psychoactive substances), characterized by the symptoms and signs such as cravings for, the development of a tolerance to, and difficulties in controlling the use of a particular substance or a set of substances, as well as showing withdrawal symptoms upon abrupt cessation of substance use.

Here now a question may arise regarding what these substances are, the use of which make one victim of one or the other psychological disorders.

By definition, a substance is any ingested material the use of which results in temporary cognitive, behavioral, or physiological symptoms within the individual. In the classification systems provided by the American Psychiatric Association and the World Health Organization, these substances are listed in the names of alcohol, caffeine, cannabis, cocaine, hallucinogens, inhalants, opioids, sedatives, stimulants, tobacco, medication drugs, and other (or unknown). However, it is the misuse of these substances, in the form of their repeated and/or excessive use known by the term *substance abuse*, that is responsible for making people first become addicted and then suffer from the agonies of substance-related addictive disorders. Let us examine how the most recent systems of classification, the DSM-5-TR and ICD-11 provided by the APA and WHO, classify the disorders falling into the category of Substance-related and Addictive Disorders:

- Alcohol-Related Disorders
- Caffeine-Related Disorders
- Cannabis-Related Disorders
- Cocaine-Related Disorders
- Hallucinogen-Related Disorders
- Inhalant-Related Disorders

- Opioid-Related Disorders
- Sedative, Hypnotic or Anxiolytic-Related Disorders
- Stimulant-Related Disorders
- Dissociative drugs-Related Disorders
- Tobacco/Nicotine-Related Disorders
- MDMA (or related drugs)-Related Disorders
- Other Specified psychoactive substances, including medications-Related Disorders

Table 13.1 Diagnostic Criteria for Disorders due to Substance Abuse

- Inability to complete or lack of participation in work, school, or home activities
- Increased time spent on activities obtaining, using, or recovering from substance use
- Impairment in social or interpersonal relationships
- Use of a substance in a potentially hazardous situation
- Psychological problems due to recurrent substance abuse
- Craving the substance
- An increase in the amount of substance used over time (i.e., tolerance)
- Difficulty reducing the amount of substance used despite a desire to reduce/stop using; and/or withdrawal symptoms

Note: Two or three symptoms indicate a mild substance abuse disorder, four or five symptoms indicate a moderate substance abuse disorder, and six or more symptoms indicate a severe substance abuse disorder.
Source: American Psychiatric Association (2022), Diagnostic and statistical manual of mental disorders: DSM-5-TR. Washington DC: American Psychiatric Association.

To Sum Up

The substance-related addictive disorders represent the type of mental and behavioral disorders found among people who resort to substance abuse to the extent of showing signs of addictive behavior toward a particular psychoactive substance, such as alcohol or a drug in the form of cravings for its consumption, the development of tolerance for its use, having a complete dependency on its use more and more irrespective of its ill consequences, and showing withdrawal symptoms upon abrupt cessation of its use. The abuse of psychoactive substances to the extent of their addiction may, thus, result in making them victims of one or the other mental and behavioral disorders specifically related to their abuse and addiction. The DSMs and ICDs have identified and described the various disorders related to substances such as alcohol, caffeine, cannabis, cocaine hallucinogens, inhalants, opioids, sedatives, stimulants, tobacco, medication drugs, and others (or unknown).

Psychoactive Substances—Types and Effects

In looking into the list of disorders classified as substance-related addictive disorders, given earlier, we see that each of these disorders is related to the abuse of one or the other types of psychoactive substances. Depending upon the nature of their effects, these psychoactive substances may, then, be classified as (A) Depressants or Sedatives, (B) Stimulants, and (C) Deliriant or mind-blowing drugs. Let us know about them.

A. Depressants or Sedatives

The substances included in this category are termed depressants or sedatives on account of their characteristics of exercising an inhibiting effect on one's central nervous system that results in diminishing the responses of the brain and nervous system and slowing down the individual's activities. As a result, these are used to relieve anxiety, stress or pain, as well as induce sleep. However, their abuse turns into a variety of problems, including one or the other types of substance-related addictive disorders. Among the psychoactive substances included in this category, alcohol is the most consumed and abused substance all over the globe. The others include the drugs classified as Opioids and Sedative-Hypnotic drugs.

Alcohol: More specifically termed ethyl alcohol or ethanol, alcohol is a psychoactive substance that is produced by the fermentation of sugars, usually in agricultural products such as fruits, cereals, and vegetables, with or without subsequent distillation. As a depressant it has an inhibiting effect on one's central nervous system, allowing the individual to relax in moments of tension and stress. It is this relaxed feeling that draws an individual to take alcoholic beverages. However, on account of the intoxicating effects, one is forced to take more and more doses for experiencing the same pleasure-giving effect, and is thus caught in the vicious cycle of falling victim to the ill consequences of alcohol abuse. The ill consequences of alcohol abuse result in the following types of impairment and damage:

- In terms of physiological damage, almost every tissue and organ of the body and its functioning is adversely affected by alcohol abuse, including the immune system of the body, making one an easy victim of diseases.
- In terms of psychological and behavioral functioning damage, alcohol abuse may cause: (i) severe deterioration in the thought processes and damage to intellectual functioning, to the extent of leading an individual to "black out" causing an inability to remember what he said or did, (ii) a quite significant deterioration in motor coordination, balance, speech, sensation and perception, (iii) deterioration in sex behavior in the form of sexual incapacity or impotence, and indulgence in sexual deviations and sex crimes, (iii) severe personality or character disorders to the extent of terming one a criminal and antisocial personality, (iv) making one victim of a number of neurological and psychotic disorders (brain syndromes) such as pathological intoxication, delirium tremens, alcoholic hallucinosis, alcoholic deterioration, and Korsakoff syndrome.

Depressants Drugs

Like alcohol, the consumption of depressant drugs begins with pleasurable experiences providing relief from anxiety, stress, and pain, and lessening of voluntary movements followed by euphoria. But these effects are short-lived and are followed by a negative phase of craving more of the drug, and consequent ill effects in terms of physiological and psychological dependence and withdrawal symptoms. There are two major categories of depressant drugs, known as (i) Opioids and (ii) Sedative-Hypnotic drugs.

Opioid is a generic term that encompasses the constituents or derivatives of the opium poppy. We may include substances like morphine, diacetylmorphine (heroin), fentanyl, pethidine, oxycodone, hydromorphone, methadone, buprenorphine, codeine, and d-propoxyphene in the category of opioids. All of these opioids possess analgesic properties and work as effective central nervous system depressants. On account of their depressant nature, all of them except heroin are prescribed for pain management and palliative care. People may also resort to their consumption non-medically for experiencing some sort of relief from anxiety-ridden stress or experiencing a state of euphoria and drowsiness. However, it is heroin that is primarily used for non-medical purposes all over the globe.

All of these opioids, while working as potential depressants, prove too harmful to individuals in the course of their abuse. Opioids also possess a unique characteristic of rapid development of tolerance to these drugs, resulting in an increased need for their consumption, and dependence on them within a short time. The highly addictive nature of opioids and resulting ill consequences lead to incalculable physiological and psychological damage, making addicted individuals highly prone to mental and psychological disorders.

Sedative-Hypnotic drugs, more commonly known as *anxiolytic drugs*, are potential depressants and sedatives, and have a unique characteristic of exercising a calming and relaxing effect on individuals. That is why these are often prescribed as pain and anxiety relief medications. We may classify these drugs as *barbiturates* (such as amytal, nembutal, and seconal) and non-barbiturates (such as bromides and paraldehyde chloral hydrate). A group of non-barbiturates known as *benzodiazepines* (including the drugs like Xanax, Ativan, and Valium) is also popular among clinicians for prescription in providing temporary relief to the anxiety-ridden individual (e.g., pre-flight or pre-surgery anxiety) or as a long term medication (e.g., generalized anxiety disorder).

However, whatever their positive primary effects may be, their abuse can result in harmful physiological and psychological damage to addicted individuals. Accordingly, addiction to opioids and hypnotics results in a number of physiological and psychological damage, including the common depressant outcomes such as loss of appetite and weight, constipation, and lack of sexual desire and social interests. However, unlike opioids, addiction to barbiturates and other hypnotics primarily affects the brain resulting in intellectual impairment and disturbance of the motor functions dependent on the cerebellum.

Moreover, the sudden withdrawal of depressants and sedatives (whether opioids or hypnotics) results in dangerous withdrawal symptoms like restlessness, nervousness, excessive perspiration, nausea, vomiting, diarrhea, severe headache, marked tremors, cardiovascular collapse, and painful muscular cramps. In the case of hypnotics, withdrawal reactions may lead to epileptic seizures and delirium. If not treated in time, seizures can cause death.

B. Stimulant Drugs

Unlike depressants that reduce the activity of the central nervous system, stimulants have the opposite effect. These drugs stimulate the brain and sympathetic nervous system resulting in alertness and an increase in response and motor activity, including the creation a feeling of euphoria and hyperactivity. The major drugs of this category are nicotine, cocaine, caffeine, and amphetamines (such as dexamphetamine, benzedrine, Dexedrine, methedrine, and methamphetamine). Let us look into them in brief.

Nicotine: Nicotine is a highly potent addictive stimulant and is the third most common psychoactive substance used worldwide, after caffeine and alcohol. It is available through the consumption of tobacco, a product available from a natural plant known as the tobacco plant. People get doses of nicotine by consuming tobacco in various ways such as chewing tobacco, inhaling its powdered stuff, and inhaling its vaporized form through cigarettes, Bidi, Hukka, or Pipe smoking, and more recently in the form of electronic cigarette smoking.

Cocaine: Cocaine is extracted from a plant known as the coca plant. It is the most potent natural central nervous system stimulant known to date (Acosta et al., 2011). It is commonly used illicitly and widely available across the world in its two main forms: cocaine hydrochloride and cocaine freebase (also known as "crack"). Cocaine is unique in that it can be ingested in various ways such as by snorting via the nasal cavity or smoking via a glass pipe. Inhaled cocaine is absorbed into the bloodstream and brain within 10–15 seconds, suggesting that its effects are felt quite instantly.

Caffeine: Caffeine is a mild psychostimulant found in the beans of the coffee plant and is a widely consumed substance in the world today. We consume it through a variety of coffee drinks, soft drinks, and energy drinks, or through the use of chocolate in our foodstuffs.

Amphetamines: The stimulants known as amphetamines are synthetically manufactured. The drugs included in the category of amphetamines may be named as Ritalin, Adderall, Benzedine, Dexedrine, Dexamphetamine, Mathedrine, Methcathinone (or ephedrine), and Methamphetamine.

These drugs can be consumed by individuals in various ways, such as injecting, snorting, smoking, or swallowing.

All these drugs classified as stimulants have the common properties of stimulating the function of the central nervous system and temporarily increasing one's level of energy and alertness, as well as providing a feeling of euphoria and confidence. As a result, these are often prescribed as medication in the treatment of certain physical ailments and mental or behavioral disorders or consumed by people for relief and positive feelings. However, irrespective of their medication or non-medication use, whenever there occurs an abuse of these drugs, it can result in serious physical and mental health problems, such as severe loss of appetite and weight, constipation, damage to bodily organs, increased anxiety and irritability, sleep deprivation, gradual impairment of intellectual functioning, and periodic episodes of delirium.

C. Deliriant or Mind-Blowing Drugs

These drugs are characterized by the effects of producing transient states resembling psychoses resulting in marked confusion, distortion in thought processes, delirium, illusions, and hallucinations. We may put the drugs classified as Hallucinogens and Cannabis in this category.

HALLUCINOGENS OR HALLUCINOGENIC DRUGS

On account of their consumption resulting in the symptoms of the state of hallucination, these drugs are known as hallucinogenic drugs. These are available in two forms—naturally derived from plants, and synthetically manufactured in laboratories. As examples of these drugs we may cite the names of LSD-25 or lysergic acid diethylamide, mescaline, psilocybin, bufotenine, methamphetamine (speed), PCP, Ketamine, and Ecstasy. Let us look into them.

(i) *LSD-25 (Lysergic acid diethylamide):* It is a chemically synthesized drug having hallucinogenic properties of an intense nature. Among the hallucinogens, it is the most popular drug that is abused all across the globe by younger generations. It is taken orally. In general, for this purpose, paper doses are placed on the tongue, where the drug is rapidly absorbed. Tablets or capsules are swallowed.

(ii) *Mescaline:* Mescaline is a hallucinogenic substance found in the fruit or button-shaped seeds that grow on the outside of certain cacti plants such as peyote cactus, which are cut off and dried and then eaten or sliced, boiled, and drunk as a tea. These buttons can also be dried and ground into an off-white powder put into a pill capsule or smoked with tobacco. It is also produced through chemical synthesis.

(iii) *Psilocybin:* Psilocybin is a hallucinogenic substance that can be availed from both fresh and dried mushrooms in varying concentrations. It can also be created in a lab. In their raw form, mushrooms are eaten fresh, cooked or brewed into tea. We can also avail psilocybin in its powdered form after drying and grinding the mushrooms for oral consumption or inhaling it through smoking, sometimes mixed with tobacco or cannabis.

(iv) Bufotenine: Bufotenune is a hallucinogenic substance isolated from several natural sources or prepared by chemical synthesis. The natural sources of its availability are (a) plant material, mostly seeds of the genus Anadenanthera (formerly Piptadenia), (b) plant organs of other genera; and (c) certain species of toads and mushrooms. It is used generally via intravenous injection and its abuse may result in severe physiological and psychological damage.

(v) *Speed (Methamphetamine):* Speed (methamphetamine), having intensive hallucinogenic properties, is a potent and addictive central nervous system stimulant. It is a synthetic chemical drug available in the form of a white, odorless, bitter-tasting powder that easily dissolves in water or alcohol. It is a synthetic chemical and it is quite cheap and easy to make from common ingredients such as the nasal decongestant pseudoephedrine. In its consumption, it is usually smoked, snorted, injected, or taken orally on the part of individuals. Prolonged use of this drug results in malnutrition, brain damage, disturbance of the heart rhythm, and dangerous impulsive, paranoid, and unpredictable behavior.

(vi) *PCP* (phenylcyclohexyl piperidine): It is a dissociative hallucinogenic drug that is capable of producing intense hallucinogenic and dissociative effects. Its abuse may result in bizarre behavior uncharacteristic of the individual, including self-harm.

(vii) *Ketamine:* It is a dissociative hallucinogenic drug that may be taken by the oral or nasal routes or injected. Despite its rare use as a medication for the treatment of certain mental disorders (e.g., treatment-resistant Depressive Disorders), it is mainly a widespread drug of nonmedical use. Its abuse results in emergent hallucinations and dissociative effects.

(viii) MDMA (Methylenedioxymethamphetamine): It is a common drug of abuse in many countries, especially among young people. It is predominantly available in tablet form known as "ecstasy" and is synthesized in a lab. It is a non-medication psychoactive drug that exercises stimulating and hallucinogenic properties.

The abuse of all these hallucinogenic drugs may result in incalculable physiological and psychological damage to drug addicts, including the causation of a number of mental and behavioral disorders specifically associated with hallucinogenic and dissociative properties. The outward symptoms of hallucinogenic drug addiction bear a strong resemblance to the behavior of schizophrenic patients. There is marked confusion, muddying of one's thinking, and the development of visual and auditory hallucinations. There is a false sense of well-being and the patient gradually develops a high tolerance and dependence on the drugs, making him or her compulsive to consume more and more doses of the drug, regardless of its consequences.

Cannabis

Cannabis is the collective term for a range of psychoactive preparations of the cannabis plant—the hemp plant. While the most powerful derivative of hemp plants is *hashish*, the most commonly known type of cannabis, marijuana, is a mixture of hemp leaves, buds, and the tops of plants (SAMHSA, 2014). It is often smoked with tobacco. As a characteristic feature, the smoking of Marijuana produces a euphoric state involving increased self-confidence and a pleasant feeling of relaxation and floating imagination. Gradually, there is a considerable distortion of the sense of time and space. In some cases, the individual becomes irritable. There is a marked impairment in motor and intellectual functioning, but the users usually think that their efficiency has increased. This false sense of adequacy gives rise to incidents of reckless driving and other antisocial episodes. In many individuals, the intoxication of marijuana may produce acute psychotic reactions, as found with hallucinogenic drugs.

In this way, we may see that the abuse of one or the other types of psychoactive substances (in the forms of alcohol and drug abuse) may result in a number of substance-related addictive disorders involving serious problems regarding one's physiological and mental well-being.

To Sum Up

Depending upon the nature of their effects, the psychoactive substances may be classified as depressants or sedatives, stimulants and deliriants, or mind-blowing.

The substances included in the category of depressants or sedatives are known for their characteristics of exercising mentionable inhibiting effects on one's central nervous, and as a result, these may be prescribed by clinicians as a medication for the relief of anxiety, stress, pain, and sleep-related problems. However, their abuse may turn into a variety of physiological and psychological problems, including mental and behavioral disorders quite specific to the effect of the particular depressant or sedative. We may include in the category of depressants or sedatives the substances (i) Alcohol, (ii) Opioids (such as morphine, heroin, fentanyl, pethidine, oxycodone, hydromorphone, methadone, buprenorphine, codeine, and d-propoxyphene) and (iii) Sedative-Hypnotic drugs in the form of barbiturates (such as amytal and seconal) and non-barbiturates (such as bromides, paraldehyde chloral hydrate, Xanax, Ativan, and Valium).

Stimulant Drugs stimulate the brain and sympathetic nervous system, resulting in alertness and an increase in response and motor activity, including the creation of feelings of euphoria and hyperactivity. The major drugs in this category are nicotine, cocaine, caffeine, and amphetamines (such as dexamphetamine, benzedine, Dexedrine, methedrine, and methamphetamine).

Deliriant or mind-blowing drugs are characterized by the effects of producing transient states resembling psychoses, resulting in marked confusion, distortion in thought processes, delirium, illusions, and hallucinations. We may put the drugs classified as Hallucinogens (such as LSD-25, mescaline, psilocybin, bufotenine, speed, PCP, Ketamine, and Ecstasy) and Cannabis (such as hashish and marijuana).

The Causes, Prevention, and Treatment of Substance-Related Addictive Disorders

There is a quite positive correlation between the abuse of one or the other substances by individuals and their consequential suffering from related mental and behavioral disorders. In fact, all intoxication and addiction to one or the other type of psychoactive substances such as alcohol and drugs may result in mental and behavior disorders of a mild to severe nature, depending on the nature and effects of the substances abused.

Therefore, the causation and etiology of the occurrence of substance-related addictive disorders are bound to depend upon the type of addiction resulting from the abuse of one or the other psychoactive substance. The same is also true for the prevention and treatment of substance-related addictive disorders. Consequently, we need to work first for the prevention of addiction to these substances (alcohol and drugs), and then seek measures for the treatment of addicted individuals (alcoholics and drug addicts).

In this way, the matter related to the causation, prevention, and treatment of substance-related addictive disorders may shift in the following pages to the discussion of the causation, prevention, and treatment measures taken for the abuse of psychoactive substance cases mainly related to the addiction of alcohol and various types of drugs.

Causation of Alcoholism—What Turns One an Alcohol Addict?

In search of the causes or factors responsible for turning people into alcoholics (alcohol addicts), we come to a factual conclusion that it is a learned phenomenon, a bad habit acquired through the interaction between the individual and his sociocultural environment. There is no one gene known as "alcohol gene" that is said to be responsible for making one alcoholic. At present, in this concern, researchers have been able to

> **Alcoholism**
>
> An addiction to the consumption of alcohol forcing an individual to indulge in excessive drinking or dependence on alcoholic beverages to the extent of disrupting life and behavior malfunctioning, and causing severe physiological, psychological, and social damage.

find a few genes such as ADH1B and ALDH2 that are known to be closely tied to the risk for problem drinking. However, there is no such findings as to say that one is born as alcoholic. In this way, by all means, it cannot be termed as a hereditary phenomenon; it is learned and acquired much like other personality traits and habit patterns by following the principles of operant conditioning. According to the theory of operant conditioning, a behavior may occur accidentally or incidentally with or without the knowledge of an organism. Its further continuance depends upon the reinforcement—positive or negative—it gets in one way or the other from the environment. Let us see how this happens in one's learning of alcohol consumption.

- We learn many things from the environment. The behavior patterns of elder members of the family and society work as a model for younger ones. Therefore, the first drink may be taken in a social gathering with other members, or secretly without the knowledge of the elders. The child or youth may be tempted to taste alcohol merely on account of curiosity or to imitate elders. Media in the form of stories, fiction, plays, and movies, as well as the observed behavior of parents and elders, can lead youth to start drinking as a learned response to develop sociability; to alleviate feelings of isolation and loneliness; to seek a readily available source of pleasure; to boost their ego, remove hesitation, and become courageous by acquiring feelings of adequacy; to seek relief from tension and worries; to remove ethical restraints to engage in undesirable, immoral, or antisocial behavior without feeling guilty; and to increase sexual interest, stimulation, and to acquire a feeling of sexual adequacy.

- After encountering their first drink, continuing with successive drinks depends upon the rein-forcement-rewarding effect they get with their liquor consumption. In fact, people learn to drink excessively as a result of its rewarding effects—positive and negative—in the manner as follows:

(i) As a sedative, alcohol is a very quick and effective method of reducing tension, and removing inhibitions. It leads to a pleasurable feeling of adequacy, relief from worries, and sociability. Such rewarding effects reinforce drinking behavior. One learns to depend upon drinking as a preferred solution to problems. The psychological dependence fur-ther aggravates the situation when the individual consumes more and more alcohol for seeking pleasure and getting relief from their unpleasant reality. Gradually, it leads to prolonged and excessive drinking, resulting in physiological, psychological, psychiatric, and social problems.

(ii) Once people become physiologically addicted to alcohol, drinking with a gradual increase in dosage amount becomes a compulsion for their physical well-being. When they decide to reduce their intake or give up the habit, negative reinforcements appear (such as electric shocks received by rats in the Skinner experiment) in terms of experiencing withdrawal symptoms like craving alcohol, tremors, perspiration, weakness, nausea, vomiting, fever, blackouts, and hallucinations. Consequently, they dare not stop drinking and this physi-ological dependence compels them to drink more and more.

Stages Reached in Becoming Hardened Alcoholics or Alcohol Addicts

The habit of excessive drinking or dependence on alcoholic beverages is perpetuated gradually. E.M. Jellinek (1942), an authority on alcoholism, has pointed out the following four stages in the development of alcoholism:

1. *Pre-alcoholic phase:* This initial phase lasts from two months to two years. Beginners who drink for social reasons or merely on account of curiosity find that it relieves them of anxiety and tension, and as a result, learn to use alcohol as a relief measure. Gradually, they begin to experience an increased tolerance for alcohol and need larger amounts to reach the same stage of sedation. This phase is characterized by a gradual shift from infrequent or light to frequent or heavy drinking.

2. *Prodromal phase:* At this stage, alcohol begins to be used more as a drug and less as a bev-erage, with dependency on it increasing and manifesting through the following behavioral phenomena:

   - The individuals become preoccupied with drinking, worrying about where and when they will have their next drink.
   - They feel guilty about drinking and usually avoid references to alcohol in conversations. At the same time, they feel a strong urge to drink and thereby often resort to surreptitious rather than open drinking.
   - There is a sudden onset of "blackouts" for some of periods of drinking.
   - There is considerable memory impairment. One may remain conscious at the time of drinking but later be unable to recall the events.

3. *The crucial phase:* The third stage is alarming. The dependency on alcohol increases to the extent that there is a danger of the individual losing everything that one values. One may lose friends and jobs, and leave the members of one's family, including children and spouse,

but not give up the habit of drinking. Thus, this behavior compels such people to withdraw from their social environment, resulting in isolation in which they drink even more heavily. In this phase, drinking is rationalized as a source of comfort. The need for liquor becomes a constant source of worry, and detrimental to diet, combined with the harmful effects of alcohol deteriorates their health, lowers their sexual drive, and makes them hostile toward their environment, ruining their harmony and peace.

4. *The chronic phase:* This is the most critical stage where individuals live only to drink. Their bodily systems become so conditioned that they must be supplied with alcohol or they suffer withdrawal reactions. In case alcohol is not available, they are ready to consume any liquid containing alcohol, like shaving lotions, hair tonics, spirits, or medical preparations. They lose control of their behavior and prolonged bouts of intoxication often lead to marked ethical deterioration (character disorders), complete neglect of personal appearance and concern for others, impairment of mental processes, and even alcoholic psychoses in some cases. In comparison with the crucial phase, the chronic phase results in the loss of tolerance for alcohol, so that even a small amount leads to intoxication. At a more advanced stage, the alcoholic admits defeat and unless provided treatment, he is unlikely to give up drinking.

To Sum Up

The substance-related addictive disorders are the exclusive product of the abuse of substances and addiction in the form of alcohol and drug addiction. Consequently, for understanding the causation and treatment of substance-related addictive disorders, we should necessarily look into the causation and treatment of alcoholism and drug addiction.

The term alcoholism refers to excessive drinking or dependence on alcoholic beverages to the extent of disrupting one's life and causing malfunctioning of the behavior, as well as severe physiological, psychological, and social damage.

The habit of excessive drinking or dependence on alcoholic beverages is perpetuated gradually under some specific phases. In this concern, the initial pre-alcoholic phase lasts from two months up to two years and is characterized by a gradual shift from infrequent or light to frequent or heavy drinking. In the second prodromal phase, alcohol is used more as a drug and less as a beverage. In the third crucial phase the dependency on alcohol increases to the extent that there is a danger of losing everything that one values. In the last "chronic phase," the individual lives only to drink.

Alcoholism costs quite dearly to alcoholics. They are likely to be ruined in terms of their physical and mental health, emotional and social relationships, and economic and moral assets. Regarding the reasons for becoming an alcoholic, it can be safely said that no person is born alcoholic and therefore the causes of alcoholism are purely environmental. Drinking is learned and acquired like many personality traits and later maintained on account of the physiological and psychological dependence that it provides.

Causation of Drug Addiction—What Turns One into a Drug Addict?

Drug addiction is caused in a similar way as alcohol addiction. The actual pattern of tolerance and physiological as well as psychological dependence on a particular drug is the result of the learning process. No one is born a drug addict but becomes so by emulating the behavior of parents, friends, and other members of society. The first dose may be taken in the form of prescribed medicine for the cure of one or the other health problem or disorder, or out of curiosity, the pursuit of fun and pleasure, looking for new thrills, and the possibility of a mystic experience. Some resort to drugs for the sake of company and others may seek escape from boredom. The behavior is reinforced and rewarded on account of the false impression of adequacy and well-being, temporary relief from anxiety, pleasant reverie, and short-lived pleasing effects or states of euphoria created by the drug. Gradually, larger and larger doses are needed for the same results and one becomes dependent physiologically as well as psychologically. Thus, what begins as an innocuous experiment ends in disaster.

Drug Addiction

A state of acute intoxication, detrimental to the individual and to society, produced by the prolonged and excessive use of a drug, is characterized by an intense craving to consume it regardless of consequences; a tendency to increase the dosage with time; physiological and psychological dependence on the effects of the drug; and the manifestation of particular withdrawal symptoms upon abrupt discontinuation of the drug use.

According to experts, stress is a great factor in turning an individual into a drug addict. The highly competitive, success-oriented style of life today creates many such odds for a large number of young people. There is a crisis of character and a deterioration of values. While the aims of life and values of elders are considered meaningless, job opportunities for youth are rare. Education can be felt to serve no purpose. All these factors may lead one to experience stressful situations. One may seek instant relief from frustration, tension, anxiety, and depression by resorting to drugs. Others use drugs to free themselves from their inhibitions, and some turn to drugs because of guilt, shame, anxiety, or disappointment in life.

In the learning, acquiring, and perpetuating of addictive behavior, the mechanism of operant conditioning plays a key role, as we have seen in the case of getting addicted to alcohol. The beginning stage of drug consumption is rewarded by positive reinforcement in the form of getting instant relief from anxiety and stress or experiencing a state of euphoria and pleasant reverie for persuading an individual to repeat and increase their drug consumption to experience the same reward. In case one tries to reduce or give up the intake of the drug, he gets punished (receives negative reinforcement) in the form of experiencing withdrawal symptoms, and this compels him to take increasing doses of the drugs, becoming helpless to the habit of consuming the drug to the extent of getting highly addicted, with considerable damage to his physical, mental, and social well-being.

To Sum Up

Regarding the causes behind one's drug addiction, it must be emphasized that it is a learned phenomenon. No one is born a drug dependent but actually becomes so by emulating the behavior of parents, friends, and other members of society, or experiencing fun and relief from anxiety or pain as a medication. The incidence of taking the first dose of a drug is reinforced and rewarded on account of the false impression of adequacy and the pleasant reverie temporarily created by the drug. Gradually, larger and larger doses are needed for the same results, and one becomes dependent, physiologically as well as psychologically, on a particular drug to the extent of turning him into a drug addict.

Treatment of Alcohol Addicts

There is no single effective way to deal with the problem of alcoholism and the resulting alcohol-related addictive disorders. In some cases, individuals may stop drinking because of the fear of being arrested and imprisoned. But alcoholism is, in fact, a medical and psychological problem rather than a law and order problem. Attempts should, therefore, be made to tackle it on medical, social, and psychological levels. When seeking treatment, one should have a clear knowledge of the symptoms of alcoholism. These may include continuous and heavy drinking or uncontrolled episodic bursts of drinking; morning drinking; blackouts; gaining no pleasure in drinking; and undesirable, uncontrolled extreme behavior. It is then time to take corrective measures such as:

1. *Institutionalization and hospitalization:* It is best to arrange for institutionalization and hospitalization for the treatment of acute alcoholic intoxication. In many cases, compulsory hospitalization is not needed, but it is important to keep alcoholics away from aversive life situations and keep their behavior under control.
2. *Clinical investigation:* This should include investigations like full blood count, chest and skull radiography, and liver function tests; as a result, proper medical treatment should be provided for the deficiency and damage.
3. *Detoxification:* The first step in treating alcoholics is detoxification—that is, the removal of alcoholic substances from the body and the treatment of withdrawal symptoms. At this stage, much care should be taken to compensate for the alcoholic's dietary deficiencies.
4. *Deterrent measures:* After detoxification, the following deterrent measures in the form of aversion therapy are commonly used for restraining patients from drinking.

   - The patients may be given drugs like disulfiram (Antabuse) or citrated calcium carbamide (Abstem) for helping them resolve not to drink. These drugs cause episodes of intense illness if the individual drinks alcohol, and thereby act as strong deterrents in preventing drinking.
   - In making the patients develop a hatred for alcohol, a substance which produces nausea and vomiting when taken with an alcoholic drink is given. With repetition, it results in a conditioned aversion to alcoholic drinks.
   - In addition, it has been well noted that many times, the shocks received from the adverse life situations may also work as an effective measure for the treatment of alcoholics by causing aversion to liquor. Sometimes the shocks received from the adverse life situations may prove valuable in treating alcoholics.

5. *Psychotherapy:* When patients have stopped drinking, they may be enrolled in group or individual psychotherapy for helping them gain insight into their behavior and develop more effective adjustment techniques other than alcohol or drug addiction. However, this measure is not recommended for alcoholics who are basically sociopathic. A therapist must work hard with alcoholics. Chronic alcoholics are usually liars and unable to keep their promises of

never drinking again. Fruitful results can be achieved by making the patient realize or learn that a life without alcohol can be more satisfying than a life completely submerged in it. In every case, the basic personality must be evaluated with the reactive events leading up to the drinking and the pattern of alcoholic behavior. The amount of support from families and whether their employment or work is still available to them requires investigation.

6. *Sociotherapy:* This treatment involves the modification of environmental situations, change in attitude, and the provision of healthy social gatherings and groups. It is directed toward counseling the patient's spouse or family and helping them make a readjustment in the family and community setting. To have their social contacts in the form of a religious gathering, social clubs emphasizing inspirational and spiritual elements may also prove useful in the treatment of alcoholics. The staging of plays, cultural programs, and showing of movies emphasizing the ill effects of alcoholism and the tranquility of life may also prove valuable. Religious gatherings purify the path of individuals. They may be helped by the Almighty or religious ideas, certainly a power greater than their own self, for admitting their mistakes and controlling their drinking with the provision of emotional support. Participation in social groups like Alcoholics Anonymous (a group composed of people who have given up drinking) may also prove useful for alcoholics to enjoy social fellowships, gain insight into their behavior, and overcome their addiction.

Duration of Treatment and Follow-Up

The duration of treatment in the case of alcoholics depends largely on the severity of the case. If they remain away from alcohol for five years, they can usually be regarded as cured. But there are many chances and incidences of relapse, especially frequent in the first two years. Great care should thus be taken in follow-up when treatment is over.

To Sum Up

Regarding the treatment provided to alcoholics for overcoming their problems including alcohol-related addictive disorders, we can observe that alcoholism is a medical and psychological problem rather than a law-and-order problem. Therefore, in dealing with it, the beginning is made with the diagnosis of early warning signals, and then resorting to measures such as (i) keeping alcoholics away from aversive life situations, (ii) subjecting them to essential clinical investigations, (iii) detoxification; (iv) using deterrent measures in the form of aversion therapy; (v) providing group or individual psychotherapy for gaining insight into their behavior and adequate adjustment, and (vi) providing sociotherapy involving modification of their environmental situation and improvement of their social adjustment.

Treatment of Drug Addiction

Drug addiction is not a law-and-order problem, as is imagined in certain circles. It is predominantly a social and psychological problem. Addicts should be distinguished from criminals who supply them with drugs and live off their misery. The irony of addicts is that they depend on drugs to the extent of pathological craving so powerful that they try and manage to get the drug regardless of legal or other obstacles. The following measures prove fruitful in the treatment of drug addicts.

1. *Compulsory hospitalization:* Compulsory institutionalization and hospitalization is a major step in the treatment of drug addicts. If the doctors wait until the patient voluntarily seeks effective treatment, they may well wait until the patient dies. Drug addicts do not want treatment—they want drugs, and in their usual surroundings and environment they refuse to be deprived of drugs. Admission into hospitals may be able to cover the following major risks:

   • Rejection by family and society that can neither understand nor manage the patient, makes the patient depressed. This situation worsens when drugs are not available during the withdrawal phase.
   • The tendency to go on to harder drugs or mixed drugs to get the desired effect may lead to disaster.
   • There is a risk of suicide by the patient on account of an accidental overdose or committing suicide when profoundly depressed or a misadventure under the intoxicating effects of a drug.
   • There is a danger of infection or other complications when the drug is injected into the body.

2. *Detoxification or "drying out" the patient:* Attempts should be made to detoxify or dry out the patient. This may be achieved through (i) the "cold turkey"'s procedure, that is, sudden total discontinuation of drugs; (ii) giving the patient progressively diminishing doses of drugs leading to complete cessation; and (iii) substituting a less addictive drug, called an agonist drug, and later seeking gradual reduction of intake. These agonist drugs provide the individual with a "safe" drug that has a similar chemical makeup to the addicted drug. One common example of this is methadone, an opiate agonist that is often used in the reduction of heroin use (Schwartz et al., 2010). However, whatever mode for detoxification is adopted, it should be adopted under the proper supervision of experts, as the cessation of the addictive drug may send the client into dangerous withdrawal symptoms.

3. *Medical measures:* With some patients, especially psychotic addicts, ECT or tranquilizing drugs may prove quite helpful. Adequate care is to be taken for the provision of antibiotics, as there is an inherent danger of possible infection. The withdrawal reactions and resulting complications should also be well guarded with the help of specific drugs. For example, epileptics may need anti-convulsants and schizophrenics may need phenothiazines. In addition, adequate dietary measures in the form of glucose and vitamins are to be ascertained for compensating for the drug deficiency, and adequate feeding and fluids should be ensured.

4. *Psychological treatment:* Psychological treatment of drug addicts requires patience and time in the form of long-term psychotherapy. The first essential step for this purpose before introducing one or the other psychotherapy on the part of the trained psychotherapist to addicts is to establish a proper therapeutic relationship with them. Then, attempts may be made to make use of the following psychotherapies:

   (i) **Use of Aversion therapy**: As a learning principle, a behavior is maintained or given up through consequences/rewards. When an individual is punished or exposed to bitter experiences after consuming a particular drug, he may develop an aversion toward the consumption of that drug. This aversion, dislike, or hatred toward the consumption of the drug may be developed through the use of the methods such as:

      • Drug addicts may be given a particular drug, edible or drinkable (effective enough to produce unpleasant and bitter experiences) along with the consumption of their addictive drug for creating an aversion toward its further consumption. As an example of an aversive drug, we may name Naloxone, which can be given to individuals with opioid abuse. It can create aversion toward the use of opioids by inhibiting the emergence of the intended euphoric effect. Similarly, the use of edible or drinkable drugs that may produce nausea and vomiting when taken with the drug dose may also result in a conditioned aversion to the use of that drug.

- In terms of shock therapy, drug addicts may be given a shock every time they think about or attempt to consume the drug for creating aversion to the use of that particular drug.

(ii) Use of Contingency management

The type of psychotherapy called contingency management is based on the principles of operant conditioning, positing that behaviors get increased or decreased as a function of immediate and directly associated consequences (rewards or punishments). We can thus make use of this method for picking up or dropping one's habits. In the treatment of drug addicts, we can use this method for (a) increasing the period of abstinence from the use of the drug on the part of a drug addict, (ii) increasing the attendance of drug addicts in a treatment program, and (iii) adherence to a prescribed medication. In general, in the adoption of contingency management therapy for the treatment of addicts, the patients are "rewarded" for demonstrating a desirable behavior (such as abstinence from substance use or compliance with a treatment program) with vouchers allowing them to gain incentives specific to their interests, such as movie tickets, sports equipment, or even cash (Mignon, 2014).

(iii) Use of Cognitive-Behavioral Therapy

Cognitive-behavioral therapy aims to train addicts to make use of cognitive as well as behavioral approaches for the adoption of desirable behavior and getting rid of undesirable behavior in the treatment of their problems. In general, it proves quite helpful in providing relapse prevention training to addicts for preventing the occurrence of a relapse. For this purpose, a therapist may proceed systematically, as follows:

- Guiding the patient to identify any interpersonal, intrapersonal, environmental, and physiological risks for relapse.
- Working with the patient on the use of cognitive and behavioral strategies such as learning effective coping strategies, enhancing self-efficacy, and encouraging mastery of outcomes for eliminating the chances of relapse.

(iv) Use of Sociotherapy

Sociotherapy is usually carried out by the clinician with the help of social workers and voluntary and non-voluntary social agencies. It consists of bringing necessary modifications in the patient's environment in order to make it appropriate for him to seek proper adjustment. The use of sociotherapy, including proper rehabilitation, is essential if the patient is to learn to face his problems and seek adjustment in society without the use of the drug. It may be achieved as follows:

- Modifying the environmental conditions: Needed modification is to be made in the environmental conditions responsible for triggering drug abuse, and the necessary support should be sought from the individual's immediate community (friends and family) for preventing relapse in the outcomes of the treatment process.
- Re-socialization: The drug addicts must learn to socialize and adjust without the consumption addiction, as well as any medication used for this purpose.

- Re-occupation: Once cured, the drug addicts should be helped in seeking employment and occupational adjustment. They need to be trained in job skills and in persistence so that they may be accepted by their employers.
- Re-housing: They should be helped in getting adequate family adjustment and re-establish themselves by learning to accommodate and fend for themselves.

The duration and extent of long-term therapeutic treatment with the use of aforementioned therapies depend upon the patient's potential and the level of maturity which the patient has reached. If adequately cared for through therapy and rehabilitation, the patient should be able to lead a full life and to develop his potential abilities.

Preventive Measures for Drug Addiction

The primary task in the prevention of drug addiction involves educating the public about its causes and consequences. There is a need to restructure unhealthy environments and reduce problems leading to frustrations, tensions, and anxieties among youth. Job opportunities must be increased and the education system reshaped to include job-oriented and employment-based courses. The energies of students and youth should be channelized into constructive and creative projects like rural reconstruction, the welfare of the society and nation, and helping the needy and the poor. This will give them a sense of purpose, and opportunities for adventure and new experiences, which they had sought by taking drugs. In outlining measures to prevent and control drug addiction, the report of a committee headed by Dr. C. Gopalan, Director-General, the Indian Council of Medical Research, has enunciated the following five basic points for this purpose:

(i)   Society can never be free of drugs, the reason being that drugs have specific individual and social purposes, and as long as they are not met by other healthier means, drug use or abuse will continue to exist.

(ii) Efforts should be made to reduce drug evils to the minimum by attacking them at various points rather than concentrating significant efforts at one point.

(iii) Drug abuse, which is a form of deviance, cannot be treated in isolation from other forms of deviance, and an attempt at creating special machinery for the control of drug abuse will be counterproductive.

(iv) One should not lose one's perspective and create gigantic and costly structures to deal with drug problems whose significance is limited in comparison to several other problems facing the country.

(v)   All the drugs form a continuum and any overzealous effort to control one drug may lead to an increase in the use of another drug.

At present, there are several central ministries in India dealing with one or the other aspects of the drug addiction problem. For controlling coordination and bringing efficiency, the committee has given the following suggestions:

- There should be integrated machinery like a national advisory board with the health minister as its chairman, and comprising representatives of all other ministries and professional organizations concerned with the problem. This will help in the formulation of a comprehensive and balanced policy to prevent and control drug abuse.
- The committee suggested legislation and a single central law instead of many laws dealing with the problem of dependence-producing drugs. The severity of control and regulation

should depend upon the extent to which the drug finds use in medical practice, its potential for abuse, and the gravity of the consequences. On this basis, it has been suggested that hallucinogens like LSD, heroin, hashish, and charas should be prohibited since these are harmful and have no medicinal value.

- The committee wants deterrent penal provisions against the smuggling of and trade in drugs on the lines of other leading countries like Japan, the United States, and Singapore. Whereas addicts should be regarded with sympathy as sick persons and should be permitted, under certain conditions, to possess specified drugs in specific quantities, the traffickers should be dealt with firmly.

To Sum Up

Drug addiction is a state of acute intoxication that is created through the prolonged excessive use of a drug, and results in serious physiological and psychological problems, including making one victim to the related addictive mental and behavioral disorders.

The causes of drug addiction are purely environmental; drug addiction is a matter of learned behavior and an inadequate adjustment to the stresses of life and style of living. *Prevention and control of drug addicts* involve measures such as: educating the public to understand the causes and consequences of drug addiction; re-structuring unhealthy environmental conditions and reduction in the problems leading to frustration, tension, and anxiety among citizens; prohibition of low medicinal value and harmful drugs; and enforcing deterrent panel provisions against the smugglers and traders of drugs.

Treatment of drug addicts involves: compulsory hospitalization; detoxification; adoption of medical measures; introduction of psychological treatment; and arranging for long-term therapy in the form of aversion therapy, contingency management, cognitive-behavioral therapy, and sociotherapy accompanied by adequate follow-up and rehabilitation measures.

Review Questions

1. What are substance-related addictive disorders? Name the various disorders listed in the latest classification systems, the DSM-5-TR and ICD-11 provided by the APA and WHO.
2. Describe the criteria mentioned in the DSM-5-TR for the diagnosis of substance-induced mental disorders.
3. Discuss in detail the different types of psychoactive substances and their consequential effects.
4. What is alcoholism or addiction to alcohol? Throw proper light on its concept and meaning along with the causes of its development.
5. How does one turn into an alcohol addict? Discuss in light of the different stages reached in turning one into a hardened alcoholic.
6. While throwing light on the causes of alcoholism, describe how alcoholism proves damaging and harmful to people and society.
7. Discuss in detail the measures employed for the treatment of alcohol addicts.
8. What is drug addiction? Throw light on its concept and meaning.

9. How is drug addiction caused? Discuss the necessary measures employed for its prevention and treatment.
10. Throw light on the causation of alcohol- and drug-induced substance-related and addictive disorders along with the measures adopted for their treatment.

References

Acosta, M., Haller, D., & Schnoll, S. (2011), Cocaine and stimulants. In R. J. Frances, A. H. Mack, & S. I. Miller (Eds.), *Clinical textbook of addictive disorders* (3rd ed. pp. 183–218), New York, NY: Guilford Press.

American Psychiatric Association (2022), *Diagnostic and statistical manual of mental disorders: DSM-5-TR*, Washington, DC: American Psychiatric Association.

Jellinek, E. M. (Ed.) (1942), *Alcohol addiction and chronic alcoholism*, New Haven, CT: Yale University Press.

Mignon, S. (2014), *Substance abuse treatment: Options, challenges, and effectiveness*, New York, NY: Springer Publishing.

SAMHSA (Substance Abuse and Mental Health Services Administration) (2014), *Results from the 2013 national survey on drug use and health: Summary of national findings*, NSDUH Series H-48, HSS Publication No. (SMA) 14–4863, Rockville, MD: SAMHSA.

Schwartz, R., Brooner, R., Montoya, I., Currens, M., & Hayes, M. (2010), A 12-year follow-up of a methadone medical maintenance program, *The American Journal on Addictions*, 8: 293–299.

Chapter 14

Sexual Deviations and Disorders

Learning Objectives

After going through this chapter, you will be able to:

- Define the term sexual deviations.
- Know about the meaning and nature of sexual deviations.
- Differentiate between the terms sexual deviation and sexual offense.
- Differentiate the term sexual deviation from the term sexual disorder.
- Discuss the major sexual deviations taking place among individuals.
- Discuss the underlying causes and treatment of sexual deviations.
- Elucidate the meaning and concept of sexual disorders.
- Throw light on the sexual disorders known as impotence and frigidity.
- Discuss the underlying causes of impotence and frigidity.
- Throw light on the measures taken for the prevention and treatment of sexual disorders.

Introduction

While looking into the systems of classification available in the forms of the Diagnostic Statistical Manuals (DSMs) and International Classification of Diseases (ICDs) brought out from time to time by the American Psychiatric Association and the World Health Organization, respectively, as discussed in Chapter 7 of the text, we see that they have mention two types of adult sex-related abnormalities known as sexual deviations and sexual disorders. Let us try to know about these deviations and disorders in this chapter.

Sexual Deviations

Deviation is a term used for explaining significant difference from the average or norm. A deviant behavior is apart from or contrary to the established or acceptable behavior in a given culture or society. Sexual deviation, in this sense, does not conform to the norms of one's

---

Sexual Deviation

The habit pattern of sexual behavior compelling an individual to seek sexual gratification from unconventional sources and means.

DOI: 10.4324/9781003398325-14

culture and society. As a term, sexual deviation has been defined by psychologists and authors in the following manner.

George *W. Kisker (1964:168):* Sexual behavior is more likely to be considered abnormal or deviant only when it interferes with personal and social adjustment—when it is self defeating or damaging to others.

Rosen et al. (1972:273): A failure of development associated with anxiety and conflict culminating in a persistent or frequently recurring preference for any form of sexual behavior that is a substitute for, and does not terminate in, genital coitus with an adult of the opposite sex, is a sexual deviation.

Anthony Storr (1964:78): Sexual deviation can only be understood as failure in the quite complicated process of learning how to love—it is the compulsive substitution of something else for heterosexual intercourse in circumstances where the latter is available.

In light of these definitions and recent researches in the field of human sexual behavior, the following conclusion may be drawn about the meaning and nature of sexual deviation.

Sex is one of the major human instinctual drives and essential needs. Although people live in spite of sexual deprivation, they may never live life to the fullest without its gratification. To enable one to gratify one's sex need may be a natural instinct but to seek its gratification in socially desirable ways is a matter of one's learned behavior. In addition to being socially acceptable, normal sexual behavior should fulfill the following conditions:

- Genital coitus is to be preferred to other modes of sexual gratification.
- It should not be engaged with in the attitude of shame, disgust, fear, guilt, or inferiority,
- It should neither cause harm to the individuals concerned nor to others.
- It should not cause personal or social maladjustment.

This means that *sexual deviation may be understood in terms of learned persistent habit patterns of sexual behavior which compel an individual to seek sexual gratification from unconventional sources and means other than the genital coitus with an adult.*

Sexual Deviation and Sexual Offense

It is important to distinguish between "sexual deviation" and "sexual offense." Although most deviations are also sexual offenses and vice versa, this is not always true. Genital intercourse with an adult member of the opposite sex is considered normal behavior. But sexual intercourse with an adult without his or her consent cannot be termed deviance but a sexual offense in the form of rape and sexual assault. In some countries, forcible intercourse even with one's spouse is termed a sexual offense. Similarly, extramarital intercourse even with a willing adult member of the opposite sex is a sexual offense, whereas it cannot be called sexual deviation or perversion in the strict sense of the term. A further distinction between these terms may be made on the ground that where there is a unique stress or persistence in habit patterns in the case of sexual deviations, an occasional departure from accepted normal behavior of the society or legal code is enough to label it as a sexual offense. Moreover, a number of sexual deviations such as anal intercourse with one's wife may not be termed sexual offense and is not punishable by law as it is not a social or legal offense.

Sexual Deviation and Sexual Disorder

Sexual deviation refers to persistent habit patterns of compulsive preference for unconventional objects or means for sexual gratification other than genital intercourse with an adult. One engages in such behavior of his own will and purpose and seeks the satisfaction of the strong sex urge or compulsion. Sexual deviation, in this way, is a psychological phenomenon.

On the other hand, sexual disorders like impotence or frigidity may involve the physiological systems too. There is a lack of coordination between the sympathetic and parasympathetic systems in impotence and frigidity. They may also be the result of psychological factors like anxiety or guilt. The individual is unable to derive gratification on account of a feeling of inadequacy or a state of incapacity caused by physiological or psychological factors. Such disorders cannot be termed sexual deviation as the individual does not deviate from the norms of sexual behavior.

To Sum Up

Sexual deviations are the learned persistent habit patterns of sexual behavior that compel an individual to seek sexual gratification from unconventional sources and means other than genital coitus with an adult.

Regarding the similarity and difference existing between the terms sexual deviation and sexual offense we may find that although most deviations may also be termed sexual offenses and vice versa, it is not always true. Genital intercourse with an adult is considered normal behavior. But sexual intercourse with an adult without his or her consent cannot be termed deviance but a sexual offense in the form of rape and sexual assault. Moreover, a number of sexual deviations such as anal intercourse with one's wife may not be termed sexual offenses and are not punishable by law, as they are not social or legal offenses.

In differentiating sexual deviation from the term sexual disorder we may see that whereas in sex deviation, individuals perform the sexually deviated acts at their own will for seeking their own gratification, in sexual disorders like impotence and frigidity, men and women are unable to derive gratification on account of psychological or physiological factors. Such disorders cannot be termed sexual deviation as the individuals do not deviate from the norms of sexual behavior.

Forms or Types of Sexual Deviations

Sexual deviations may take various forms. In some cases a child, close relative, or a corpse is used as an object for the sexual act. In others, although the partner may be adult, genital intercourse is avoided and another act substituted for it. Likewise, other cases, no second person is directly involved, but sexual gratification is obtained from objects other than people or from observing the sexual activities of others or exhibiting one's genital organs. In other cases, the person himself acts as an object for deviation as found in autoerotic masturbation.

The following are some of the major sexual deviations:

1. *Pedophilia:* In this type of deviation, the adult deviant takes a child, girl or boy, for any sexual activity—masturbatory, oral, and/or genital. The deviant is usually male and may

be of a passive or aggressive nature. The passive type desires the child as a love object and often persuades the child for a willing partnership. An aggressive type inflicts sexual abuse on the child while sadistically hurting or punishing the child. Pedophilia is dangerous as it leads to physical violence and psychological damage to the victim.

2. *Oralism and analism:* In this type of deviation, the individual does not perform genital intercourse but tries to seek sexual gratification with the exclusive reliance on the anus instead of the vagina for penile insertion. Such behavior is termed sexual analism. When the deviant depends exclusively on oral-genital contact for gratifying his or her sex needs, such behavior is referred to as sexual oralism and may take the following forms:

   • Masturbation
   • Cunnilingus, the application of the mouth to the female genitals
   • Fellatio, the application of mouth to the male genitals
   • Exclusive reliance on foreplay at the cost of displeasing the partner

4. *Sadism and masochism:* The term "sadism" is used to describe the sexual deviation in which erotic excitement or pleasure is derived from the infliction of pain upon the partner. The pain may be inflicted physically by such means as biting, pinching, whipping, mutilating, and even committing murder, or psychologically by means of abuse or criticism. The term "masochism," on the other hand, refers to the deviation in which sexual gratification is achieved by being punished or experiencing pain.

   The pain and punishment in these deviations become the source of erotic excitement and pleasure. Engaging in minor sadistic or masochistic behavior or rituals cannot be termed deviation. It is only when such behavior is extreme or divorced from sexual intercourse that it can be termed a deviation. A true sadist or masochist obtains sexual gratification from the sadistic or masochistic practice irrespective of the consequences. Sadistic behavior is often more dangerous than masochism. The sadist wants to hurt while the victim is unwilling and the offender is often violent.

5. *Fetishism:* The term fetishism is applied to a sexual deviation in which magic appears to reside, not in a whole person but in a part of the person, or an object connected with the person. The fetishist feels a compulsive and irrational sexual attraction toward an inanimate object such as an undergarment, shoe, fur, or glove, or is fascinated by some part of the body other than the genitals such as the buttocks, thighs, feet, breasts, or hair. In extreme forms of fetishism, such body parts or inanimate objects become the most preferred source of sexual attraction and gratification. A fetishist has no desire and gets no pleasure from genital intercourse or other forms of lovemaking with a partner of the same or opposite sex.

6. *Zoophilia or bestiality:* In this type of deviation, animals are used for the achievement of sexual excitation and gratification. The actual sexual pattern may involve masturbation by rubbing against the body of the animal, oral-genital contacts, masturbation or actual sexual intercourse.

7. *Necrophilia:* In this deviation, sexual excitation and gratification is sought through viewing or actually having sexual relations with a dead body. This is a comparatively rare deviation observed in psychopathological males.

8. *Incest:* This deviation is sexual activity between close blood relations, prohibited in a given culture or society, such as between a brother and a sister, father and daughter, mother and son, man and granddaughter or wife of his son, woman and her grandson or husband of her daughter, and so on. Such incest taboos are essential to prevent disruption of community and family life.

9. *Exhibitionism:* Exhibitionism is a sexual deviation in which gratification is obtained by exposing the genitals publicly, usually to members of the opposite sex or to children, who

are involuntary observers or complete strangers. It is more exclusively a male deviation; for although females may expose the genitals or may appear nude or semi-nude in an advertisement, film, or other public shows, this is done at the behest of and for the pleasure of others and is rarely resorted to by females as a means of obtaining sexual gratification.

The urge to expose oneself can be overwhelming and virtually uncontrollable, and occurs again and again, usually in the same place and at the same time of the day in spite of penalties and treatment. Although a male exhibitionist hurts his victim, his behavior is not as threatening and aggressive as in the case of sadism or sexual assault, molestation, or rape. His gratification comes from observing her reaction, which is a mixture of surprise, fear, disgust, and resentment.

10. *Voyeurism or scopophilia:* In this deviation, sexual gratification is obtained through clandestine peeping and observation of the genitals or sexual behavior of others. The curiosity to see the genital organs of the opposite sex and watch other people or animals engaged in sexual activity is so widespread that it seems difficult to label voyeurism as a sexual deviation. It may be regarded as a deviation when it is substituted for other conventional methods of gratification, preferred even to coitus or indulged in at serious risk.

11. *Frotteurism:* In this deviation, sexual satisfaction is obtained by rubbing or pressing against a member of the opposite sex. Often in crowded or lonely places, males try to seek sex gratification by rubbing or pressing the buttocks, hips, breasts or genitals of females or by rubbing their own genitals against the body of the female without engaging in sexual intercourse.

To Sum Up

There are several forms and types of sexual deviations, such as:

(i) Pedophilia (the deviant behavior in which an adult uses a child, girl or boy for sexual activity), (ii) Oralism (the dependence on oral-genital contact for gratifying sex needs), *(iii)* Analism (the exclusive reliance on the anus instead of the vagina for penile insertion), (iv) Sadism (sexual gratification from the infliction of pain upon the sexual partner), (v) Masochism (sexual gratification from being punished or experiencing pain), (vi) Fetishism (a compulsive and irrational sexual attraction and obtaining sexual gratification from inanimate objects or part of the body other than the genitals), (vii) Bestiality (using animals for the achievement of sexual excitation and gratification, (viii) Necrophilia (obtaining sexual gratification through viewing or actually having sexual relations with a dead body), (ix) Incest (sexual activity between close blood relations), (x) Exhibitionism (the sexual gratification obtained by exposing the genitals publicly usually to member of the opposite sex or to children who are involuntary observers or complete strangers), (xi) Voyeurism (the sexual gratification obtained through peeping, observation of the genitals or sexual behavior of others, and (xii) Frotteurism (the sexual gratification obtained by rubbing or pressing against a member of the opposite sex.

Causes of Sexual Deviation

It is often thought that sexual deviations result on account of defective biological makeup—chromosomal abnormalities or abnormalities of endocrine functions—but it has not been proved true, as no consistent abnormalities have been observed in any group of sexual deviants. So far, the most reasonable and satisfactory causes of sexual deviations are provided by the interaction of several psychological factors. The dynamics of these factors may involve the following patterns.

1. *Pathogenic family environment:* All learning begins at home. The pathogenic family environment is the primary source of causing abnormalities in sexual behavior. The child may copy the abnormal sex behavior of his parents or elders in the family. He may be shocked at the disharmony and frequent quarrelling between his parents, or may develop a distaste or unconscious fear for natural sexual behavior on account of the uncongenial home environment and unpleasant relationships. His natural behavior may deviate on account of parental rejection or isolation from other children. The needs related to his psychological or biological satisfaction may lead him to be trapped in sexual deviation when he finds opportunities to do so.

2. *Early traumatic sex experiences:* Many times, early sexual experiences and episodes start the process of deviation. Sexual assault of a minor girl by an adult may prove damaging to her normal sexual behavior and thus lead her toward sexual deviations.

3. *Generalized inhibitions and sexual ignorance:* Sex is regarded taboo in most societies. There is a natural craving for seeking information on account of the sex-related curiosities among children and youth. This craving, coupled with adventurism, may lead them to unusual experimentation, wrong notions and practices about sex. Sex ignorance may be responsible for many sexual complications, fears and complexes, ultimately resulting in abnormal sexual behavior.

4. *Deprivation of outlet for normal sex behavior:* Sex is a powerful basic urge. It begins to dominate one's behavior especially after attaining puberty. The denial of satisfaction of this basic need through normal ways may force an individual to seek gratification in unconventional objects or methods. A lonely father, deprived of a sexual relationship, may seek his preadolescent daughter for his gratification. Under similar conditions or deprivation, an adult may be persuaded to adopt exhibitionism, voyeurism, pedophilia, homosexuality, bestiality, or even necrophilia as a substitute for conventional sexual behavior. The individual involved in abnormal behavior on account of deprivation rarely likes to abandon the deviation at a later stage.

5. *Fear and complexes associated with the opposite sex and normal sex behavior:* Many times, abnormal sex behavior is caused by the fear and complexes associated with members of the opposite sex and the establishment of normal sexual behavior with them. Whenever an individual is ridiculed, rebuffed, and humiliated in his efforts to approach members of the opposite sex or suffers failures and frustrations in his sex advances or sex acts, he may turn toward other safer sources of affection and sexual outlets. A traumatic experience with a natural sexual outlet may lead to a number of complexes and feelings of inferiority about one's sexual adequacy and may lead the individual to avoid the conventional outlets for gratification. Heterosexual frustrations may lead to fear and excessive anxiety concerning sexual behavior with members of the opposite sex or partner. These fears, anxieties, and complexes end in a unique distaste for normal sexual behavior.

6. *Conditioning to abnormal patterns of sex behavior:* Prolonged deprivation of natural sexual outlets or feelings of hostility, apathy, and fear toward conventional sexual practices may lead an individual to seek a convenient and safer pattern of abnormal sexual behavior. When such opportunities become available, or he is helped by older deviants or incidental situations, he may find himself engaging in his first abnormal behavior. The perpetuation of the sexual deviation now depends upon the result of this first experience. If he gets rewards in terms of sexual gratification, his behavior is reinforced. Gradually, he learns to use similar objects or methods for the satisfaction of his sexual needs.

7. *Fixation of abnormal sex behavior:* Encouraged by or satisfied with adopted abnormal patterns of sexual behavior, one becomes habituated to using it for sexual gratification. This behavior gets fixed on account of the following reasons:

- One may think of it as a convenient means of meeting sex needs.
- One may resort to it for avoiding possible sex failures and frustrations.
- One may consider it as a safer means of hiding sexual inadequacies and in-competencies.
- One may find it the most pleasurable act.

Repeated acts of abnormal sexual behavior condition an individual to depend completely on one or more patterns of abnormal sexual behavior for the gratification of sex needs. The individual is no longer inclined toward conventional sex objects or methods and if provided opportunities, is compelled to prefer unconventional ones to conventional ones. When that happens, we may label the individual as sexually deviated or perverted.

Treatment of Sexual Deviations

The treatment of sexual deviations is no different from the treatment of other types of abnormal behavior. This behavior, caused by fears, anxieties, and complexes related to sex, is the result of the learning of maladaptive responses through early conditioning and fixation at later stages. The causes are more psychological than anything else and therefore the treatment measures have to be psychological. Various psychotherapies designed to help the patient gain insight into his motivations, change his basic attitudes, and work out more acceptable patterns of sexual behavior are used. Individual and group psychotherapies yield encouraging results for correcting sexual deviants.

In most cases, behavior therapy proves effective in alleviating the fear, anxiety, and complexes related to the opposite sex and normal sexual patterns. Appropriate counseling providing adequate information and proper sex techniques proves beneficial for the majority of sexual deviants. As a result, the inhibited deviant may be helped to be less prudish. One may be persuaded to shift from an undesirable object or method to a desirable one.

It is important to note that sexual deviation or perversion cannot be treated through punitive measures. It is a behavioral problem and therefore attempts should be made for effective psychological treatment with an adequate follow-up program of proper rehabilitation.

To Sum Up

Regarding the causes underlying sexual deviations, it can be seen that to a great extent, these are produced by the interaction of several psychological factors, such as (i) pathogenic family environment, (ii) early traumatic sexual experiences, (iii) generalized inhibitions and sexual ignorance, (iv) deprivations of outlets for normal sexual behavior, (v) fear and complexes associated with the opposite sex and normal sexual behavior; and (vi) conditioning and fixation on abnormal patterns of sexual behavior.

The treatment measures for sexual deviations are mostly psychological. Psychotherapies like behavior therapy, analytical therapy, and group therapy prove effective in dealing with sexual deviants. These psychological treatments should be followed through by an adequate follow-up program of proper rehabilitation.

Sexual Disorders

The term sexual disorders refers to those psycho-physiological disturbances that interfere with the full enjoyment of conventional sexual relations. As a result, genital intercourse, the most lovable and enjoyable sex act, becomes an unhappy, un-enjoyable ritual for one or both partners. Impotence and frigidity are the two main sexual disorders of such nature.

Impotence

Impotence refers to that psycho-physiological disturbance in the sexual behavior of a man which causes an impairment in his desire for sexual gratification or an inability to achieve it. This sexual disorder or inadequacy takes the following forms:

> **Impotence**
>
> The sexual disorder experienced on the part of men causing impairment in their desire for sexual gratification or an inability to achieve it.

Primary impotence: It refers to the case where the male has never been able to achieve an erection sufficient for successful intercourse, either heterosexual or homosexual.

Situational secondary impotence: It refers to the case where a male finds himself unable to achieve an erection sufficient for successful intercourse, either heterosexual or homosexual, but has been able to do so in the past.

Incidental permanent impotence: It refers to the case where a person previously able to get an erection and maintain sexual relations, incidentally develops a permanent impairment in his sexual potency on account of some chronic illness, drug addiction, injuries to the genitalia, or disease of the nervous system.

Ejaculatory impotence: In this type of impotence or sexual inadequacy, the man is unable to inhibit ejaculation long enough for his female partner to have an orgasm or sexual satisfaction. In some cases, he ejaculates even without an erection or intromission, and in others, during penetration or just after intromission. In some rare disorders, he is unable to ejaculate intravaginally, although erections and intromissions are normal.

Frigidity

Frigidity is the most common sexual disorder found in females. It is the counterpart of male impotence. Frigid women show a considerable lack of interest in the desire for sexual gratification or find it difficult to achieve it in their sexual behavior. This sexual disorder may take some of the following forms.

> **Frigidity**
>
> The sexual disorder found in females resulting in a considerable lack of interest in their desire for sexual gratification or making it difficult for them to achieve it in their sexual behavior.

Primary frigidity: This refers to the case where a woman has never had an orgasm (ability to get sexual gratification as experienced) from either masturbation or intercourse. In a more severe case, she experiences no desire for sexual gratification.

Situational secondary frigidity: This refers to the case where a woman is unable to have orgasms or responds negatively to erotic responses in a specific situation.

Causes of Impotence and Frigidity

Impotence and frigidity are often accompanied by a lack of desire for sexual gratification, but this is not always true. Sometimes, despite one's desire to seek sexual gratification, one fails to achieve it on account of his own failure or failure on the part of his or her partner. The possible causes of these disorders may be listed as follows:

Physiological factors: Impotence and frigidity may be attributed to physical damage to the sex organs or nervous system on account of disease, physical injuries, and physiological malfunctioning. In many cases drugs, are held responsible for impotence and frigidity. These are phenothiazines (especially Melleril). Similarly, monoamine oxidase inhibitors with tricyclic antidepressants decreases libido. Contraceptive pills also decrease sexual activity. Many illnesses, especially serious infections, diabetes, chronic tuberculosis, cancer growth and malignancy may lead to serious sexual inadequacies on account of the damage to sexual organs or the nervous system. Aortic disease may affect the presacral nerves and therefore cause the failure of erection. Similarly, clitoral, vaginal, or penile infection, biological deformities of the sex organs, and malfunctioning of the sex glands may cause sexual apathy and inadequacy.

Psychological factors: The cases of impotence and frigidity on account of physiological factors are quite rare. They are often caused on account of psychological causes resulting from the interaction of one's self with the circumstances and situations in one's environment. The major psychological factors may be grouped as follows:

- Sexual guilt
- Fear and complexes surrounding sex
- Depression
- Lack of emotional closeness or affection between sex partners
- Sex frustrations
- Sexual perversion or deviation
- Bedroom mistakes/faulty techniques

The psychological reasons leading to a feeling of inadequacy in males or females is a learned response. It may be the result of faulty earlier training or experiences for a female who comes to know about sexual relations as dirty, bad, lustful, evil, and harmful. For a male, the fear and anxiety related to inadequacy may work as a potent factor for causing impotency. The lack of emotional closeness to one's sex partner may result in sexual failure causing disappointment, anxiety, and self-devaluation to one or both partners. In some cases, the feelings of hostility give rise to a lack of sexual desire and non-cooperation in the sex act, leading to frigidity or impotence. A failure and dissatisfaction in a single act of erotic love and intercourse may either lead to unnecessary hostility and resentment toward the other partner or it may develop fear and anxiety related to one's inadequacy. A vicious cycle thus starts; the fears and doubts about one's inadequacy and hostility or frustration may make one feel less adequate and more hostile or apathetic toward one's partner.

Prevention of Sexual Disorders

It is difficult to control sexual disorders caused by physiological factors like physical injuries to the sex organs, damage to the nervous system, or severe disturbances of body chemistry. The preventive measures may prove useful in such cases but not always. The permanent damage done on account of physical factors is incurable and therefore much attention must be paid to sexual disorders caused by psychological factors. The following measures prove fruitful in the prevention of psychological impotence and frigidity:

- Proper sex education of parents and other members of the society
- Proper sex education of the youngsters and adults before marriage
- Proper sex education of the married couple for maintaining an ideal sexual relationship, emphasizing the knowledge and skill of lovemaking and sex techniques.

Treatment

The only effective means of treatment of impotence and frigidity consists of the establishment of a stable, intimate, affectionate relationship involving confidence, security, and love. A number of psychological therapies like analytical psychotherapy, behavior therapy, client-centered therapy, family and couple therapy, gestalt therapy, and group psychotherapy may be attempted for this purpose.

In attempting treatment, a therapist must take it for granted that, leaving aside a few exceptions, there are no truly impotent men or frigid women. They are the victims of situations and events. Their behavior is a consequence of unhappy sexual experiences and inadequate sex knowledge. Therefore, it is a matter of sexual re-education, de-conditioning of unhappy experiences, removal of unnecessary fear complexes and feelings of inadequacies, and eliminating the mental blockages responsible for the lack of adequate sex response that is to be aimed for in any therapeutic measure suitable in a particular case of impotence or frigidity.

To Sum Up

Sexual disorders are psycho-physiological disturbances that interfere with the full enjoyment of conventional sexual relations. Impotence and frigidity are the two main disorders of such nature.

Impotence causes impairment in the desire for sexual gratification in a man or an inability to achieve it. Frigidity, the counterpart of impotence, is found in females. It creates in them a lack of interest and desire for sexual gratification or difficulty in achieving it.

Regarding the underlying causes, we may see that in some cases, impotence and frigidity may be attributed to physical damage to sex organs or the nervous system. But more often, these disorders are learned responses involving factors such as sexual guilt, fear, complexes, depression, conflicts, frustrations, sexual perversion, and bedroom mistakes.

Preventive measures for sexual disorders need to be adopted for the avoidance of physical injury to the sex organs and nervous system. In psychological measures of prevention, proper sex education of parents and adult members (before and after marriage) may prove fruitful.

The treatment of sexual disorders often consists in establishing a stable, intimate, affectionate relationship involving confidence, security, and love. A number of psychological therapies like behavior, analytical, family, and couple therapy may be successfully attempted for this purpose.

Review Questions

1. While defining the term sexual deviation, throw light on its meaning and nature.
2. Differentiate the term sexual deviation from the terms sexual offense and sexual disorder.
3. What are sexual deviations? Name and discuss the major sexual deviations found among individuals.
4. Discuss the underlying causes and treatment of sexual deviations.
5. What are sexual disorders? Throw light on their meaning and concept.
6. What are impotence and frigidity as sexual disorders found among individuals? Discuss their nature and implications.
7. What may be the causes underlying the existence of impotence and frigidity among men and women? Discuss.
8. Throw light on the measures taken for the prevention and treatment of sexual disorders.

References

Kisker, G. W. (1964), *The disorganized personality* (3rd International Students ed.), New York, NY: McGraw-Hill.

Rosen, E., Fox, R., & Gregory I. (1972), *Abnormal psychology* (2nd International Student ed.), Philadelphia, PA: Saunders.

Storr, A. (1964), *Sexual deviation*, London: Penguin Books.

Chapter 15

Elimination and Eating Disorders

Learning Objectives

After going through this chapter, you will be able to:

- Know about the meaning, nature, and types of elimination disorders found among children.
- Describe what enuresis is.
- Throw light on the identification and diagnosis of enuresis by taking cognizance of the criteria laid down in the DSM-5.
- Discuss the underlying causes and methods of treating enuresis.
- Know about the meaning, nature, and symptoms of encopresis.
- Throw light on the identification and diagnosis of encopresis by taking cognizance of the criteria laid down in the DSM-5.
- Discuss the underlying causes and methods of treating encopresis.
- Know about the meaning, nature, and types of eating disorders.
- Tell, what is anorexia nervosa?
- Tell about the identification and diagnosis of anorexia nervosa in light of the criteria laid down in the DSM-5.
- Know about the meaning and nature of bulimia nervosa.
- Throw light on the identification and diagnosis of bulimia nervosa in view of the criteria laid down in the DSM-5.
- Elucidate the meaning and nature of the eating disorder known as binge eating disorder.
- Throw light on the identification and diagnosis of binge eating disorder in view of the criteria laid down in the DSM-5.
- Discuss, how do the three eating disorders—anorexia nervosa, bulimia nervosa, and binge eating disorder—differ from each other?
- Describe in detail the causes underlying eating disorders.
- Throw light on the treatment measures carried out for the treatment of cases related to eating disorders.

Introduction

As we have seen in Chapter 7 of this text, the classification of mental disorders DSM-IV-TR (2000), provided by the American Psychiatric Association, has included and described

DOI: 10.4324/9781003398325-15

Elimination and Eating Disorders in the category of "Disorders usually first diagnosed during infancy, childhood, or adolescence." In its latest revisions—the DSM-5 published in 2013 as well as the DSM-5-TR in 2022—both of these developmental disorders have been classified on their own in two separate classification categories: (i) Elimination Disorders and (ii) Feeding and Eating Disorders. Let us discuss some essentials about these disorders associated with the development and life of children and adolescents.

Elimination Disorders

What are Elimination Disorders?

Nature has made the proper provision of providing outlets for the elimination of the waste products such as urine and feces in a regular way from our bodies. Newborns may be seen to urinate and pass feces from the provided outlets in natural ways found convenient to them. Young children often urinate or pass feces in their clothes, in bed, on the laps of others, or on the floor. After reaching a certain age, babies are provided toilet training for urinating and passing feces in a socially desirable manner in a proper way in proper places. Moreover, as they grow in age and develop, they are able to exercise necessary control over their bladders and bowl.

> **Elimination Disorders**
>
> The type of disorder in which children are found to urinate and pass feces involuntarily in the ways and means as well as at the time and places they find convenient to do so, even after reaching an age at which they are expected to exercise needed control over their elimination organs.

However, the practice of urinating and passing feces does not go so smoothly with some children, even after reaching an age at which they are expected to exercise needed control over their elimination organs. Contrarily, they may be found to urinate or pass feces involuntarily in the ways and means as well as at the places they find convenient to do so. Moreover, this does not at all relate to any physical illness suffered by them, nor does it happen to them accidentally and occasionally. It is repeatedly performed any time during the day, but more often at night during sleep, and causes a great amount of distress to them and others. The children experiencing this sort of unwelcome behavior regarding the elimination of urine and feces from their bodies are termed as children suffering from elimination disorders.

Types of Elimination Disorders

There are two types of elimination disorders, Enuresis and Encopresis, described subsequently.

Enuresis

The word enuresis is derived from a Greek word (*enourein*), which means "to void urine." Accordingly, the term enuresis stands in the clinical and psychological world for a type of elimination disorder related to the passing of urine on the part of individuals. In defining this disorder, we may say that

> **Enuresis**
>
> An elimination disorder relating to an abnormal behavior (involuntary or purposeful) of toilet-trained developing children (more than four years old) or adults in which they are found to urinate repeatedly in their clothes and beds at night during sleep or even during the day.

Enuresis is a type of elimination disorder that relates to abnormal behavior (involuntary or purposeful) of toilet-trained developing children (more than four years old) or adults in which they are found to urinate repeatedly in their clothes and beds. It typically occurs to them at night during sleep but may also occur during the day.

The emotional impact of enuresis on a child and family can be considerably damaging. Children with enuresis are commonly punished and are at risk for emotional and physical abuse. Research evidences have demonstrated a number of damaging effects experienced on the part of children suffering from enuresis, such as embarrassment, anxiety, loss of self-esteem, and effects on self-perception, interpersonal relationships, quality of life, and school performance.

Identification and Diagnosis of Enuresis

As far as its identification and diagnosis are concerned, children suffering from enuresis or bedwetting are no different than normal children in appearance or other observable symptoms. Their problem lies in the inability to exercise control over the bladder, making them urinate in their clothes or bed. Therefore, their wet clothes or bed are the only way to tell about their urination-related disorder.

For helping in the diagnosis and identification of Enuresis, the American Psychiatric Association has laid down the distinctive criteria in the DSM-5 (2013), as shown in Table 15.1.

Causes Behind the Development of Enuresis

What causes enuresis among developing children is not very clear to clinicians and researchers. A number of possible factors in their various combinations are considered to cause this elimination disorder among children, including:

1. *Genetic Factor*—Enuresis is said to be linked to genetic inheritance. Those with enuresis typically have a close relative (parent, sibling) who has had or will have the same disorder.
2. *Biological Factor:* In the views of physiologists and biologists, children become victims of enuresis because they have a small bladder capacity or weak bladder muscles for holding the amount of urine produced.

Table 15.1 DSM-5 Criteria for the Diagnosis of Enuresis

1. Repeated voiding of urine into bed or clothes, whether involuntary or intentional
2. The behavior either (a) occurs at least twice a week for at least three consecutive months or (b) results in clinically significant distress or social, functional, or academic impairment
3. The behavior occurs in a child who is at least five years old (or has reached the equivalent developmental level)
4. The behavior cannot be attributed to the physiologic effects of a substance or other medical condition

Enuresis can be further divided into the following three subtypes on the basis of the time of occurrence:
• Nocturnal (i.e., during sleep)
• Diurnal (i.e., during waking hours)
• Nocturnal and diurnal

Source: American Psychiatric Association (2013), Diagnostic and Statistical Manual of Mental Disorders, Fifth Edition, (DSM-5), Washington, DC: APA.

3. *Developmental Factor:* According to the developmental psychologist, on account of the delay in acquiring the necessary maturity, some children do not acquire the needed level of maturity to make them feel that (i) their bladder is full and they should go to the toilet, as well as (ii) to arouse them from sleep for the activity.

4. *Psychodynamic Factor:* According to psychodynamics theorists, repressed wishes and underlying conflicts as well as anxiety may be potent causes for generating enuresis.

5. *Behavioral and Sociocultural factor:* Psychologists, mainly behaviorists and social psychologists, view enuresis as an outcome of disturbed family interactions, faulty upbringing, and improper, unrealistic, or coercive toilet training.

Whatever reason may be there for the germination of the problem related to enuresis out of the factors pointed out above, one thing is certain: the problem gets precipitated by stressful events, uncongenial home and school environment, and maltreatment— particularly the physical or psychological abuse experienced by children at one or the other occasions.

Treatment of Enuresis

Children usually "grow out" of their elimination disorders by the time they reach their teens. If treatment is necessary, the most effective choice for enuresis is behavior modification, which involves a special pad that the child bears on at night. If the pad gets wet, an alarm goes off and the child is directed to go to the bathroom.

Since the prevalence of enuresis decreases with age, most younger children suffering from enuresis usually correct themselves even without treatment by the time they grow as adolescents. However, for speeding up the process or dealing with some complicated cases, the treatment method or therapy known as behavior modification therapy is considered the most workable and effective. In its applied form it can be used in the ways specified ahead (Comer, 2015).

1. In dealing with the problem of enuresis, behavior therapy may make use of a specific technique termed "the bell-and-battery technique." In this technique, a bell and battery are wired to a pad consisting of two metallic foil sheets, and the entire apparatus is placed under the child at bedtime. Whenever the child urinates during his or her sleep, a single drop of urine sets off the bell, awakening the child as soon as he or she starts to wet. Thus the bell (unconditioned stimulus) paired with the sensation of a full bladder (conditioned stimulus) produces the response of waking. Conditioned in this way, eventually, a full bladder alone is able to awaken the child for going to the toilet.

2. Another effective behavioral treatment method is dry-bed training. Here, children with enuresis are provided with necessary training in cleanliness and retention control. The training schedule adopted for this purpose includes (i) awakening the child periodically during the night, (ii) making him or her go to the bathroom for passing urine, and (iii) reinforcing such proper behavior through suitable rewards.

To Sum Up

Developmental disorders such as elimination and eating disorders are found to show their presence among individuals first during infancy, childhood, or adolescence.

In general, children experiencing abnormal and unwelcome behavior regarding the elimination of urine and feces from their body are termed as children suffering from the elimination disorders classified as enuresis and encopresis.

Enuresis is a type of elimination disorder that relates to an abnormal behavior (involuntary or purposeful) of toilet-trained developing children (more than four years old), or adults who urinate repeatedly in their clothes and beds. It typically occurs to them at night during sleep but may also occur during the day. The emotional impact of enuresis on a child and family can be considerably damaging. The disorder related to enuresis can be diagnosed and identified on the basis of the children's inability to exercise control over the bladder, making them urinate in their clothes or bed.

A number of possible factors in their various combinations classified as Genetic, Biological, Developmental, Psychodynamic, Behavioral, and Sociocultural factors may be considered to cause and intensify elimination disorders among children. Regarding the treatment of enuresis, it can be seen that most younger children suffering from enuresis usually correct themselves even without treatment by the time they grow as adolescents. If needed, then, it remains quite useful to make use of behavioral therapy techniques such as (i) the bell-and-battery technique, and (ii) the dry-bed training method.

Encopresis

The word Encopresis has its root in Greek signifying involuntary defecation. In this sense, as a mental disorder, Encopresis stands for a type of abnormal behavior (involuntary or purposeful) demonstrated by toilet-trained developing children (more than four years old) or adults in which they are found passing feces repeatedly in places other than the toilets, such as in their clothing or bed, or anywhere at their convenience.

> **Encopresis**
>
> An elimination disorder relating to an abnormal behavior (involuntary or purposeful) of toilet-trained developing children (more than four years old) or adults in which they are found passing feces repeatedly in places other than toilets, such as in their clothing or bed, or anywhere at their convenience.

Symptoms of Encopresis

In addition to defecating in improper places, children suffering from encopresis may demonstrate a number of physiological, physical, and psychological symptoms such as:

1. There are disturbances and problems in their digestive system, including complaints of (i) abdominal pain, (ii) loss of appetite, (iii) constipation and/or hard stools, (iv) inability to retain feces (bowel incontinence), (v) loose, watery stools (bowel movement), and (vi) the need to scratch or rub the anal area due to irritation from watery stools.
2. They may show a strange behavior characterizing (i) decreased interest in physical activity, (ii) remaining aloof by withdrawing from friends and family, (iii) avoiding socially

interactive situations such as going on picnics, camping, or even attending functions and classes in the school, (iv) secretive behavior associated with the act of having a bowel movement, (v) nervousness and anxiety for their bowel difficulty, and (vi) feelings of shame and embarrassment on account of their wet and spoiled clothes.

Identification and Diagnosis of Encopresis

In addition to gathering information derived through observation and reporting the presence of the symptoms (outlined above) associated with encopresis, the identification and diagnosis of children suffering from encopresis may be further assured with the use of the diagnostic criteria available in the DSM-5 published by the American Psychiatric Association in 2013, as shown in Table 15.2.

In order to get further certainty regarding the diagnosis of encopresis among children, a complete medical examination including the evaluation of their medical history is needed on the part of trained physicians and clinicians. They may make use of certain tests for ruling out other possible causes in the form of physical disorders involving constipation and digestive problems. If no physical disorder or somatic cause is found, then they may definitely associate the problem with the mental disorder known as Encopresis.

Causes Behind the Development of Encopresis

A number of factors—biological, physiological, physical, and psychological—may work in one or the other combinations for causing Encopresis in the manner outlined ahead.

1. **Physiological and Physical factors:** The most common cause of encopresis is chronic (long-term) constipation—the inability to release stools from the bowel. This may happen on account of factors such as (i) unhealthy food habits—especially a diet low in fiber, (ii) lack of sufficient amounts of water, (iii) lack of exercise, (iv) pain caused by a sore in or near the anus, (v) inconsistent bathroom routines, (vi) fear or reluctance to use unfamiliar bathrooms, (vii) not taking the time to use the bathroom, and (viii) a physical problem related to the intestine's ability to move stool.
2. **Psychological factors:** Apart from the physiological factors, encopresis is also caused and intensified on account of the level of anxiety, stress, or frustrations suffered by the child in his or her sociocultural environment on account of (i) improper and hard ways of toilet-training, (ii) stressful events in the child's life such as quarreling and disputes between parents, family illness, maltreatment of the child, or even the arrival of a new sibling

---

Table 15.2 DSM-5 Criteria for the Diagnosis of Encopresis

1. Patient's chronological age must be at least four years;
2. A repeated passage of feces into inappropriate places, e.g., clothing or floor. This can be either intentional or involuntary;
3. At least one such event must occur every month for at least three months;
4. The behavior is not attributable to the effects of a substance, e.g., laxative, or another medical condition, with the exception of a mechanism involving constipation.

Source: American Psychiatric Association (2013), Diagnostic and Statistical Manual of Mental Disorders, Fifth Edition, (DSM-5), Washington, DC: APA.

Treatment of Encopresis

Encopresis is found to affect fewer children than enuresis, and is more common in boys than in girls. Like enuresis, it also gets better as the child gets older, although the problem can come and go for years. In order to have better treatment, we may employ a number of therapies or treatment measures capable of addressing the physiological, physical, behavioral, and emotional issues associated with this disorder. In general, it remains advantageous to concentrate on measures like the following for this purpose.

1. **Physiological and Medical treatment:** Since constipation and irregular bowel functioning are the major issues with children suffering from encopresis, sincere efforts should be made to help children in overcoming these issues by resorting to the means such as:

   - Clearing any feces that has become impacted in the large intestine.
   - Providing a fiber-rich diet.
   - Using stool softeners such as mineral oil, laxatives, and lubricants for stimulating regular bowel functioning.
   - Introducing physical activities and exercise in the daily schedule of the child.
   - Taking help of suitable medication, if necessary, for dealing with the issues of constipation, irregular bowel, digestion and intestine functioning-related problems.
   - Providing biofeedback training to help children to be conscious of passing feces when needed and bring improvement to the habit of making scheduled trips to the bathroom.

2. **Behavioral and psychological treatment:** Since encopresis is very much associated with psychological and emotional factors, its treatment also requires fighting the battle on this front. In this concern, it should be well remembered that punishment in any way is not typically effective, and usually increases rather than decreases the problems related to this disorder. As a result, it remains beneficial to make use of treatment measures involving behavioral and psychological therapies such as:

   - Behavior modification techniques involving classical and operant conditioning, schedule of reinforcement, and shaping of the behavior.
   - Psychotherapy (a type of counseling) for helping the child cope with the shame, guilt, or loss of self-esteem associated with the disorder.
   - Planning and providing suitable psychological interventions to the affected children and their families for dealing with the problems related to the disorder.
   - Parental training and family therapy for dealing with the issues related to the disorder.
   - Cognitive behavioral therapy and psychotherapy for dealing with the symptoms of anxiety, depression, and frustrations associated with the disorder.

To Sum Up

The elimination disorder encopresis may be defined as a type of abnormal behavior (involuntary or purposeful) demonstrated by toilet-trained developing children (more than four years old) or adults in which they are found passing feces repeatedly in places other than toilets, such as in their clothing, bed, or anywhere at their convenience.

In the diagnosis and identification of encopresis, attempts should first be made to derive information from observation of the physiological, physical, and psychological symptoms related to this disorder, and then these observations should be consulted against standard diagnostic criteria, such as the DSM-5 criteria provided by American Psychiatric Association and medical reports available for this purpose.

A number of factors—physiological, physical, and psychological—may work in one or the other combinations for causing Encopresis. However, chronic, long-term constipation and the increased level of anxiety and stress that accompany it are found to play a major role in encopresis.

Like enuresis, encopresis also gets better as the child gets older. For seeking its treatment, a number of treatment measures classified as (i) physiological and medical treatment and (ii) behavioral and psychological treatment may be used for addressing the physiological, physical, behavioral, and emotional issues associated with this disorder.

Feeding and Eating Disorders

What are Feeding and Eating Disorders?

Feeding and Eating Disorders are disorders caused by problems related to feeding and eating habits. For the formal definition of the term, let us look into its interpretation in the latest classification systems, the DSM-5 and DSM-5-TR, provided by the American Psychiatric Association (APA).

Feeding and Eating Disorders

The type of developmental disorders making individuals experience severe disturbances in their feeding and eating behaviors in the form of remaining pre-occupied with food and their body weight.

DSM-5: Feeding and Eating disorders are illnesses in which the people experience severe disturbances in their eating behaviors and related thoughts and emotions. People with eating disorders typically become pre-occupied with food and their body weight (APA, 2013).

DSM-5-TR: [Feeding and eating disorders are] . . . characterized by a persistent disturbance of eating or eating related behavior that results in the altered consumption or absorption of food and that significantly impairs physical health or psychosocial functioning (APA, 2022).

Consciousness and preoccupation with food and body weight for looking attractive has always been a great craving on the part of youngsters and adolescents. However, it has gained great momentum during the modern age of fashion and glamor. The excessive inclination to become more and more thin and lean (especially on the part of young girls and women) has led to intensifying a number of serious health-related problems and behavioral disorders designated as feeding and eating disorders.

Types of Feeding and Eating Disorders

Feeding and Eating disorders affect several million people, at a given time—most often women between the ages of 12 and 35. Within the DSM-5 (2013) and DSM 5-TR (APA, 2022), six disorders are classified under the Feeding and Eating Disorders category. These are pica, rumination disorder, avoidant/restrictive food intake disorder, anorexia nervosa, bulimia nervosa, and binge eating disorder. In this chapter, we will cover the latter three, the most generalized ones among adolescents and young adults.

Anorexia Nervosa

Anorexia Nervosa is the most pronounced, difficult, and dangerous disorder among all three major eating disorders found in individuals. The peak age of its onset has been found between 14 and 20 years. Females are more affected by this disorder than their male counterparts, as about 90 to 95% of all cases of anorexia nervosa reported are females. The desire to become thin by losing weight through dieting makes the whole story of the commencement of this disorder and gradually it may drive the individual to the point of starving and even to the extent of completely ruining his or her health and life, to the extent of suicide. How this happens, and what goes in Anorexia nervosa, may be better revealed through the information derived from the case histories as follows.

Julie: The thinner, the better

Julie was 17 years old when she first came for help. She looked emaciated and unwell. Eighteen months earlier she had been overweight, weighing 140 pounds at 5 feet and 1 inch. Her mother, a well-meaning but overbearing and demanding woman, nagged Julie incessantly about her appearance. Her friends were kinder but no less relentless. Julie, who had never had a date, was told by a friend she was cute and would have no trouble getting dates if she lost some weight. So she did! After many previous unsuccessful attempts, she was determined to succeed this time.

After several weeks on a strict diet, Julie noticed she was losing weight. She felt a control and mastery that she had never known before. It wasn't long before she received positive comments, not only from her friends but also from her mother; Julie began to feel good about herself. The difficulty was that she was losing weight too fast. She stopped menstruating. But now nothing could stop her from dieting. By the time she reached our clinic, she weighed 75 pounds. Her parents were worried about her. Julie did not initially seek treatment for her eating behavior. Rather, she had developed numbness in her left lower leg and a left foot drop—an inability to lift up the front part of the foot—that a neurologist determined was caused by peritoneal nerve paralysis believed to be related to inadequate nutrition. The neurologist referred her to our clinic.

Like most people with anorexia, Julie said she probably should put on a little weight, but she didn't mean it. She thought she looked fine, but she had "lost all taste for food," a report that may not have been true because most people with anorexia crave food at least

---

some of the time but control their cravings. Nevertheless, she was participating in most of her usual activities and continued to do extremely well in school and her extracurricular pursuits. Her parents were happy to buy her workout videotapes, and she began doing one every day—and then two. When her parents suggested she was exercising enough, and perhaps too much, she worked out when no one was around. After every meal, she exercised with a workout tape until, in her mind, she burned up all the calories she had just taken in.

Source: Durand and Barlow (2013:289)

On the basis of things revealed from case histories like the one above as well as the conclusions arrived at from research findings, individuals affected by Anorexia Nervosa have been found to be characterized as follows:

1. Becoming thinner and thinner by losing weight is a key goal for individuals with anorexia nervosa.
2. Typically, the disorder begins with a desire of becoming thin on the part of individuals, especially on the part of young and adolescent girls slightly overweight or of normal weight (intending to look more attractive and acceptable by others).
3. They resort to dieting (observing fasting and putting severe restrictions on their food intake) for reducing weight and becoming thin. However, the desire of reducing weight and becoming thin is soon converted into an obsession about becoming thinner and thinner, as well as feeling haunted by a morbid fear of gaining weight and losing control over eating.
4. In the process of going through their obsession with weight reduction, they pick up a variety of means other than fasting or severe food restrictions, such as

   • Heavy exercising and physical activities.
   • Trying to throw out their food intake by vomiting or taking large doses of laxatives (the drugs or medicines tending to stimulate or facilitate the evacuation of the bowels).

5. Strangely enough with their desire as well as attempts to avoid food intake, people with anorexia are preoccupied with food, demonstrable through their behaviors such as

   • Spending considerable time thinking and even reading about food and planning their limited meals.
   • Cooking elaborate meals for others while eating nothing themselves.
   • Reporting that they feel fed while seeing the food items or eating them by others in real encounters or even in pictures or videos.

6. Persons with anorexia nervosa have such low opinions of their body shape that they are never satisfied with the results obtained through the measures taken on their part in this concern. The perception of a girl suffering from Anorexia Nervosa reveals this fact in the manner given below:

   I look in a full-length mirror at least four or five times daily and I really cannot see myself as too thin. Sometimes after several days of strict dieting, I feel that my shape is tolerable, but most of the time, odd as it may seem, I look in the mirror and believe that I am too fat.

(Comer, 2015:35)

7. On account of their craving for becoming thin and dissatisfaction with the results of this concern, as well as their possession of a distorted perception on their part about their body image, it is quite usual for persons with anorexia nervosa to consider themselves fat (still needing to lose some weight from some parts of the body), while others view them as emaciated, sickly; a frame of skins and bones in a state of semi-starvation.

8. People with anorexia nervosa may also be found to be affected by a number of psychological, social, and behavioral problems and typical behaving patterns such as:

   (i) They usually suffer from depression, anxiety, low self-esteem, and insomnia or other sleep disturbances.
   (ii) Many of them may grapple with substance abuse.
   (iii) They may display typical obsessive-compulsive behavior patterns such as setting rigid rules for food preparation and even cutting food into specific shapes, as well as prioritizing exercise over most other activities in their lives.
   (iv) Behaving as a perfectionist, a characteristic that typically precedes the onset of the disorder.

9. People with anorexia nervosa, eventually, suffer from a number of medical problems on account of their persistent obsession with becoming thinner, such as:

   • Suffering from significant problems on account of poor nutrition, such as losing hair from the scalp, and getting rough, dry, and cracked skin, as well as brittle nails and blue feet.
   • Having a low body temperature, low blood pressure, body swelling, reduced bone mineral density, and slow heart rate.
   • Development of amenorrhea, the absence of menstrual cycles on the part of women.
   • Suffering from problems related to metabolic and electrolyte imbalances causing death by heart failure or circulatory collapse.

Identification and Diagnosis of Anorexia Nervosa

The observation and reporting of symptoms and characteristics of individuals suffering from anorexia nervosa provide a lot of evidence and clues regarding the presence of such an eating disorder. For diagnostic certainty, further help may be taken from the criteria provided in the DSM-5 by American Psychiatric Association (2013), as shown in Table 15.3.

Table 15.3 DSM-5 Criteria for the Diagnosis of Anorexia Nervosa

1. Individual purposely takes in too little nourishment, resulting in a body weight that is very low and below that of other people of similar age and gender.
2. Individual is very fearful of gaining weight, or repeatedly seeks to prevent weight gain despite low body weight.
3. Individual has a distorted body perception, places inappropriate emphasis on weight or shape in judgments of herself or himself, or fails to appreciate the serious implications of her or his low weight.

Source: American Psychiatric Association (2013), Diagnostic and Statistical Manual of Mental Disorders, Fifth Edition, (DSM-5), Washington DC: American Psychiatric Association.

> ## To Sum Up
>
> Anorexia nervosa is an eating disorder in which people pursue extreme thinness and lose dangerous amounts of weight. The central features of this disorder are a drive for thinness, intense fear of weight gain, disturbed body perception, and other cognitive disturbances. Typically, the disorder begins after a person who is slightly overweight or of normal weight has been on a diet, and females are more affected by this disorder than males. In terms of its outcomes, people with this disorder are found to develop various medical and health problems regarding the skin, metabolism, and heart—particularly amenorrhea (the absence of menstrual cycles in women).

Bulimia Nervosa

A less difficult but quite dangerous and harmful eating disorder in the name of Bulimia nervosa is often visible among individuals. Like Anorexia nervosa, it also occurs mostly in females, again in 90 to 95% of cases. It also begins in adolescence or early adulthood and often lasts for years, with periodic letup. In perfect similarity to Anorexia nervosa, it is also dominated by a morbid fear of gaining weight and extreme consciousness and craving for appearing thin and slim. However, for becoming thin where people suffering from anorexia nervosa resort to fasting until the point of starving, people with bulimia nervosa, while avoiding regular meals, also go on frequent eating binges, quite often secretly, and then force themselves to vomit or take other extreme steps to keep from gaining weight. On account of its distinguishing feature, eating binges and then purging afterward, the bulimia eating disorder is also known as binge-purge syndrome. In all its functioning and outcomes, bulimia nervosa and individuals suffering from bulimia nervosa are found to be characterized as follows:

1. The hallmark of bulimia nervosa is to engage in repeated, out of control, episodes of binges, i.e., eating a large amount of food at once quite rapidly with minimal chewing —typically, junk food (usually sweet, high-calorie foods with a soft texture, such as ice cream, cookies, doughnuts, and sandwiches). Here the person eats much more food than most people would eat during a similar time span.
2. Another distinguishing feature of Bulimia nervosa is that people with this disorder repeatedly perform attempts to compensate for such eating and potential gain by forcing themselves to vomit; misusing laxatives, diuretics, or enemas; fasting; or exercising excessively.
3. The third important diagnostic characteristic of bulimia nervosa is an excessive preoccupation with body shape and weight. Accordingly, they feel that their continuing popularity and self-esteem would largely be determined by the weight and shape of their body. They are weight-conscious and, like people with anorexia nervosa, they also remain haunted by the fear of weight gain. But unlike them, who get success in losing weight, the weight of people with bulimia nervosa usually stays within a normal range or fluctuates markedly within that range even after going through a lot of purging and other compensatory measures.
4. As with anorexia nervosa, a bulimic pattern typically begins during or after a period of intense dieting, often one that has been successful and earned praise from family members and friends.
5. The behavior related to falling prey to binge episodes is usually preceded by feelings of great tension. However, as a tension reliever and pleasurable act in itself, it soon develops into an obsessive as well as compulsive act performed by the individual as a secret mission.

6. Failure to achieve the mission of losing weight results in (i) inducing the feelings of extreme self-blame, shame, guilt, and depression, and (ii) intensifying fears related to the gaining of weight and disclosure of the secret binge episodes.

7. Although people with either disorder—anorexia and bulimia—worry about the opinions of others, those with bulimia nervosa tend to be more concerned about pleasing others, being attractive to others, and having intimate relationships.

8. Individuals suffering from chronic bulimia nervosa, besides suffering from a host of psychological problems particularly related to anxiety, depression, obsession-compulsion, and mood disorders, are also found to suffer from a number of medical consequences such as the following (Durand and Barlow, 2013:288):

- Women with bulimia nervosa may also suffer from irregular menstrual periods, such as suffered by those with anorexia nervosa—however, to a lesser extent.
- The exposure of teeth and gums to hydrochloric acid in the process of repeated vomiting may result in serious dental problems such as erosion of the dental enamel on the inner surface and tearing of the esophagus, of the front teeth, and even loss of teeth.
- The act of frequent purging may also result in (i) enlargement of salivary glands and (ii) upsetting of the chemical balance of bodily fluids, including sodium and potassium levels, leading to serious medical complications such as disrupted heartbeat, seizures, and kidney failure.
- Binge eating and laxative abuse may result in a number of indigestion and intestine problems, such as severe constipation or permanent colon damage.

Identification and Diagnosis of Bulimia Nervosa

The observation and reporting of symptoms and characteristics of individuals suffering from Bulimia Nervosa provide a lot of evidence and clues regarding the presence of this eating disorder. For diagnostic certainty, further help may be taken from the criteria for diagnosing them provided in the DSM-5 by the American Psychiatric Association (2013), as shown in Table 15.4.

Table 15.4 DSM-5 Criteria for the Diagnosis of Bulimia Nervosa

1. Repeated binge eating episodes.
2. Repeated performance of ill-advised compensatory behaviors (e.g., forced vomiting) to prevent weight gain.
3. Symptoms take place at least weekly for a period of three months.
4. Inappropriate influence of weight and shape on appraisal of self.

Source: American Psychiatric Association (2013), Diagnostic and Statistical Manual of Mental Disorders, Fifth Edition, (DSM-5), Washington DC: American Psychiatric Association.

To Sum Up

Similar to anorexia nervosa, bulimia nervosa is also dominated by a morbid fear of gaining weight. However, for becoming thin, instead of resorting to rigorous fasting, people with bulimia nervosa, while avoiding some regular meals, before others go on frequent eating binges, quite often secretly, and then force themselves to vomit or take other extreme steps to keep from gaining weight. The binges are often in response to increasing tension and are followed by feelings of guilt and self-blame. In terms of consequences, people with bulimia nervosa are found to be affected by a number of psychological problems (particularly related to anxiety, depression, obsession-compulsion, and mood disorders) and medical problems associated with their teeth and gums, indigestion and intestine disturbances, and menstrual cycle problems in women.

Binge Eating Disorder

Binge eating disorder is the latest addition to the list of eating disorders. It is less common, cumbersome, and problematic than both of its counterparts—anorexia and bulimia nervosa eating disorders. Only two to seven percent of the total population is estimated to be affected by Binge eating disorder. It is also notable that while anorexia nervosa and bulimia nervosa usually occur in females, binge eating disorder is evenly distributed among both sexes. The main distinguishing features and symptoms related to Binge eating disorder may be outlined as follows:

1. The chief characteristic of this disorder is an overwhelming, all-encompassing drive to be thin, much similar as experienced in the other two nervosas—bulimia and anorexia.
2. Moreover, like people with bulimia nervosa or anorexia nervosa, those with binge eating disorder typically are preoccupied with food, weight, and appearance; base their evaluation of themselves largely on their weight and shape; misperceive their body size and are extremely dissatisfied with their body; struggle with feelings of depression, anxiety, and perfectionism; may abuse substances; and typically first develop the disorder in adolescence or young adulthood (Comer, 2015:358).
3. For their binge eating behavior it may be said that, much like those with bulimia nervosa, people with binge eating disorder engage in repeated eating binges during which they feel no control over their eating.
4. However, in contrast to the other eating disorders, anorexia nervosa and bulimia nervosa, Binge eating disorder has been found to be characterized by special features and symptoms such as:

   - Individuals with binge eating disorder do not demonstrate inappropriate compensatory behavior like purging, excessive exercising, and resorting to misuse of drugs and laxatives after eating binge.
   - The binge eating disorder does not necessarily begin with efforts at extreme dieting.
   - Although aspiring to limit their eating, people with binge eating disorder are not as driven to thinness as those with anorexia nervosa and bulimia nervosa.
   - People suffering from binge eating disorder are more social and sexually active than those with anorexia nervosa and bulimia nervosa.

5. It has also been found that where most overweight people do not have binge eating disorder, two-thirds of those with binge eating disorder become overweight or even obese.
6. It has also been found that about half of individuals with binge eating disorder try dieting before bingeing, and half start with bingeing and then attempt to diet. Those who began bingeing first become more severally affected by binge eating disorder and are more likely to have additional disorders (Durand and Barlow, 2013:291).

Identification and Diagnosis of Binge Eating Disorder

The observation and reporting of symptoms and characteristics of individuals suffering from Binge eating disorder provide a lot of evidence and clues regarding the presence of such an eating disorder. For diagnostic certainty, further help may be taken from the Diagnostic Criteria provided by the American Psychiatric Association (2013) in its DSM-5, as shown in Table 15.5.

Table 15 5 DSM-5 Criteria for the Diagnosis of Binge Eating Disorder

Binge Eating Disorder—Recurrent binge eating episodes
1. Binge eating episodes include at least three of the following features
    (i) Unusual fast eating, (ii) Absence of hunger, (iii) Uncomfortable fullness, (iv) Secret eating due to a sense of shame, (v) Subsequent feelings of self-disgust, depression, or severe guilt
3. Significant distress
4. Binge eating episodes take place at least weekly over the course of three months
5. Absence of excessive compensatory behaviors.

Source: American Psychiatric Association (2013), Diagnostic and Statistical Manual of Mental Disorders, Fifth Edition, (DSM-5), Washington DC: American Psychiatric Association.

To Sum Up

Binge eating disorder is an eating disorder in which people have frequent binge eating episodes but do not display inappropriate compensatory behaviors. Although most over-weight people do not have binge eating disorder, two-thirds of those with binge eating disorder become overweight. Unlike anorexia nervosa and bulimia nervosa, this disorder is evenly distributed among males and females.

In the description carried out in the previous pages about all three types of eating disorders, all essentials about their meaning, nature, functioning, and outcomes have been highlighted. How do these three main disorders differ from one another? Drawing a summarized conclusion in this concern Comer (2015:350) writes:

> In the former two eating disorders (anorexia nervosa and bulimia nervosa) there lies a morbid fear of gaining weight and extremely consciousness and craving for appearing thin and slim. Here the sufferers of anorexia nervosa are very much convinced that they need to be extremely thin, and they lose so much weight that they may starve themselves to death. People with bulimia nervosa go on frequent eating binges, during which they uncontrollably consume large quantities of food, and then force themselves to vomit or take other extreme steps to keep from gaining weight. A third eating disorder, binge eating disorder, in which people frequently go on eating binges but do not force themselves to vomit or engage in other such behaviors, appears to be on the rise. People with binge eating disorder do not fear weight gain to the same degree as those with anorexia nervosa and bulimia nervosa, but they do have many of the other features found in those disorders.

What Causes Eating Disorders?

Eating disorders of one or the other kind are said to be the function of a multiplicity of causes governed by biological, psychological, and sociocultural factors. Let us know about their impacts in generating and perpetuating these disorders.

Biological Factors

Biological and genetic theorists talk about the role of biological and genetic factors in causing eating disorders among people and in their support put forward the following research evidence and arguments:

- Like most psychological disorders, eating disorders are found running in families and thus seem to have a genetic component. Family history studies conducted in this concern reveal that relatives of people with eating disorders are found six times more likely than other people to develop the disorders themselves.
- It has been also found that in case one identical twin has one or the other eating disorder, the other twin also develops the disorder in as many as more than 50% of the cases. However, in contrast, the rate for fraternal twins, (who are generally less similar in comparison to identical twins), for showing such similarity is quite less than for identical twins.
- There has been a link found between eating disorders and the genes responsible for the production of one of the neurotransmitters, known as serotonin, the lower level of which in an individual has been seen as responsible for contributing to eating disorders by, for example, leading to depression and obsessive-compulsive disorders that are associated with eating disorders, and also by causing the body to crave and binge on high carbohydrate foods.
- Apart from such genetically based evidence, biological processes are also quite active in the regulation of eating and thus of eating disorders, and substantial evidence points to the hypothalamus as playing an important role in the development of eating disorders.

  However, whatever evidence may exist for substantiating the role of genetic and biological components in generating eating disorders, they remain quite hollow and weightless, as researchers and biologists have not been able to point out a single pair of defective genes, or inherited biological apparatus responsible for transmitting or causing eating disorders or abnormalities to the next generation. Moreover, eating disorders, like all other mental or psychological disorders and behavior abnormalities, are the results of ongoing maladjustments on account of what has happened in the past or is happening at present to him or her in the available sociocultural environment. Let us, therefore, look for the related psychological and sociocultural factors for the explanation of eating disorders.

Psychological Factors

The clinical observations and research evidences have suggested a number of psychological factors working behind generating and perpetuating eating disorders among children and adolescents. These may be named as (i) low self-esteem, (ii) a diminished sense of personal control and confidence in their own abilities accompanied by a distorted self-perception of body image, and (iv) an increased level of anxiety and depression.

Children and adolescents who lack self confidence and self-reliance are more prone to being victimized by the abnormalities of eating disorders. Such children and adolescents are easily influenced by the opinions of others about their body appearance and then are driven toward dieting or other food restrictions for their ego defense. Their distorted perception of their own body image, accompanied by their increased level of anxiety about becoming thin, then pushes them to pick up a strange obsession and compulsion for looking thin in the eyes of others and the self in the shape and form of one or the other eating disorders. To throw light on the strange situation faced by growing children and adolescents in this concern, Bruch (1978:128) writes:

> There is a peculiar contradiction—everybody thinks you're doing so well and everybody thinks you're great, but your real problem is that you think that you are not good enough. You are afraid of not living up to what you think you are expected to do. You have one great fear, namely that of being ordinary, or average, or common-just not good enough. This peculiar dieting begins with such anxiety. You want to prove that you have control, that you can do it. The peculiar part of it is that it makes you feel good about yourself, makes you feel "I can accomplish some- thing." It makes you feel "I can do something nobody else can do."

As a major psychological factor, an increased level of anxiety converted into a mood and depressive disorder may also prove a potent factor in causing one or the other types of eating disorders. The claim that depressive disorder sets the stage for eating disorders may be supported by four kinds of evidences put forward by Comer (2015:362), as follows:

> First, many more people with an eating disorder qualify for a clinical diagnosis of major depressive disorders than do people in the general population. Second, the close relatives of people with eating disorders seem to have a higher rate of depressive disorders than do close relatives of people without such disorders. Third, many people with eating disorders, particularly bulimia nervosa, have low activity of the neurotransmitter serotonin similar to the serotonin abnormalities found in depression. And finally, people with eating disorders are often helped by some of the same depressants drugs that reduce depression.

Sociocultural Factors

There are sociocultural factors and things inherent in one's sociocultural environment that may contribute to the origin and development of one or the other abnormalities and problems related to eating disorders. Even what we know as psychological factors such as ego deficiency, lack of confidence, low self-esteem, distorted self-perception of body image, and aroused levels of anxiety and depression may be said to be byproducts of the maladjustment and negativity experienced by individuals in their sociocultural environments at home, family, school, and in their community as well as social and cultural settings. Let us look into the role of sociocultural factors in the development of eating disorders:

1. Hilde Bruch, a pioneer in the study and treatment of eating disorders, has claimed that disturbed mother-child interactions lead to serious *ego deficiencies* in the child (including a poor sense of independence and control) and to severe *perceptual disturbances* that jointly help produce disordered eating (Bruch, 2001).
2. A defective style of parenting may lead to a lack of genuine self-reliance and self-confidence among growing children, so that they become incapable of having faith in their abilities,

or accepting of their self (including their body shape) in their present form. It may also make them unable to exercise proper control over their needs and impulses, reflected in their uncontrollable binge eating and compensatory behavior.

3. The uncongenial and improper environment available at home may play a damaging role in germinating as well as perpetuating eating disorders. Besides pushing the child to anxiety and depression symptoms, it can provide incentives as well as role models for learning and practicing behaviors associated with one or the other eating disorders. The description provided here below by a 16-year-old girl may reveal how the behavior of a mother may drive a child into developing an eating disorder.

When I was a kid, say six or seven, my Mom and I would go to the drug store all the time. She was heavy and bought all kinds of books and magazine on how to lose weight. Whenever we talked, like after I got home from school, it was almost always about dieting and how to lose weight. . . . I (went) on diets with my Mom, to keep her company. I just got better at it than she did. My eating disorder is my mother's therapy. . . . It's also the way we have time together—working on the diets and exercise and all of that. We've stopped talking about diets since I got anorexia, and now I don't know what we can talk about.

Source: Zerbe (2008:20–21)

---

4. The sociocultural trend available in today's society in the form of remaining thin for looking good is found to play a substantial role in putting societal pressure on individuals, especially adolescents and young women, toward eating disorders. In learning an eating disorder-related behavior, the craving for becoming thin directly results in intense dieting, the first dangerous step down the slippery slope to anorexia and bulimia nervosa (Durand and Barlow, 2013:294). The trend of looking attractive by becoming thin is so universal that it is not uncommon to find a number of performers, models, cine stars, and even athletes around the globe in the race of getting thinner and thinner, and thus getting victimized as patients of eating disorders.

Treatment of Eating Disorders

Treatment of eating disorders is a difficult task in its actual operation. The various therapies and treatment procedures involve hospitalization, medical and drug therapy, supportive psychotherapy, behavioral therapy, group therapy, and family therapy. However, no royal road or uniform procedure can be followed in the treatment of all eating disorders. Treatment differs for each of the disorders classified as Anorexia nervosa, Bulimia nervosa, and Binge eating disorder. Let us discuss the procedure and methods adopted for their treatment one by one.

Treatments for Anorexia Nervosa

Anorexia nervosa is the most dangerous in its consequences among all three eating disorders. There may be considerable weight loss, and in case it is quite severe for an individual (say 40% or more below their normal weight), dehydration, serve chemical imbalances, and possible organ damage may result. We must provide them with medical treatment as early as possible.

The difficulty here may arise on account of the unwillingness of the affected individuals. People with anorexia nervosa rarely ask for nor agree to treatment, as they consider themselves fine in all aspects. Sometimes, after hearing comments or concern about their thinness, their disorder-related behavior is reinforced and they go further in their slimming efforts. In such a situation, a single alternative lies in getting them compulsorily hospitalized or providing them with needed medical therapy before reaching the dangerous point. For providing such treatment, one must proceed in the manner as follows:

1. In dealing with severe and life-threatening cases of anorexia nervosa, clinicians may need to force tube and intravenous feedings on a patient who refuses to eat.
2. At the next stage, attempts should be made in the form of helping patients with anorexia nervosa gain weight quickly and return to health within weeks. The popular weight restoration technique known as a *nutritional rehabilitation program* may be effectively used for treating patients. Here, the services of a trained nurse are employed for this purpose. She is supposed to (i) gradually increase a patient's diet over the course of several weeks, and (ii) educate patients about the program, track their progress, provide encouragement, and help them recognize that their weight gain is under control and will not lead to obesity.

Restoring weight is thus the main and only aim of the treatment performed through medical measures. However, initial weight gain is a poor predictor of long-term outcomes in anorexia nervosa. Without attention to the patient's underlying dysfunctional attitudes about body shape and interpersonal disruptions in his/her life, the patient will almost always relapse (Durand and Barlow, 2013:302). After providing necessary medical treatment, therefore, the focus of attention should shift to helping him or her through other treatment measures such as the use of cognitive behavioral therapy and family therapy.

Use of Cognitive Behavioral Therapy: Cognitive behavioral therapy represents a treatment measure involving a perfect combination or synthesis of two types of interventions—cognitive and behavioral. While providing cognitive intervention, the use of this therapy is meant for bringing the needed change in their mindset by making them able to (i) identify their "core pathology" (the deep-seated belief that they should be judged by their shape and weight and by their ability to control these physical characteristics), (ii) learn alternative ways of coping with stress and solving problems, (iii) recognize their need for becoming independent and learn more appropriate ways to exercise control, and (iv) better identify their internal sensations and feelings and develop trust in them.

On the other side, in providing behavioral intervention in this therapy, patients are encouraged to (i) learn monitoring of their feelings, hunger levels, and food intake in a better way along with a proper understanding of their mutual relationship, (ii) bring needed changes in their attitudes about eating and weight, (iii) remove their maladaptive assumptions and fears associated with anorexia nervosa, such as "our weight and shape determine our worth and value in the society," or "for being perfect, I should lose weight and appear lean and thin."

In this way, as a whole, cognitive behavioral therapy through cognitive and behavioral interventions brings changes to the mindset and maladaptive and abnormal eating behavior of patients.

Although cognitive behavioral techniques are often of great help, it is best to supplement them with other approaches, such as family therapy.

Use of Family Therapy: What is done by the clinicians and therapists in the form of providing medical or cognitive behavioral treatment to the patients of anorexia nervosa must be supplemented and followed by the help received through other approaches or therapies such as family therapy.

In the approach related to the use of Family therapy, a therapist, behavioral psychologist, or professional must work with family members to educate them about the rehabilitation of the anorexia nervosa patient. The attempts made in this direction focus on bringing attitudinal and functional changes in the behavior of the family toward the child/adolescent along with his or her distinctive eating disorder issues. For realizing this goal, the family therapist may proceed in the following manner:

- He meets with the family as a whole in its natural functioning situations and tries to find out what is going on in the family related to the disorder of the affected child. He then acquaints the family members with the troublesome family patterns responsible for creating difficulties for the affected child and helps the members and family as a whole to bring needed modifications to the family environment and behavior.
- In addition, every effort is made by him to include the family to accomplish two goals. First, negative and dysfunctional communication in the family regarding food and eating must be eliminated, and meals must be made more structured and reinforcing. Second, attitudes toward body shape and image distortion are discussed at length in family sessions. Unless the therapists attend to these attitudes, individuals with anorexia nervosa are likely to face a lifetime preoccupation with weight and body shape, struggle to maintain marginal weight and social adjustment, and be subject to repeated hospitalization. Family therapy directed toward the goals mentioned here seems to be effective, particularly with young girls (Durand and Barlow, 2013:302).

Treatments for Bulimia Nervosa

Treatment programs for Bulimia nervosa, much like Anorexia nervosa, involve practices such as medical approaches, cognitive behavioral therapy, and family therapy for the treatment of people suffering from bulimia nervosa. However, the treatments carried out with these methods may differ in some ways in their application and outcomes in the ways discussed ahead.

Medical treatment or Therapy: People with bulimia nervosa seldom require emergency services of getting hospitalized like anorexia nervosa sufferers. Still, it is recommended to utilize the services of eating disorder clinics and professionals for helping the sufferers for coming out of their troubles and difficulties. The treatment programs carried out in these clinics are aimed to serve two types of objectives— immediate and general. In serving immediate goals, attempts are made for helping clients to eliminate their binge-purge patterns and establish good eating habits. The serving of the general goal focuses on eliminating the underlying causes of bulimic patterns. Here help may also be taken with the use of drug therapy.

The use of drug therapy, which is of limited help to people with anorexia nervosa, appears to be quite effective in many cases of bulimia nervosa. For this purpose, clinicians and therapists often prescribe one or the other antidepressant drugs similar to those considered effective for the treatment of mood disorders and anxiety disorders.

Although the clinical treatment and use of drug therapy may be seen to serve the goal of providing immediate and temporary relief to the affected individual, these measures must be accompanied and followed by cognitive behavioral therapy for deriving long-lasting effects.

Cognitive behavioral Therapy: The use of cognitive behavioral therapy has been found particularly effective and helpful in treating individuals suffering from bulimia nervosa—perhaps even more so than those suffering from anorexia nervosa. It is particularly aimed at bringing needed modifications in the problematic eating behavior (binge eating and purging) and associated attitudes about the overriding importance and significance of body weight and shape known to be associated with the eating disorder bulimia nervosa.

A general procedure involved in the use of cognitive behavioral treatment or therapy may involve activities such as the following (Durand and Barlow, 2013:302):

- Teaching patients the consequences of binge eating and purging and the ineffectiveness of vomiting and laxative abuse for weight control.
- Educating patients about the adverse effects of dieting.
- Scheduling them to eat small, manageable amounts of food five or six times per day, aimed at eliminating the alternating periods of overeating and dietary restriction—the hallmarks of bulimia.
- Focusing on altering dysfunctional thoughts and attitudes about body shape, weight, and eating.
- Teaching them to make use of coping strategies for resisting the impulse to binge and purge besides getting them preoccupied with useful activities for denying them spare time to engage in binge eating.

In order to bring desired modifications in the behavior and attitudes of bulimia nervosa patients, one or the other useful behavioral modification techniques and psychotherapies may also be utilized by counselors and therapists. Talking about such treatment measures, Comer (2015:374) writes:

Cognitive behavioral therapists may also use the behavioral techniques of exposure and response prevention to help break the binge-purge cycle. This approach in general involves exposing people to situations that would ordinarily raise anxiety and then preventing them from performing their usual compulsive responses until they learn that the situations are actually harmless and their compulsive acts unnecessary. For bulimia nervosa, the therapists require clients to eat particular kinds and amounts of food and then prevent them from vomiting to show that eating can be a harmless and even constructive activity that needs no undoing. Typically, the therapist sits with the client while the client eats the forbidden foods and stays until the urge to purge has passed studies find that this treatment often helps reduce eating—related anxieties, bingeing, and vomiting.

The use of Family and Group Therapy: The techniques and measures related to the use of family therapy for the treatment of people suffering from bulimia nervosa may be successfully taken along the lines of providing treatment and follow-up help to victims of anorexia nervosa. In addition, here in dealing with cases of bulimia nervosa, we can also make use of group therapy as an approach to their treatment. Group therapy is delivered in a group setup rather than on an individual basis, as done in medical, cognitive behavioral, and other psychotherapies. In one of the approaches adopted in group therapy, the therapist may begin with the formation of self-help groups composed of sufferers of bulimia nervosa. In these groups, victims of bulimia nervosa get valuable opportunities for sharing their concerns and experiences with one another. This helps them to acquire valuable information, self-confidence, and self-help lessons for dealing with their eating disorder problems. For example, here they may learn that (i) their disorder is not unique or shameful, (ii) their binge eating behavior is quite common in their companions and there is no need to maintain secrecy for it, (iii) their obsessive-compulsive behavior patterns related to their disorder can be successfully controlled if approached properly. In their group, all are on the same footing, suffering from the same problems, therefore there is no need for them to hide their weaknesses, or fear about getting exposed and criticized by others. They are free to give and receive support to each other in the form of honest feedback and insight by sharing their difficulties and measures proving helpful to them in overcoming their difficulties.

Treatment for Binge Eating Disorder

Unlike Bulimia nervosa, the newly discovered Binge eating disorder is characterized as "bingeing without purge." Here the affected individual, although practicing an obsessive-compulsive behavior of binge eating, does not engage in purging. However, except purging, many other behavioral characteristics are significantly alike in both these disorders. Perhaps it is the reason that for the treatment of patients suffering from Binge eating disorder we at present are employing the same techniques and methods of treatment or therapies as followed in the treatment of Bulimia nervosa discussed previously, in the forms of drug therapy, family therapy, group therapy, and behavior modification therapies such as cognitive-behavioral therapy or other forms of psychotherapy. It has been found that the use of such therapies and treatments certainly helps in reducing or eliminating binge eating patterns, besides bringing needed changes in the attitude of the affected individuals particularly related to overconcern with weight and shape. It has also been noted that all such treatment measures, therapies, and interventions, cognitive or behavioral, provide only short-term help. There is a relatively high risk of relapse for binge eating disorder patients who have been treated. Moreover, it is also not uncommon to find treated patients becoming overweight and obese, a problem that requires further attention. Thus, in all its dimensions and forms, the treatment as well as follow-up programs chalked out for people with binge eating disorder need further study for accomplishing their goals.

To Sum Up

Regarding the *causes underlying eating disorders* of one or the other kind we may say that their occurrence is the function of a multiplicity of causes governed by biological, psychological, and sociocultural factors. In this concern, where biological and genetic theorists talk about the role of biological and genetic factors in causing eating disorders, psychologists and behaviorists blame psychological factors such as ego deficiency; lack of self-confidence and self-reliance; and increased levels of anxiety, depression, and stress for the development of these disorders. The sociocultural perspective in this concern asserts that it is the defective upbringing, uncongenial environment, and faulty role models available at home, school, and in the community that lead to the development of psychological problems responsible for the germination as well as perpetuation of eating disorders.

The treatment of eating disorders involves the use of several therapies and treatment procedures such as hospitalization, medical and drug therapy, supportive psychotherapy, cognitive behavioral therapy, group therapy, and family therapy. However, treatment in its actual operation differs for each of the disorders. In treating patients of Anorexia nervosa, the priority lies in getting them hospitalized and taking measures to help them gain weight and return to normal health. Afterward, the focus of attention should shift to helping them through other treatment measures such as the use of cognitive behavioral therapy and family therapy, with the objective of bringing changes to the patient's mindset and modifying as well as normalizing the maladaptive and abnormal eating behavior of the patients. Treatment programs for Bulimia nervosa aim to help patients in eliminating their binge-purge patterns and establishing good eating habits. For carrying out these objectives, a combination of treatment procedures involving the use of medical therapy (including the use of antidepressant drugs and medication), cognitive behavioral and other alternative psychotherapies, as well as family and group therapy may be employed. For the treatment of patients suffering from Binge eating disorder, we at present are employing the same techniques and methods of treatment or therapies as being followed in the treatment of Bulimia nervosa in the forms of drug therapy, family therapy, group therapy, and behavior modification therapies such as cognitive-behavioral therapy and other forms of psychotherapy. It has also been noted that all such treatment measures, provide only short-term help, and the possibility of them becoming obese cannot be ruled out.

Review Questions

1. What do you understand by the term elimination disorders? Name the types of elimination disorders and discuss any one of them in detail.
2. What is enuresis? How can we identify and diagnose it in light of the criteria laid down in the DSM-5?
3. Discuss the underlying causes and methods of treatment of cases related to enuresis.
4. What is encopresis? Discuss its symptoms visible among affected children.
5. Throw light on the identification and diagnosis of encopresis in cognizance of the criteria laid down in the DSM-5.
6. Describe in detail the underlying causes and methods of treatment of cases related to encopresis.
7. What are feeding and eating disorders? What are their different types? Discuss any one of them in detail.
8. What is anorexia nervosa? How can it be identified and diagnosed? Discuss in light of the criteria laid down in the DSM-5
9. What is bulimia nervosa? Throw light on the identification and diagnosis of bulimia nervosa in view of the criteria laid down in the DSM-5.
10. What is binge eating disorder? How can it be identified and diagnosed? Answer in view of the criteria laid down in the DSM-5.

11. Describe, how do all the three feeding and eating disorders-anorexia nervosa, bulimia nervosa, and binge eating disorder, differ from each other?
12. Discuss in detail the causes underlying feeding and eating disorders.
13. Throw light on the measures taken for the treatment of cases related to each of the three feeding and eating disorders—anorexia nervosa, bulimia nervosa, and binge eating disorder.

References

American Psychiatric Association (2013), *Diagnostic and statistical manual of mental disorders* (5th ed.), Arlington, VA: American Psychiatric Publishing.

American Psychiatric Association (2022), *Diagnostic and statistical manual of mental disorders: DSM-5-TR*, Washington, DC: American Psychiatric Association.

Bruch, H. (1978), *Eating disorders: Obesity; anorexia nervosa and the person within*, New York, NY: Basic Books.

Bruch, H. (2001), *The golden age: The enigma of anorexia nervosa*, Cambridge, MA: Harvard University Press.

Comer, R. J. (2015), *Abnormal psychology* (9th ed.), New York, NY: Worth Publishers (A Macmillan Education Imprint).

Durand, V., & Barlow, D. (2013), *Essentials of abnormal psychology* (6th ed.), Wadsworth: Cengage Learning.

Zerbe, K. J. (2008), *Integrated treatment of eating disorders beyond the body betrayed*, New York, NY: W.W. Norton.

Sleep Disorders

Introduction

In the classification of mental disorders provided by the American Psychiatric Association, sleep disorders have been specially mentioned as one of the prominent psychological disorders by assigning them a full-fledged separate category. While in the DSM-IV TR (2000), this category has been named "Sleep Disorders," in the later classifications of the DSM-5 (2013) and DSM-5-TR (2022), it has been named Sleep-Wake Disorders. Let us know the essentials about our sleeping behavior and the consequences of it turning into a behavioral disorder.

Our Sleeping Behavior

Our sleeping behavior is a natural behavior that is closely associated with the satisfaction of one of our essential biological needs—sleep—after long hours of daily activity. The satisfaction of this need in an appropriate way is quite necessary for keeping us in good health, much in the same capacity as the consumption of food, drinking of water, and inhaling of oxygen in a proper amount supports our physical well-being. Apart from physical, it also affects our psyche and mental health in a variety of ways, and this is why normality maintained in our sleeping behavior

DOI: 10.4324/9781003398325-16

keeps us normal in our functioning and overall well-being. Any abnormality or irregularity in our sleeping behavior in terms of sleep disturbances, deprivations, and disorders may result in one or the other types of psychophysical, neurotic, and psychotic abnormalities and disorders. Let us examine the different ways one can fall victim to such disturbances, abnormalities, and disorders. But before doing this, let us first look at what happens with us usually during our night sleep.

The Types and Stages of Our Sleep

Normally, people who remain awake for long hours during the day fall asleep during the night hours, ranging from five to eight hours. During this duration of their night sleep, they are found to go through several different stages of sleep, involving two types of sleep—REM (Rapid eye movement) sleep and Non-REM (Non-rapid eye movement) sleep. While falling asleep, people first go through an episode of NREM sleep, involving three initial stages called (i) the transitory or lightest stage of sleep, (ii) the stage of light sleep, and (iii) the stage of deep sleep. Then they enter the fourth stage of their night sleep characterized by REM.

NREM sleep aims to provide complete rest, relaxation, and healing to the body and mind, especially through the third stage of deep sleep. REM sleep associated with the fourth stage of one's sleep is characterized by the rapid movement of one's eyes in different directions. Being an active type of sleep, it is unable to provide such rest and peace as available in NREM sleep. In comparison to NREM sleep, it is popularly known as the dreaming stage of one's sleep, as 90% of one's total dreams are experienced in this stage of sleep. Besides this, awakening, as well as arousals, can occur more easily in this type of sleep. However, voluntary muscles are generally paralyzed during REM sleep, and hence, one's body is unable to act upon the dreams experienced in REM dreams (bad dreams and nightmares) in the way as happens in NREM dreams involving night terrors and sleepwalking.

To Sum Up

Our night sleep involves two types of sleep known as REM (Rapid eye movement) sleep and NREM (Non-rapid eye movement) sleep. While falling asleep, people first go through an episode of NREM sleep involving three initial stages characterized as lightest, light, and deep sleep. They then enter the fourth stage of their REM type of sleep. NREM sleep aims to provide complete rest, relaxation, and healing to the body and mind, especially through the third stage of deep sleep, REM. Awakening as well as arousals can occur more easily in the fourth stage of sleep—REM sleep.

Sleep Disorders—Concept and Types

Sleep disorders represent irregularities, disturbances, and abnormalities, occurring in one's night sleep. These disorders have been identified and categorized by researchers and clinicians into two major categories, known as Dyssomnias and Parasomnias.

Dyssomnia sleep disorders: In this category, we include sleep disorders that are mainly associated with disturbances occurring in the amount, timing, or quality of one's sleep. People suffering from such sleep disorders are found complaining in the following manner: (i) I am unable to get enough sleep, (ii) I feel difficulty in falling asleep when I need or desire so,

(iii) My sleep is disturbed with a slight noise or sometimes with no reason, (iv) I don't feel refreshed even after sleeping the whole night, and so on.

Dyssomnia sleep disorders, on account of their varying characteristics, may be further categorized as (a) Primary insomnia, (b) Primary hypersomnia, (c) Narcolepsy, (d) Breathing-related sleep disorder, and (e) Circadian rhythm sleep disorder (sleep-wake schedule disorder).

Parasomnia sleep disorders: In this category, we may include sleep disorders that are mainly associated with disturbances in arousal and sleep stage transitions from one stage of sleep to another that intrude upon the sleep process. People suffering from such sleep disorders are found to demonstrate abnormal behaviors in their sleep (both NREM and REM), such as nightmares, night terrors, and sleepwalking. In this way, parasomnia sleep disorders are not problems with sleep itself but abnormal events that occur either during sleep or during that twilight time between sleeping and waking. Parasomnia sleep disorders may be further categorized into two distinct types: (i) those that occur during REM sleep such as nightmares and (ii) those that occur during NREM sleep such as night terrors and night sleepwalking.

The aforementioned types or categorizations and sub-categorizations of various Sleep disorders suffered by people during their sleep are illustrated in Figure 16.1.

To Sum Up

Sleep disorders represent irregularities, disturbances, and abnormalities, occurring in one's night sleep. These disorders have been categorized into two broad categories, known as Dyssomnias (disturbances in the amount, timing, or quality of one's sleep) and Parasomnias (disturbances in arousal and sleep stage transition from one stage of sleep to another). Dyssomnias are further sub-categorized as Primary insomnia, Primary hypersomnia, Narcolepsy, Breathing-related sleep disorder, and Circadian rhythm or sleep-wake schedule disorder. Parasomnias are further sub-categorized into two distinct types: (i) those occurring during REM sleep such as nightmares and (ii) those occurring during NREM sleep such as night terrors and night sleepwalking.

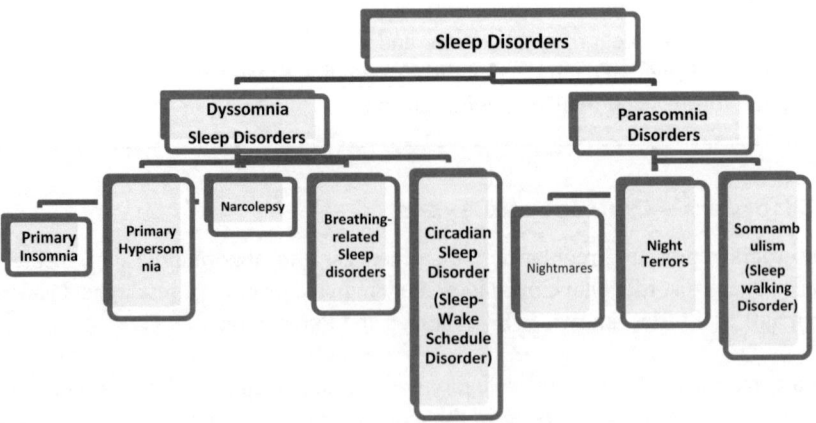

Figure 16.1 The categorizations and sub-categorizations of sleep disorders

Let us look into the essentials regarding the nature and characteristics of these sleep disorders classified above. For this purpose, let us first discuss the sleep disorders falling in the category of Dyssomnias.

Primary Insomnia

The term insomnia means the inability to sleep. It may imply that a person suffering from such a sleeping disorder may be found awake all the time. However, a total lack of sleep is not possible, as a high degree of its occurrence may eventually lead to death. In its practical application, the term primary insomnia is found to be associated with some typical problems and difficulties arising in one's night sleep, characterized as:

(i) *Difficulty initiating sleep:* People suffering from primary insomnia may complain that it becomes too difficult for them to fall asleep despite their best efforts in doing so. They have to wait for it continuously for hours.

(ii) *Difficulty in maintaining sleep:* They may complain that they are unable to enjoy sound sleep for a satisfactory duration. They wake up frequently during their night sleep and once awakened, it becomes difficult for them to go back to sleep.

(iii) *Nonrestorative sleep:* They may complain that their night sleep is not fulfilling the required restorative function, as even after spending a reasonable number of hours in their night sleep, they are unable to feel fresh for doing activities the next day.

These problems and difficulties arising in one's night sleep can be more clearly visualized through the case history given ahead.

Sonja was a 23-year-old law student with a history of sleep problems. She reported that she never really slept well, both having trouble falling asleep at night and awakening again in the early morning. Since she started law school last year, her sleep problems had grown even worse. She would lie in bed awake until the morning hours thinking about school, getting only three to four hours of sleep on a typical night. In the morning, she had a great deal of difficulty getting out of bed and was frequently late for her early-morning class. Sonja's sleep problems and their interference with her schoolwork were causing her to experience increasingly severe depression. In addition, she recently reported having a severe anxiety attack that woke her in the middle of the night. All of these difficulties caused her to be increasingly isolated from family and friends, who finally convinced her to seek help.

Source: Adapted from Durand and Barlow (2013:311)

Identification and Diagnosis of Primary Insomnia

The American Psychiatric Association has provided the following criteria for the identification and diagnosis of the sleeping disorder Primary insomnia in the DSM-5.

Table 16.1 Diagnostic Criteria for Primary Insomnia

- A predominant complaint of dissatisfaction with sleep quantity or quality, associated with one (or more) of the following symptoms:
  (i)   Difficulty initiating sleep
  (ii) Difficulty maintaining sleep, characterized by frequent awakenings or problems returning to sleep after awakenings
  (iii) Early-morning awakening with inability to return to sleep.
- The sleep disturbance causes clinically significant distress or impairment in social, occupational, educational, academic, behavioral, or other important areas of functioning.
- The sleep difficulty occurs at least three nights per week, is present for at least three months, and occurs despite adequate opportunity for sleep.
- The insomnia is not better explained by and does not occur exclusively during the course of another sleep-wake disorder.
- Coexisting mental disorders and medical conditions do not adequately explain the predominant complaint of insomnia.
- The insomnia is not attributable to the physiological effects of a substance (e.g., a drug of abuse, a medication).

Source: APA (2013)

Primary Hypersomnia

Hypersomnia sleeping disorder runs quite contrary to insomnia sleeping disorder, both in its nature as well as functioning. The difference between these disorders is evident through the prefixes "hyper" and "in" appearing in their word composition. In their usual meanings, "hyper" stands for a great amount or abnormal excess of a thing or phenomenon, while the prefix "in" stands for lacking or without. Accordingly, while people suffering from primary insomnia are not getting enough sleep, people suffering from hypersomnia, on the other hand, grapple with the problem of sleeping too much. Besides sleeping for a greater amount and duration in the night, these people are also found to fall asleep several times during the day.

Clinically speaking, the causation of primary hypersomnia is linked with some or the other dysfunction of one's central nervous system. In its symptomology, it is revealed through major sleep episodes and excessive sleepiness consisting of prolonged (one-to-two-hour) episodes of non-rapid eye movement sleep. It has a similar presentation to narcolepsy but is not generally associated with cataplexy or sleep-onset rapid eye movement. In its outcomes, it is known as one of the serious sleep disorders, often disrupting the work, family life, and interpersonal ties of the sufferers. The characteristic feature of this sleeping disorder may be properly revealed through a case history provided ahead.

A 32-year-old Caucasian woman came to us with complaints of excessive daytime sleepiness (EDS). She had no problems with her sleep or general health until two years before, when she began to experience excessive daytime fatigue. Her condition progressed and at the time of presentation, she was able to sleep for extended periods of time (up to two to three days at a stretch) and still be hyper somnolent during the day. On questioning, she denied cataplexy, hypnagogic hallucinations, or sleep paralysis. There was no prior history of closed head injury, meningitis, or any focal cerebrovascular symptoms. During her initial diagnostic work for fatigue, she was found to have a mildly elevated TSH level. She was started on thyroxine, but her symptoms persisted (in spite of her TSH value subsequently returning to normal). She had been working in an office setting, but quit her job a month before on account of her EDS and difficulty in concentrating. She stopped driving because she had found herself in the wrong lane on occasion, unsure of how she got there. She is married with two children and there is no family history of excessive daytime sleepiness.

Source: John et al. (2007)

Identification and Diagnosis of Primary Hypersomnia

The American Psychiatric Association has provided the following criteria for the identification and diagnosis of the sleeping disorder Primary Hypersomnia in the DSM-5, as shown in Table 16.2.

Narcolepsy

In the category of Dyssomnia sleep disorders, narcolepsy is considered a quite serious and chronic sleep disorder usually characterized by features like (i) excessive daytime sleepiness, (ii) sleep attacks, and (iii) rapid eye movement (REM) sleep abnormalities such as cataplexy, sleep paralysis, and hypnagogic hallucination.

On account of their appearance in the abnormal behavior of other disorders, the symptoms of narcolepsy cited above may often be misdiagnosed, for example:

- The excessive daytime sleepiness of narcolepsy patients may be mistaken for identifying them as suffering from primary hypersomnia or with the fatigue of atypical depression,
- The cataplexy exhibited in the functioning of the narcolepsy patients may be mistaken for considering them as suffering from epilepsy, and
- The vivid hypnagogic hallucinations exhibited in the behavior of narcolepsy patients may be mistaken for them being affected with hallucinations of a psychotic disorder.

Table 16.2 Diagnostic Criteria for Primary Hypersomnia

Diagnostic criteria for Primary Hypersomnia (named as hypersomnolence in DSM-5)
- Self-reported excessive sleepiness (hypersomnolence) despite a main sleep period lasting at least seven hours, with at least one of the following symptoms:
  (i) Recurrent periods of sleep or lapses into sleep within the same day.
  (ii) A prolonged main sleep episode of more than nine hours per day that is non-restorative (i.e., un-refreshing).
  (iii) Difficulty being fully awake after abrupt awakening.
- The hypersomnolence occurs at least three times per week, for at least three months.
- The hypersomnolence is accompanied by significant distress or impairment in cognitive, social, occupational, or other important areas of functioning.
- The hypersomnolence is not better explained by and does not occur exclusively during the course of another sleep disorder.
- The hypersomnolence is not attributable to the physiological effects of a substance (e.g., a drug of abuse, a medication).
- Coexisting mental and medical disorders do not adequately explain the predominant complaint of hypersomnolence.

Source: APA (2013)

However, Narcolepsy differs from the other so-mentioned disorders in its possession of a unique characteristic signifying the presence of all three REM sleep abnormalities—cataplexy, sleep paralysis, and hypnagogic hallucination—besides being loaded with the symptom of excessive sleepiness and sleep attacks. Let us know about the nature and characteristics of all these three REM sleep abnormalities visible in Narcolepsy patients.

By the term cataplexy, we mean a sudden loss of muscle tone at the time of their REM sleep on the part of narcolepsy patients for a duration ranging from several seconds to several minutes. It is usually preceded by a strong emotion such as anger or happiness. As an example of the negative outcomes of cataplexy (sudden loss of muscle tone) experienced on the part of narcolepsy patients, we may cite instances such as suddenly falling asleep (for a brief duration) while cheering your favorite team, or collapsing to the floor in a sound sleep, while having heated verbal argument with someone. In seeking reasons for such behavior Durand and Barlow (2013:315) write:

> Cataplexy appears to result from a sudden onset of REM sleep. Instead of falling asleep normally and going through the four non-rapid eye movement (NREM) stages that typically precede REM sleep, people with narcolepsy periodically progress right to the dream-sleep stage almost directly from the state of being awake. One outcome of REM sleep is the inhibition of input to the muscles, and this seems to be the process that leads to cataplexy.

The second REM-sleep-related characteristic or terrifying experience demonstrated by narcolepsy patients in their abnormal behavior is known as sleep paralysis. Here, they are subjected to a paralysis-like attack in their REM sleep and are unable to move or speak for a brief period immediately after their awakening.

The third REM-sleep-related characteristic visible in narcolepsy patients is passing through terrifying experiences in the shape of hypnagogic hallucinations, such as experiencing vivid illusions of being caught in a fire or flying through the air.

The characteristic features of Narcolepsy may be properly revealed through a case history provided ahead.

A 22-year-old woman consulted with our department because of her excessive daytime sleepiness and sleep attacks. Her daytime sleepiness began when she was around 13 years old and it had been getting worse. When she was in high school, she couldn't stay awake during her classes or exams. When she worked at a department store as a saleswoman after graduating from high school, she frequently dozed off standing up, and for this, she was dismissed. She also got into a collision while driving due to a sudden sleep attack. Cataplexy developed as her daytime sleepiness got worse, and after the age of 19, it would occur almost every day. Cataplexy occurred when she laughed, got angry, or exchanged jokes. It even occurred when she was excited, surprised, and embarrassed, and when she reminisced about happy moments. Her knees would suddenly buckle and her jaws sagged. She also complained of seeing ghosts or animals and hearing her name called when she was lying down at night. She experienced realistic and often scary dreams throughout the night; when she awoke, she was unable to move. There was no history of trauma to the head or any psychiatric illnesses. However, her father did suffer from constant sleepiness and fatigue, and also occasional sudden muscle weakness in both knees when laughing. Although he consulted various hospitals, they told him nothing was out of the ordinary, but they recommended that he see a psychiatrist. The psychiatrist prescribed him 37.5 mg of venlafaxine and 0.75 mg of alprazolam for depression. However, he was still sleepy and languid in spite of those medications.

Source: Yoon-Kyung Shin et al. (2007)

Identification and Diagnosis of Narcolepsy

The American Psychiatric Association has provided the following criteria for the identification and diagnosis of the sleeping disorder Narcolepsy in the DSM-5, as shown in Table 16.3.

Table 16.3 Diagnostic Criteria for Narcolepsy

- Excessive daytime sleepiness to occur at least three times per week for at least three weeks.
- The presence of at least one or more of the following:
  (i)   Cataplexy (brief, bilateral loss of muscle tone)
  (ii) A deficiency of the hormone hypocretin, as indicated by levels in cerebrospinal fluid
  (iii) A formal nocturnal sleep study or multiple sleep latency test (MSLT) that shows abnormal REM sleep latency (elements of REM sleep at the beginning or end of the sleep cycle that may result in sleep paralysis).

Source: APA (2013)

Breathing-Related Sleep Disorders

The term breathing-related sleep disorders is used for the type of sleep disorders in which there lie some physical origin—namely problems with breathing while asleep, causing them to experience widely disrupted sleep at night and excessive sleepiness (insomnia) during the day. Their breath-related problems are uniquely harmful and damaging in their nature and consequences. Let us look into the origin and nature of these problems.

It is quite natural for our muscles in the upper airway to relax during sleep. Such relaxation of the muscles causes the constriction of the air passage and may create difficulty and hurdles in our breathing. However, in the case of individuals known to grapple with breathing-related disorders, the constriction of these muscles, during their sleep, is in such a great amount that it may stop their breathing altogether for a period of 10 to 30 seconds. This phenomenon is known as sleep apnea in the world of medicine and abnormal psychology.

There are three types of sleep apnea—obstructive, central, and mixed sleep apnea—each causing a distinctive type of breath-related sleep disorder among affected individuals. Let us see how.

Obstructive sleep apnea: In this type of sleep apnea, there occurs a short-term stoppage of breathing despite the normal functioning of one's respiratory system. It happens due to some obstruction caused to one's breathing on account of the narrowness of the airway or the interference caused to the ongoing efforts of breathing by some abnormality or damage to breathing organs. The sleep disorder caused by such sleep apnea is distinguished in the form of people's loud and frightening snoring at night. Here, the affected person remains quite unaware of his or her snoring problem despite troubling others present in the vicinity. Obstruction sleep apnea, however, may create a lot of obstruction and difficulties in the continuity of their sound sleep and they may wake up frequently during their night sleep. In addition to snoring and frightening episodes of interrupted breathing and disrupted sleep, the other noticeable symptoms found in the behavior of the persons suffering from obstructive sleep apnea are (i) partial or complete cessation of breathing during sleep, (ii) reduction in blood oxygen levels, (iii) heavy sweating during the night, (iv) morning headaches, and (v) excessive daytime sleepiness or insomnia.

People of all ages, including children, may be affected by obstructive sleep apnea. However, generally, overweight adults (particularly men rather than women) are found to be affected with this disorder in a greater proportion, snoring heavily and showing other visible symptoms of obstructive sleep apnea.

Central sleep apnea: In this type of sleep apnea, there occurs the total cessation of respiratory activity for brief periods. It is alleged to be caused by disorders or diseases related to one's central nervous system, such as cerebral vascular disease, head trauma, and degenerative disorders (Durand and Barlow, 2013:315). Like obtrusive sleep apnea, people suffering from central sleep apnea are also found to experience obstruction and interruption in their sound sleep. They may wake up frequently during the night. However, in its consequences this sleep disorder differs a lot from obtrusion-related sleep apnea in the sense that (i) the people suffering from this disorder do not report excessive daytime sleepiness or insomnia, (ii) it does not exhibit major breathing problem symptoms such as abnormal snoring, (iii) it does not cause many difficulties or problems to the sufferers in their daily life, and as a result, they seldom come forward for seeking treatment to this disorder.

Mixed sleep apnea: True to its name, this type of sleep apnea is a combination of both obstructive and central sleep apnea. The persons suffering from this type of sleep disorder thus may exhibit a combination of symptoms and face the difficulties of both obstructive and central apnea patients. As a whole, they may experience breathing difficulties interrupting their sleep, resulting in symptoms similar to those of insomnia.

Identification and Diagnosis of Breathing-Related Sleep Disorders

The American Psychiatric Association has provided the criteria shown in Table 16.4 for the identification and diagnosis of Breathing-related sleep disorders in its DSM IV TR.

Table 16.4 Diagnostic Criteria for Breathing-related sleep disorders

- Sleep disruption, leading to excessive sleepiness or insomnia, that is judged to be due to sleep-related breathing condition (e.g., obstructive or central sleep apnea syndrome, central alveolar hypoventilation syndrome)
- The disruption is not better accounted for by another mental disorder and is not due to the direct physiological effects of a substance or another general medical condition.

Source: APA (2000), DSM-IV-TR

Circadian Rhythm Sleep Disorders

The term Circadian Rhythm Sleep Disorders is used for the type of sleep disorders in which affected individuals are found to experience disturbances and interruptions in their night sleep on account of some or the other types of shift in their sleep-wake schedule. With a close association to the sleep-wake schedules of affected individuals, these disorders are also known as sleep-wake schedule disorders. The American Psychiatric Association (2000) in its DSMIV-TR has named them as a product of the mismatch between the sleep-wake schedule required by a person's environment and his or her circadian sleep-wake cycle. Let us look into the possibilities of witnessing such a mismatch or shift in the sleep-wake schedule of affected people.

1. One possibility may arise in experiencing a jet-lag-related situation in one's day-to-day living. When we visit a different time zone, we may experience sleep-related problems in a distinctive form. In the United States, for example, it is day time when it is night time in our country, and vice versa. As a result, when in a different time zone we may find ourselves falling asleep during the daytime and getting awakened during the night, according to our sleep-wake schedule. Such difficulty and disturbance experienced in our sleep cycle is known as the jet lag type of circadian rhythm sleep disorder.
2. The other possibility of becoming victim to a circadian rhythm sleep disorder may arise in the situation where the type of work done or duties performed in an occupation requires individuals to remain awake during the sleeping hours of the night and sleep during day hours, in contradiction to their habitual sleep-wake pattern. The situation gets worsened or complicated when they have to work only sometimes at night and other times during the day, as demanded by their work environment. Such alterations and fluctuations in one's work schedule make people to fall prey to the unwanted outcomes of the atypical type of sleep disorder known as shift work type sleep disorder.
3. In addition to these two well-known types of circadian rhythm sleep disorders, Durand and Barlow have mentioned the presence of a third type of circadian rhythm sleep disorder existing among affected persons, described as follows:

In contrast with jet lag and shift work sleep-related problems, which have external causes such as long-distance travel and job selection, several circadian rhythm sleep disorders seem to arise from within the person experiencing the problems. Extreme night owls, people who stay up late and sleep late, may have a problem known as delayed sleep phase type. Sleep is delayed or later than the normal bedtime. At the other extreme, people with an advanced sleep phase type of circadian rhythm disorder are "early to bed and early to rise" Here sleep is advanced or earlier than normal bed-time.

(Durand and Barlow, 2013:316)

The characteristic features of circadian rhythm sleep disorder may be revealed through a case history provided ahead.

A 24-year-old male patient reports difficulty falling asleep, followed by daytime sleepiness, a pattern that has persisted for about five years since his days as a student. His excessive sleepiness has become more severe during the past year due to the 8 AM starting time for his work shift. He recently needed to take two personal days off from work due to an inability to report on time. Once asleep, he does not have difficulty staying asleep. His bedtime ranges from 11:30 PM to 1:00 AM, with the time required to fall asleep averaging two hours. His wake time is scheduled for 6:45 AM on workdays. Weekday mornings are particularly difficult. The patient feels "out of it" until about noon. He has fallen asleep while driving to work and has had several near-miss traffic accidents in the past month. His blood pressure is stable at 130/80 mm Hg, and he has a body mass index (BMI) of 26. His mother and brother both suffer from similar types of insomnia symptoms.

Source: Zee (2011)

Identification and Diagnosis of Circadian Rhythm Sleep Disorders

The American Psychiatric Association has provided the following criteria in Table 16.5 for the identification and diagnosis of circadian sleep disorders in its DSM-5.

Table 16.5 Diagnostic Criteria for Circadian Sleep disorders

- A persistent or recurrent pattern of sleep disruption that is primarily due to an alteration of the circadian system or to a misalignment between the endogenous circadian rhythm and the sleep-wake schedule required by an individual's physical environment or social or professional schedule.
- The sleep disruption leads to excessive sleepiness or insomnia, or both.
- The sleep disturbance causes clinically significant distress or impairment in social, occupational, and other important areas of functioning.
- The disturbance does not occur exclusively during the course of another sleep disorder or other mental disorder
- The disturbance is not due to the direct physiological effects of a substance or a general medical condition.

Source: APA (2013)

To Sum Up

In the category of dyssomnia sleep disorders, *Primary insomnia* represents the sleep disorder in which people are found to experience problems and difficulties in their night sleep, such as difficulty in initiating and maintaining sleep and the unfulfillment of the required restorative function by their night sleep.

Hypersomnia sleeping disorder runs on the other hand quite contrary to the insomnia sleeping disorder both in its nature as well as functioning. While people suffering from primary insomnia are not getting enough sleep, people suffering from hypersomnia, on the other hand, grapple with the problem of sleeping too much. Besides sleeping for a greater duration in the night, these people are also found to fall asleep several times during the day.

In the category of Dyssomnia sleep disorders, *Narcolepsy* is considered a serious and chronic sleep disorder usually characterized by features like (i) excessive daytime sleepiness, (ii) sleep attacks, and (iii) rapid eye movement (REM) sleep abnormalities such as cataplexy (a sudden loss of muscle tone resulting into the abnormal behavior such as falling asleep for a brief duration while cheering a favorite team), sleep paralysis (inability to move or speak for a brief period immediately after awakening in REM sleep), and hypnagogic hallucination (passing through terrifying experiences such as experiencing a vivid illusion of being caught in a fire or flying through the air).

The term *Breathing-related sleep disorders* is used for the type of sleep disorders in which there lie some physical origin—namely problems with breathing while asleep, causing them to experience widely disrupted sleep at night and excessive sleepiness (insomnia) during the day. Their breathing problems are reflected in experiencing a phenomenon of the stoppage of their breathing altogether for a period of 10 to 30 seconds, referred to as sleep apnea in the world of medicines and abnormal psychology. There are three types of sleep apnea (known as obstructive, central, and mixed sleep apnea), each causing a distinctive type of breath-related sleep disorder among affected individuals.

The term *Circadian Rhythm Sleep Disorder* is used for the type of sleep disorder in which affected individuals are found to go through a persistent or recurrent sleep disruption leading to excessive sleepiness or insomnia on account of a mismatch between the sleep-wake schedule required by their environment and their circadian sleep-wake cycle, such as what happens in experiencing jet-lag while visiting a county in a different time zone, or providing night shift duty in the work schedule.

Parasomnia Sleep Disorders

Let us now look into all three parasomnia sleep disorders—nightmares, night terrors, and night sleepwalking, one by one.

Nightmares

As told earlier, nightmares in the form of bad dreams occur during one's REM or dream sleep. These may be experienced in the form of a peculiar type of bad dreams by all persons of all ages, but are more common with children and tend to decrease with age. These are distinguished from bad dreams in the sense that, where nightmares are defined as disturbing dreams that awaken the sleeper, bad dreams are those that do not awaken the person experiencing them. Moreover, to qualify as a nightmare disorder, these bad dream experiences must be so distressful and terrifying that they impair a person's ability to carry on normal activities; for instance, making a person too anxious to try to sleep at night (Durand and Barlow, 2013:320). Other distinguishing features of nightmares come in the forms of (i) not making people move around, as happens to them in the NREM sleep-related disorders, night terror and sleepwalking, and (ii) vivid dream recollection immediately upon waking.

The above cited characterized features of the nightmare sleep disorder may be properly revealed through a case history provided below:

David was a 70-year-old retired lorry driver. He sought help at the insistence of his adult daughter after she witnessed what she thought was her father having a seizure one night. David admitted to a seven-year history of disturbed sleep. Every two to three weeks he experienced a night where his dreams were vivid and violent, involving being chased by animals or attacked by strangers.

The dreams manifested themselves in physical actions such as David punching the wall or flinging himself out of bed. These actions were carried out while still asleep but would jerk him awake. Sleepwalking was never a feature of his. He did not feel unduly tired after one of these disturbed nights but had suffered minor bruising. On other nights, he would get approximately eight hours of unbroken sleep. David prided himself on keeping fit, undertaking some kind of activity every day. He had no past medical history and was taking no regular medications.

Source: Topp (2009)

Table 16.6 Diagnostic Criteria for Nightmares

- Repeated occurrences of extended, extremely dysphoric, and well-remembered dreams that usually involve efforts to avoid threats to survival, security, or physical integrity and that generally occur during the second half of the major sleep episode.
- On awakening from the dysphoric dreams, the individual rapidly becomes oriented and alert.
- The sleep disturbance causes clinically significant distress or impairment in social, occupational, or other important areas of functioning.
- The nightmare symptoms are not attributable to the physiological effects of a substance (e.g., a drug of abuse, a medication).
- Coexisting mental and medical disorders do not adequately explain the predominant complaint of dysphoric dreams.

Source: APA (2013)

Identification and Diagnosis of Nightmares

The American Psychiatric Association has provided the following criteria in Table 16.6 for the identification and diagnosis of the sleeping disorder Nightmares in its DSM-5.

Night Sleep Terrors

Night sleep terrors are also termed bad dreams and may resemble nightmares in some ways, such as the child crying and feeling frightened. However, unlike nightmares, they have a distinction of (i) involving a state of panic (e.g., inability to move, breathe) experienced by the dreamers in their sound sleep, (ii) occurring during one's NREM deep sleep, (iii) making dreamers act upon their dreaming experience in the form of sitting up, screaming, running around the bedroom, and defending the self from an unseen attacker while remaining under the state of their sound sleep, (iv) providing no chance to awake and comfort the terrified child, as is possible during a nightmare, and (v) no remembering on the part of the child of what happened to them during the night terror episode.

The characteristic features of sleep terrors visible among children affected may be more clearly understood by a glimpse of the case history of a sleep terror-affected child given ahead.

We report a case of sleep terror in a four-year-old boy. The parents observed that for the past month, after the child goes to sleep, he wakes up in the middle of the night. This behavior occurs once or twice a week. On these occasions, the child is found standing somewhere in the house, crying, and seemingly disoriented, with rapid breathing and profuse sweating. When the parents attempt to comfort him or return him to his room, he becomes quite upset, striking out at them and screaming loudly. He continues to scream and fight for several minutes, followed by spontaneous cessation. Once the child is calmed, the parents can put him back in his bed, and he sleeps through the rest of the night without incident. In the morning, he wakes up in his usual happy mood and does not remember what occurred the previous evening. The parents are worried that he might be having seizures or developing a severe behavioral problem. Lab bloodwork is solicited, including an electroencephalogram (EEG). All returned normal results.

Source: Guzman and Wang (2008)

Table 16.7 Diagnostic criteria for Sleep terror disorders

- Recurrent episodes of abrupt terror arousals from sleep, usually occurring during the first-third of the major sleep episode and beginning with a panicky scream.
- There is intense fear and signs of autonomic arousal, such as mydriasis, tachycardia, rapid breathing, and sweating, during each episode. There is relative unresponsiveness to efforts of others to comfort the individual during the episodes.
- No or little (e.g., only a single visual scene) dream imagery is recalled.
- Amnesia for the episodes is present.
- The episodes cause clinically significant distress or impairment in social, occupational, or other important areas of functioning.
- The disturbance is not attributable to the physiological effects of a substance (e.g., a drug of abuse, a medication).
- Co-existing mental and medical disorders do not explain the episodes of sleep terrors.

Source: APA (2013)

Identification and Diagnosis of Sleep Terrors

The American Psychiatric Association has provided the following criteria in Table 16.7 for the identification and diagnosis of sleep terror disorders in its DSM-5.

Sleepwalking or Somnambulism

Sleepwalking, as the name signifies, represents the state of a person in which he or she is seen to walk or engage in one or the other type of activities while sleeping. Like sleep terrors, the sleepwalking phenomenon occurs during one's NREM sleep. The occurrence of this phenomenon during NREM sleep naturally implies that when people walk and engage in activities in their sleep, they are probably not acting out a dream. Moreover, since it occurs during the deepest stages of NREM sleep, waking someone during the sleepwalking episode is difficult; if the person is somehow awakened, he or she typically will not remember what has happened. Besides sleepwalking, some somnambulism patients are found to commit serious offenses and engage in undesirable social behavior and violence, including homicide and suicide. There are instances where people suffering from sleepwalking disorders have travelled a long journey in their deep sleep and committed offenses like murder, stealing, and dacoity, and were later acquitted from the charges on account of their innocence of doing these acts under the influence of uncontrollable sleep disorder.

In this way, somnambulism, the sleepwalking disorder, is characterized by atypical distinguishing features, making it a unique sleep disorder visible among some people. The nature and outcomes of this disorder may be made clearer to you by going through the following case history.

A male child aged eight years and ten months, a student in the fourth grade, hailing from a Hindu nuclear family of middle socioeconomic status and an urban background, presented to our center with the complaint that he had been walking in his sleep for the past five months. After going to bed at about 11 PM, he would get out of bed between 12 midnight and 3 AM and perform a variety of activities—go to the toilet and urinate, recite pieces of conversation, act out a scene from a TV serial, and so on. During this period, he would never attempt to leave the room and never injure himself. He would walk with his eyes open, but he did not respond to the calling out of his name. Each episode would last for five to seven minutes and would end with the patient returning to his bed and resuming his sleep. Only one episode would occur in a single night and these would occur once every one to two weeks. The patient had no recollection of the episode on waking up. In the month prior to his presentation at the clinic, the episodes had increased to once every alternate night. There was no history suggestive of any daytime interference in the scholastic and interpersonal functioning of the child. The child's past history was unremarkable and he had attained normal developmental milestones. There was a family history of psychotic illness in a cousin and alcohol dependence in a paternal uncle. There was no family history of sleepwalking or epilepsy. No stressors could be identified and the mental status examination was unremarkable. The child's mean intelligence quotient (IQ) at the time of the detailed assessment was 116.

Source: Bhardwaj Rahul and Suresh Kumar (2007)

Identification and Diagnosis of Sleepwalking Disorder

The American Psychiatric Association has provided the following criteria shown in Table 16.8 for the identification and diagnosis of sleepwalking disorder in its DSM-5.

Table 16.8 Diagnostic Criteria for Sleepwalking Disorder

- Repeated episodes of rising from bed during sleep and walking about usually occurring during the first third of the major sleep episode.
- While sleepwalking, the individual has a blank, staring face; is relatively unresponsive to the efforts of others to communicate with him or her; and can be awakened only with great difficulty.
- No or little (e.g., only a single visual scene) dream imagery is recalled.
- Amnesia for the episodes is present.
- The episodes cause clinically significant distress or impairment in social, occupational, or other important areas of functioning.
- The disturbance is not attributable to the physiological effects of a substance (e.g., a drug of abuse, a medication).
- Co-existing mental and medical disorders do not explain the episodes of sleepwalking

Source: APA (2013), DSM-5

To Sum Up

In the category of parasomnias sleep disorders, *Nightmares* represent the type of disorders in which people are found to experience bad dreams occurring during one's REM or dream sleep, in contrast to two other parasomnias type disorders—sleep terror and sleepwalking—which occur during NREM sleep. They differ from normal bad dreams in terms of getting the individual awakened, and proving too distressful or terrifying to impair a person's ability to carry on normal activities, i.e., making a person too anxious to try to sleep at night. Other distinguishing features of nightmares are known in the form of (i) not making people move around, as happens to them in the NREM sleep-related disorders—night terrors and sleep-walking—and (ii) vividly remembering the dreams immediately upon waking.

Night sleep terrors, while appearing similar to nightmares, differ from them in the sense of (i) occurring during one's NREM deep sleep, (ii) representing a state of panic (e.g., unable to move, breathe) experienced by the dreamers, (iii) making dreamers act upon their dreaming experience while remaining under the state of their sound sleep, (iv) providing no chance to awake and comfort the terrified child, as is possible during a nightmare, and (v) no remembering on the part of children of what happened to them during the night terror episode.

Sleepwalking represents the state of a person in which he or she is seen to walk around or engage in other activities such as eating in the kitchen, as well as committing serious acts such as murder, stealing, suicide attempts, and so on during their sleepwalking.

The Underlying Causes of Sleeping Disorders (Dyssomnias and Parasomnias)

There has been little knowledge and understanding about the exact causes behind the occurrence of the various sleeping disorders. However, a number of theories or viewpoints have been put forward for this purpose by researchers and practitioners from time to time, depending upon their own theoretical grounds and research findings. As a result, genetic, psychoanalytic, biological and medical, psychological, and environmental maladjustment have thus been blamed for the causation of sleep disorders. For example, while emphasizing the possibility of a genetic component involved in the causation of sleep disorders, hereditarians talk about the higher incidence of their occurrence among identical twins and within families. The psychoanalyst and socio-psychological scientists, in this concern, blame unfulfilled wishes, maltreatment, and maladjustment received by the children in their sociocultural environment, extreme fatigue, anxieties and stresses, sleep deprivation, or the use of sedative or hypnotic drugs for the causation of these sleep disorders. The biologists and medical professionals on the other hand here name biological and constitutional defects as well as illnesses and diseases for the outcomes of these sleep disorders; i.e., the failure of the brain mechanism (that normally inhibits the voluntary muscles) for doing various undesirable acts under the influence of somnambulism.

To Sum Up

Regarding the causation of one or the other sleep disorders—dyssomnias and parasomnias—while hereditarians talk about the higher incidence of their occurrence among identical twins and within families, the psychoanalyst and socio-psychological scientists blame unfulfilled wishes, maltreatment, and maladjustment received by children in their sociocultural environment, extreme fatigue, anxieties and stresses, sleep deprivation, or the use of sedative or hypnotic drugs for this purpose. Biologists and medical professionals, on the other hand, here name biological and constitutional defects as well as illnesses and diseases for the outcomes of these sleep disorders.

Treatment Measures for the Sleep Disorders (Dyssomnias and Parasomnias)

The Treatment of Dyssomnias

The list of Dyssomnias we described previously included the sleep disorders known as primary insomnia, hypersomnia, narcolepsy, breathing-related disorders, and circadian rhythm sleep disorders. The treatment measures applied to all these dyssomnias may be classified as medical measures, environmental measures, and psychological measures. Let us discuss the use of these measures in the treatment of such sleep disorders.

Medical Measures

The use of medicine or medical treatment is one of the widely used practices for seeking remedy to any disturbance—physical or mental—in the human body. In this sequence, clinicians and physicians may prescribe a number of suitable medicines shown in Table 16.9 for the treatment of various dyssomnias.

Table 16.9 Medication Used for the Treatment of Various Dyssomnias

Type of Dyssomnia sleep disorder	The prescribed medicine or medical measure for treatment
Primary Insomnia	One of several benzodiazepines including (i) Short-acting drugs such as triazolam (Halcion), zaleplon (Sonata), and zolpidem (Ambien) and (ii) long-acting drugs like flurazepam (Dalmane).
Primary Hypersomnia	Stimulants such as methylphenidate (Ritalin) or modafinil.
Narcolepsy	Antidepressant drugs to deal with cataplexy (loss of muscle tone) attacks.
Breathing-related sleep disorders	(i) Recommending weight loss to obese patients. (ii) Using a mechanical device called the continuous positive air pressure (CPAP) machine for improving breathing in people suffering from obstructive sleep apnea. (iii) Recommending surgery to help remove blockage in parts of the airways.
Circadian rhythm sleep disorders	There is no usual practice to recommend medications for the treatment of these sleep disorders.

Practically speaking, the use of medication, especially the prescription of drugs, is generally made to treat insomnia (trouble sleeping). However, the use of drugs is severally criticized on account of the drawbacks or ill consequences resulting from their use, such as the following.

- The use of drugs may intensify the problem by causing excessive sleepiness.
- It can make people dependent on them.
- People may be found to misuse them deliberately or non-deliberately.
- These medications have a limitation to work for the short-term treatment (not longer than four weeks) of insomnias. They do not work well for the treatment of long-term chronic sleep problems. Moreover, in their longer use, there lies an inherent danger of promoting dependence and rebounding insomnia.
- According to the latest researches, the use of some medications prescribed for the treatment of insomnia have a possibility of increasing the likelihood of sleepwalking and other problems such as sleep-related eating disorders.

Environmental Measures

For the treatment of Dyssomnias, a certain type of special measure involving environment modifications or changes in the patient's prevalent circumstances are also used by practitioners and professionals on a number of occasions. The use of such measures can help much in seeking treatment for the cases affected with circadian rhythm sleep disorders.

In making environmental setting adjustments for dealing with circadian rhythm sleep disorder problems, one may be advised to follow certain measures like:

1. It remains always better to move bedtime later than to move bedtime earlier. In case you feel sleepy in the daytime while staying in the United States, it will be better for you to delay your sleeping until the scheduled hours of night bedtime. In this way, people can best readjust their sleep patterns by going to bed several hours later each night until bedtime is at the desired hour. Similarly, scheduling shift changes in a clockwise direction (going from a day to an evening schedule) seems to help workers adjust better to their sleep-wake cycle.
2. The use of phototherapy (bright light) is also found to help greatly in dealing with circadian rhythm-related problems. While making use of this therapy, the affected people are typically asked to sit in front of a bank of fluorescent lamps that generate light greater than an amount significantly different from normal indoor. Several hours of exposure to this bright light have successfully reset the circadian rhythms of many individuals (Durand and Barlow, 2013:319).

Psychological Measures

The abnormality of behavioral functioning lies at the roots of dyssomnias, which is why their appropriate remedy lies in making use of one or the other psychological treatments chiefly based on behavior modification techniques or therapies.

We can name the important ones as (i) Cognitive behavioral therapy, (ii) Guided imagery therapy, (iii) Meditation therapy, (iv) Progressive-relaxation therapy, and (v) Stimulus control therapy.

Cognitive behavioral therapy (CBT): Treatment carried out in this behavioral approach aims to bring changes in the defective cognitive functioning of the affected people particularly related to their dysfunctional beliefs and unrealistic expectations about their sleep lying at the roots of their chronic insomnias, such as (i) having over concern about the total sleep duration (i.e., "I must get eight hours of sleep each night, and if I get less than eight hours of sleep, it will make me ill"), (ii) anxiety about the disorder ("excessive sleepiness or insomnia is dangerous; it may lead to insanity"), and so on. CBT aims to replace these views with more adaptive substitutes. For this purpose, the therapist tries to bring alterations to the unrealistic beliefs and attitudes of patients about sleeping by discussing topics such as normal amounts of sleep, our ability to compensate for lost sleep, providing the correct information about sleeping behavior in terms of normal amounts of sleep needed, the ability to compensate for lost sleep, and the removal of any misperceptions in this concern.

Guided Imagery Therapy: The term imagery stands for the process of creating an experience/image in the mind of an individual in the absence of any external stimuli. In the treatment of insomnia, the therapists try to make use of suitable and appropriate imageries, putting the affected individuals to experience the act of sleeping in their mind. The experience of such imagery on their part helps in providing them relaxation and relief from the anxiety associated with their difficulty sleeping.

Meditation therapy: Anxiety- and stress-related situations and an unfavorable attitude developed by individuals about their sleep may work as strong factors in creating hurdles and difficulties sleeping. The meditation technique practiced by affected people may work wonders in bringing relief and remedy in this situation. The practice of meditation such as transcendental meditation proves helpful in providing the needed relaxation for seeking remedy to the anxiety regarding the difficulty sleep of affected people.

Progressive relaxation therapy: The technique of progressive relaxation may be successfully used in the treatment of anxiety- and stress-ridden sleep problems. In its practical application, progressive relaxation begins with the affected person lying on his back with arms extended to the side. One by one, major muscle groups of the body are first tensed and then slowly relaxed. This is aimed to assist in the identification of the various muscle systems within the body and to help the affected individual to learn how to discriminate between tensed and relaxed muscle conditions. The step-by-step relaxation of the tensed muscles then helps the affected individual to seek a remedy to his or her sleep difficulty.

Stimulus control therapy: This type of behavioral therapy is based on the assumption that stimuli present in one's sleeping environment play a key role in the quantity and quality of one's sleep. Therefore, due care should be taken for exercising the necessary control over these stimuli for ensuring trouble-free sleep. Thus, the main focus of this therapy lies in helping patients learn how to exercise control over the environmental stimuli affecting their sleep. For this purpose, due attention in this therapy is given to helping patients learn the art of (i) re-associating their bedtime and the sleep environment with their sleeping and (ii) seeking correction of learned maladaptive behaviors that disrupt their sleep. A therapist while making use of this therapy may work for instructing and advising the concerned patients to adapt to the following schedule and practices in their sleeping behavior.

- They should avoid making use of their bed and bedroom for anything other than sleeping, such as reading, eating, laying idle on the bed or watching TV.
- It should be made their habit to go to bed only when sleepy.
- In case, they are unable to fall asleep in a reasonable duration, say 20 or 30 minutes, then they should not unnecessarily struggle for it. It remains better for them to get up and go to another room. Stay up as long as they wish and then return to the bedroom to sleep.

- They should be made to follow a set sleep-wake schedule for helping their body acquire a consistent sleep rhythm. For this purpose, they should be advised to set the alarm and get up at the same time every morning regardless of how much sleep they received during the night.
- They should be advised to avoid napping during the day for enjoying uninterrupted scheduled sleep at night.
- It should also be made a habit to avoid any recovery sleep in the day to compensate for the loss of sleep during the previous bad night.

The Treatment of Parasomnias

Treatment for parasomnias (nightmares, sleep terrors, and sleepwalking) usually begins with a recommendation to ignore infrequent episodes of such disorder as well as wait and see if they disappear on their own. However, in case these are persistent, lead to the potential for injury, are disruptive to family members, or result in embarrassment, sleep disruption, or extreme daytime sleepiness to the individual, then attempts should be made for the necessary treatment suiting the nature and seriousness of the disorder faced. In their practical application, these treatment approaches usually focus on promoting safety and eliminating causes or triggers associated with such sleep disorders. We can try to adopt one or the other approaches mentioned as follows.

1. *Treating the underlying condition or cause*: In adopting this approach, therapists and professionals first try to find out the underlying conditions or inherent causes lying behind parasomnias (nightmares, sleep terrors, and sleepwalking). In cases where these are associated with an underlying medical or mental health condition or another sleep disorder (such as obstructive sleep apnea or restless legs syndrome), then treatment should be planned to overcome this problem. Similarly, if these are the result of a particular medication, then attempts should be made to bring alterations to the dosage or prescription to eliminate this unwanted side effect.
2. *Addressing anxiety, stress, and depression:* In the causation of parasomnia-related sleep disorders, an increased level of stress, anxiety, and depression is often found to contribute in a big way. It is therefore quite natural for affected persons to take help from counselors and therapists in getting due relief from the anxiety, stress, and depression associated with their disorder. The therapists and counselors may make use of a number of strategies to relieve stress, tension, and depression, involving cognitive behavioral therapy, hypnosis, biofeedback, or relaxation therapy, including meditation.
3. *Scheduled awakening:* This approach involves waking the person who has episodes of Parasomnias (nightmares, sleep terrors, or sleepwalking) at a scheduled time—say 15–20 minutes before a typical episode of these disorders occurs (they usually occur at the same time each night)—and keeping them awake for a suitable duration.
4. *Seeking self-help:* In getting rid of a problem, self-help is always considered the best help. Therefore, attempts need to be made for encouraging patients to seek prevention and treatment of parasomnias by learning and practicing the measures of self-help, such as (i) keeping a regular wake-sleep schedule, (ii) engaging in regular exercise including yogic asanas, breathing practices, and meditation, (iii) practicing good sleep hygiene for preventing sleep deprivation, (iv) practicing the methods of self-hypnosis, (v) caring about night sleep environment, such as making one's bedroom a relaxing place reserved for sleep, and (vi) avoiding the use of alcohol, caffeine, cocaine, and nicotine.
5. *Seeking medical treatment and medication:* The help of medical treatments in the form of surgery or other suitable means may be taken for the necessary correction of the physiological and neurological abnormalities and defects responsible for causing parasomnia-related problems

among individuals. In addition, suitable medication or drugs may be prescribed as needed for the treatment of parasomnias, focusing on getting the nightmare, sleep terror, or sleepwalking problem under control and helping the sufferer get a better night's rest. The various types of drugs often prescribed by medical professionals for this purpose may be cited as follows:

(i) Antidepressants such as Trazodone or Benzodiazepines
(ii) Sedative drugs such as Prosom, and
(iii) Anticonvulsants such as Klonopin.

All of these medications can be helpful in reducing the frequency and severity of nightmare, sleep terror, or sleepwalking episodes. However, the decision regarding the suitability of the particular one must be taken by the medical professional caring for the patient. Moreover, the decision regarding drug-related treatment should be taken with necessary caution, as all of these drugs have their own side effects and are not meant for long-term use.

To Sum Up

The treatment measures applied to all dyssomnia-type disorders may be classified as medical measures, environmental measures, and psychological measures. In this sequence, where medical measures are found to make use of one or the other suitable drugs, and medication prescribed by qualified professionals for taking control of dyssomnias, environmental measures modify the patient's environment for seeking relief and treatment. The psychological measures used in the form of a number of behavioral therapies such as Cognitive behavioral therapy, Guided imagery therapy, Meditation therapy, Progressive relaxation therapy, and Stimulus control therapy may prove quite effective in controlling and treating persons affected by one or the other dyssomnias.

The treatment measures applied to all the parasomnias —nightmares, night terrors, and sleepwalking—follow the policy of first waiting and watching for their disappearance on their own. In case of their persistence and seriousness, the measures adopted may be named as (i) treating the underlying condition or cause associated with the disorder, (ii) addressing anxiety, stress, and depression by making use of cognitive behavioral therapy, hypnosis, biofeedback, or relaxation therapy including meditation, (iii) scheduled awakening, say 15–20 minutes before a typical episode of these disorders, (iv) seeking their prevention and treatment by learning and practicing self-help measures, and (v) seeking medical treatment and using medication or drug therapy.

Review Questions

1. Discuss what happens with us usually during our night sleep, especially mentioning the types and stages of our sleep in the form of REM and NREM sleep.
2. What do you understand by the term sleep disorders? Throw light on their meaning and nature.
3. What are dyssomnia sleep disorders? Name their different types and discuss any two of them in detail.
4. What is primary insomnia? Discuss its characteristic features and ways of identification and diagnosis in full cognizance of the criteria laid down by the APA in its DSM-IV-TR.

5. What is primary hypersomnia? How does it differ from primary insomnia? Discuss its underlying causes.
6. Discuss the characteristic features and ways of identification and diagnosis of the sleep disorder known as primary insomnia.
7. What is narcolepsy? Throw light on its characteristic features and tell how one might identify and diagnose it in affected individuals.
8. What is a breath-related sleep disorder? How does it affect an individual in his night sleep? Throw light on the ways of its identification and diagnosis in light of the criteria laid down by the APA in the DSM-IV-TR.
9. What is circadian rhythm sleep disorder? Throw light on its characteristic features and describe its identification and diagnosis among affected individuals.
10. What are parasomnia sleep disorders? Name their different types and discuss any one of them in detail.
11. What are nightmares, night terrors, and sleepwalking sleep disorders? Throw light on their characteristic features and ways of identification and diagnosis in light of the criteria laid down by the APA in its DSM-IV-TR.
12. What are sleep disorders? Discuss the underlying causes of sleep disorders.
13. Throw light on the measures taken for the treatment of sleep disorders.

References

American Psychiatric Association (2000), *The diagnostic and statistical manual of mental disorders (DSM-IV-TR)*, Washington, DC: American Psychiatric Association.

American Psychiatric Association (2013), *Diagnostic and statistical manual of mental disorders* (5th ed.), Washington, DC: American Psychiatric Association.

American Psychiatric Association (2022), *Diagnostic and statistical manual of mental disorders: DSM-5-TR*, Washington, DC: American Psychiatric Association.

Bhardwaj, R. and Kumar, S. (2007), Somnambulism: Diagnosis and treatment, *Indian Journal of Psychiatry*, 49(2): 123–125, retrieved from www.ncbi.nlm.nih.gov/pmc/articles/PMC2917078/

Durand, V. M., & Barlow, D. H. (2013), *Essentials of abnormal psychology* (6th ed.), Belmont, CA: Wadsworth.

Guzman, C. S., & Wang, Y. P. (2008), Sleep terror disorder: A case report, *Brazilian Journal of Psychiatry*, 30(2), retrieved from www.scielo.br/scielo.php?script=sci_arttext&pid=S1516-44462008000200016

John, D. J., Manoharan, A., & Varghese, R. (2007), A case of primary hypersomnia, *Annals of Indian Academy of Neurology*, 10: 58–60.

Shin, K. Y., Hong, S. C., Cho, Y. J., Jeong, Jinhyun, Han, J. H. & Lee, S. P. (2007), Case study of a narcoleptic patient with a family history of narcolepsy, Department of Neuropsychiatry, St. Vincent's Hospital, Korea, *Psychiatry Investigation*, 4: 121–123, retrieved from www.psychiatryinvestigation.org/upload/pdf/0502007022.pdf

Topp, J. (2009), Case study-disturbed sleep and vivid nightmares, retrieved from www.gponline.com/case-study-disturbed-sleep-vivid-nightmares/neurology/article/965128

Zee, P. C. (2011), Case histories in circadian rhythm sleep disorders, *MedScape*, retrieved from www.medscape.org/viewarticle/745357

Old Age or Degenerative Disorders

Introduction

It is natural to experience a considerable decrease in physical and mental strength and capacity with the increase in age during an individual's older years. As a result, we may find the old aged

DOI: 10.4324/9781003398325-17

falling victim to physical and mental weaknesses and developing one or the other physiological and mental disorders and diseases. Besides becoming patients of certain physical illnesses and diseases, it is quite common for old aged people to suffer from a number of neurocognitive disorders and diseases, demonstrating visible symptoms of abnormal and disruptive behavior, such as Delirium, Dementia, Alzheimer's disease, Pick's disease, Parkinson's disease, and Huntington's disease. All these disorders have been classified and described in the category of Neurocognitive disorders in the latest classification systems, the DSM-5 and DSM-5-TR, of the American Psychiatrist Association. Let us look into some essentials of these disorders and diseases in detail.

Delirium

Etymologically, the word delirium is derived from the Latin words de (meaning "out of") and lira (meaning "track"). The term delirium may thus stand for "being off-track or deviating from the usual state or condition of the mind," resulting in a state of utter confusion or clouding of one's consciousness. This is why delirium is also known as an acute state of confusion or clouding of one's consciousness.

> **Delirium**
>
> A neurocognitive disorder particularly more common in older persons representing an acute state of confusion or clouding of one's consciousness, leading to misinterpretations, illusions, and, on occasion, hallucinations.

The acute state of confusion representing delirium typically develops over a short period of time, usually hours or days. In its developed form it is characterized by some distinguishable symptoms such as:

- Extreme trouble focusing attention, making them unable to concentrate and think in an organized way, leading to misinterpretations, illusions, and on occasion, hallucinations.
- Profound disturbances in the sleep-wake cycle resulting in making them drowsy during the day yet awake and agitated at night, and experiencing vivid dreams, nightmares, and sleep terrors in a greater amount on their part.
- Major disturbances in their orientation to environment and perception resulting in such incidents as making them believe that it is morning in the middle of the night, that they are home when actually they are in the hospital room, and also committing blunders such as mistaking the unfamiliar with the familiar, and an inability to tell what day it is and who they are.
- Major disturbances and difficulties in speech and communication, making them impossible to engage with in proper conversation nor speak in a clearly understanding ways.
- Memory impairment, especially for recent events, is common among them.
- A lot of incoherency and swings in their activity and mood display, resulting in some or the other typical behavior such as ripping one's clothes in one moment and sitting lethargically the next, looking quite alert and happy at one moment, and then lost, careless, and sad in the next moment.
- Demonstrating a lot of emotional instability in their behavior, such as switching rapidly from one emotion to another, and negativity involving depression, anxiety, anger, euphoria, and irritability.

- A common presence of certain physical symptoms such as a flushed face, dilated pupils, tremors, rapid heartbeat, elevated blood pressure, and incontinence of urine and feces. Moreover, they may also be found to become soporific and lethargic if their delirium gets worsened.
- People of any age are subject to detect delirium, but it is more common among children and older adults. Among older adults, it is particularly common in nursing homes and hospitals (Kring et al., 2012:461).

Elderly hospitalized patients frequently develop altered mental status as a complication of their illness, exemplified in the case history of an older hospitalized woman given ahead.

Delirium in an Older, Hospitalized Woman

An 86-year-old woman, admitted with complaints of shortness of breath and cough, was found to have pneumonia. Her past medical history included cataract surgery, hypertension controlled with medications, and type 2 diabetes controlled by diet. She was ambulatory, lived alone, and at baseline completed all activities of daily living independently. According to her daughter, the patient was never disoriented. At admission, the patient appeared mildly dehydrated on physical examination. Her oxygen saturation was 94% on 2 liters of oxygen by nasal cannula, and an arterial blood gas showed a normal $pCO2$ of 40 mmHg. Her daughter requested to spend the night at the bedside but was told she could not stay.

Overnight, the patient was noted to be disoriented by the nursing staff. She began pulling at her intravenous lines and attempting to get out of bed. The covering physician was called and ordered that the patient be placed in four-point restraints.

The following morning, the daughter returned to find her mother in restraints, speaking incoherently, and severely short of breath. Upon finding her mother confused, the daughter asked the nurse what had happened and reiterated to the nurse that her mother had never been confused before.

Source: Deborah D'Avolio (2018)

Identification and Diagnosis of Delirium

The American Psychiatric Association (2013) has provided the following criteria shown in Table 17.1 for the identification and diagnosis of the Neurocognitive disorder delirium in the DSM-5.

Causes of Delirium

Delirium, by its very definition, is known as an organically caused decline from a previous baseline level of mental function that develops over a short period of time (APA, 2013). This leads us to conclude that delirium is secondary to an underlying medical condition, deterioration in one's physical and mental health, and concurrent diseases and illnesses suffered by the individual in

Table 17.1 Diagnostic Criteria for Delirium

A. A disturbance in attention (i.e., reduced ability to direct, focus, sustain, and shift attention) and awareness (reduced orientation to the environment).

B. The disturbance develops over a short period of time (usually hours to a few days), represents a change from baseline attention and awareness, and tends to fluctuate in severity during the course of a day.

C. An additional disturbance in cognition (e.g., memory deficit, disorientation, language, visuospatial ability, or perception).

D. The disturbances in Criteria A and C are not better explained by another preexisting, established, or evolving neurocognitive disorder and do not occur in the context of a severely reduced level of arousal, such as coma.

E. There is evidence from the history, physical examination, or laboratory findings that the disturbance is a direct physiological consequence of another medical condition, substance intoxication or withdrawal (i.e., due to a drug of abuse or to a medication), or exposure to a toxin, or is due to multiple etiologies.

Source: APA (2013), DSM-5

the course of his or her life. The things and factors representing such deterioration and underlying medical conditions may be briefly named and categorized as follows:

- Fever and certain diseases (like shock, heart attacks, hypoxia, anemia, hyperthyroidism, cancer, etc.)
- Infections (like pneumonia, urinary tract infections)
- Neurological disorders (like head trauma or seizures)
- Drug addiction and drug-withdrawal reactions
- Medication misuse, whether deliberate or inadvertent
- Intoxication by certain substances, such as side effects of prescribed drugs or changes in drug prescription
- Strokes and stress (including the trauma of surgery)
- Metabolic and nutritional imbalances (as in dehydration, uncontrolled diabetes, thyroid dysfunction, kidney or liver failure, congestive heart failure, or malnutrition)
- Brain damage and dementia

Treatment of Delirium

As we know, the course of a remedy or treatment lies in taking care of the causes behind the problem. Therefore, while taking measures for the treatment of delirium, due attention should be paid to the things responsible for causing delirium. Beginning in this direction, efforts should thus be made to have a thorough examination of the patient for all possible underlying causes of the disorder, such as drug intoxication, fever, infections, diseases, strokes and stresses, metabolic and nutritional imbalances, and so on, and then suitable treatment should be planned accordingly in view of treating the underlying medical conditions. Besides taking the course of such treatment for delirium patients, urgent supporting measures may be employed in the shape of a prescription of one or the other suitable drugs for treating delirium symptoms. These may usually include antipsychotic drugs (to treat agitation and hallucinations and to improve sensory problems) such as (i) Haloperidol, (ii) Risperidone, (iii) Olanzapine, and (iv) Quetiapine. However, in case the patient has an alcohol or drug withdrawal problem, then it remains useful to prescribe benzodiazepines (such as diazepam, lorazepam, chlordiazepoxide, or oxazepam) for this purpose.

To Sum Up

In the category of neurocognitive disorders, delirium represents a disorder in which the affected person feels a major disturbance in his or her attention (such as the inability to concentrate and think in an organized way), and orientation to the environment, accompanied by the clouding of consciousness leading to a state of utter confusion (i.e., memory impairment, misinterpretations, illusions and, on occasion, hallucinations, such as mistaking the unfamiliar with the familiar, and inability to tell about what day it is and who they are).

Regarding the causation of delirium, it is said to be caused and progressed through organic or underlying medical conditions such as deterioration in one's physical and mental health, and concurrent diseases and illnesses suffered by the individual in the course of his or her life.

Suitable treatment for delirium should be planned in view of treating the underlying medical conditions causing delirium in the patient. Besides this, urgent as well as supporting measures may be employed by prescribing suitable drugs for treating delirium symptoms.

Dementia

Etymologically, the word dementia is derived from the Latin words de (meaning "without") and mens (meaning "mind"), which join together to mean "without mind" or "senseless." However, in its practical use in the medical and psychological world, the

---

Dementia

A Neurocognitive disorder representing an acute deterioration in one's cognitive abilities resulting in multiple cognitive deficits including impairment in memory.

---

term is used for "an acute deterioration in one's cognitive abilities affecting one's functioning in a variety of ways." It is in this sense that in the DSM-IV-TR and DSM-5, the term dementia has been categorized and defined as "a Neurocognitive disorder that results into multiple cognitive deficits including impairment in memory." The WHO's classification in the ICD-10, however, has provided more elaborate explanation by terming dementia as

a syndrome due to disease of the brain, usually of a chronic or progressive nature, in which there is disturbance of multiple higher cortical functions, including memory, thinking, orientation, comprehension, calculation, learning capacity, language, and judgment. Consciousness is not clouded. The impairments of cognitive functions are commonly accompanied, and occasionally preceded, by deterioration in emotional control, social behavior or motivation.

In conclusion, by the term dementia, we may hereby refer to a disorder or a disturbed state of one's mind representing the deterioration of one's cognitive abilities to the point that his or her overall functioning gets impaired in a variety of ways including a great memory loss.

The distinguishable characteristics and features of dementia in light of the definitions and explanations provided in the DSMs and ICDs may be briefed as follows:

- A great memory loss demonstrable in terms of one's difficulty remembering things, especially recent events, such as (i) leaving the task unfinished on account of forgetting what was to be done, (ii) inability in remembering the names of familiar objects in their environment i.e., the name of a daughter or son and their own day-to-day belongings, (iii) forgetting about their daily routines, such as taking a bath or dressing properly, (iv) getting lost themselves even in their day-to-day familiar surroundings.
- A great deterioration in one's cognitive abilities and functioning related to several cognitive domains including, thinking, reasoning, problem-solving, making judgments, drawing conclusions and inferences, difficulty comprehending situations and making plans or decisions, learning new things, making computations and calculations of a simple nature, and so on.
- There appears no clouding of consciousness turning one into a state of acute confusion as happens with patients of delirium.
- Accompanying or preceding the impairment of cognitive functioning is a deterioration in emotional control and social behavior, reflected in abnormal behavior such as losing control of their impulses, using coarse language in conversation, making inappropriate jokes, shoplifting, and making sexual advances to strangers.
- Demonstrating the symptom of behaviors related to depression, delusions, delirium, and hallucination.
- Defined as mental deterioration of organic or functional origin, dementia is known to be caused on account of one or the other types of strokes and diseases of the brain, usually of a chronic or progressive nature.

Moreover, the course of dementia may be progressive, static, or remitting, depending on the cause. Many people with progressive dementia eventually become withdrawn and apathetic. In the terminal phase of illness, the personality loses its sparkle and integrity. Relatives and friends say that the person is just not himself or herself anymore. Social involvement with others keeps narrowing. Finally, the person is oblivious to his or her surroundings (Kring et al., 2012).

These typical features found in old aged people suffering from dementia may be sometimes seen even in the younger adults as visualized through the case history of a patient suffering from Alzheimer's type dementia provided ahead.

Alzheimer's type dementia in a patient

A 37-year-old male patient visited an outpatient clinic with complaints of gradual cognitive decline which had started three years earlier. Working as an industrial researcher, he started to make serious calculation mistakes that made him quit his job, and he began working as a manager in a company. However, his frequent forgetfulness, along with aggravation in recent memory impairments hampered him from fulfilling his duties, making him change jobs frequently. Apraxia and apathy had started two years before his visit to our clinic, and his disorientation to time and person was worsened to a degree that it became impossible to commute daily between his workplace and home. At the time of his visit to our clinic, not only was he fired from his recent job, but also, he needed frequent reminders from his family to maintain his hygiene. His sleep disturbance became prominent, frequently waking up middle of the night talking to himself. Before his visit to our clinic, he had visited two hospitals for evaluation and management of his symptoms, but to no avail. For a thorough examination of his symptoms, he was immediately admitted to our psychiatric ward. His laboratory findings did not reveal any abnormalities, and his tests for human immunodeficiency virus and syphilis turned out to be negative. In his cognitive tests, in contrast to his relatively preserved language function, he displayed serious impairments in free recall, 20-minute delayed recall, and recognition.

Source: Yoo et al. (2017)

Identification and Diagnosis of Dementia

The American Psychiatric Association has provided the following criteria for the identification and diagnosis of the old age disorder dementia in its DSM IV TR, as shown in Table 17.2.

Table 17.2 Diagnostic Criteria for Dementia

- Development of multiple cognitive deficits that include memory impairment and at least one of the following cognitive disturbances:
  - (i)   aphasia (the loss or impairment of the power to use words as symbols of ideas)
  - (ii) apraxia (the loss or impairment of the ability to execute movements without muscular paralysis)
  - (iii) agnosia or a disturbance in executive functioning (the loss of the ability to recognize familiar objects by seeing, hearing, or touching)
- The cognitive deficits must be sufficiently severe to cause impairment in occupational or social functioning and must represent a decline from a previously higher level of functioning.

Source: APA (2000), DSM-IV-TR

Distinction Between Delirium and Dementia

Delirium and dementia, both falling in the category of neurological disorders in late life, have a number of overlapping features and symptoms making the task of differentiation between them a little difficult. Each of them may be misdiagnosed in the presence of the other in a patient. However, both have sufficient uniqueness to distinguish them from each other. In a simple way, we may safely distinguish between the terms delirium and dementia on the basis of being named respectively as "a deterioration of cognitive abilities" and "a state of mental confusion." In this regard, Knight (1996) has offered a useful suggestion for the required distinction between them in the following words.

The clinical "feel" of talking with a delirium patient is rather like talking to someone who is acutely intoxicated or in an acute psychotic episode. Whereas the demented patient may not remember the name of the place where she or he is, the delirious patient may believe it is a different sort of place altogether, perhaps mistaking a psychiatric ward for a used car lot.

(pp. 96–97)

In further helping with the task of distinguishing between dementia and delirium, Kring et al. (2012) have listed a variety of features comparing them in the following way.

Table 17.3 Comparative Features of Dementia and Delirium

Dementia	Delirium
Gradual deterioration of abilities	Rapid onset
Deficits in memory for recent events	Trouble concentrating and staying with a train of thought
Caused by disease processes that are directly influencing the brain	Secondary to another medical condition
Usually progressive and nonreversible	Fluctuations over the course of a day
Treatment offers only minimal benefit	Usually reversible by treating underlying condition, but potentially fatal if cause (e.g., infection or malnutrition) is not treated
Prevalence increases with age	Prevalence is highest in the very young as well as the old

Source: Kring et al. (2012:461)

Types of Dementia

There are many different types of dementia. These may be divided into the following categories on the basis of their etiology (Kring et al., 2012:454):

- Dementia of the Alzheimer's type
- Vascular Dementia
- Dementia due to other general medical conditions
- Substance-induced persisting Dementia
- Dementia due to multiple etiologies
- Dementia not otherwise specified; when cause cannot be determined.

Causes of Dementia

Dementia is caused by damage to or loss (death) of nerve cells and their connections in the brain. Depending on the area of the brain that is affected by the damage, dementia can affect people differently and cause different symptoms, giving rise to various types of dementia. This damage or loss of nerve cells may be caused either by (i) a head injury, a stroke, or a brain tumor, or by (ii) a neurodegenerative disease (progressive brain cell death that happens over time). Such damage or loss of nerve cells, in turn, puts obstacles in the path of ongoing communication among the brain cells. This lack of communication between brain cells is responsible for adversely affecting the thinking, feeling, and acting behavior of the affected persons in their own ways. As we know, the human brain has many distinct regions, each of which is responsible for different functions (for example, memory, judgment, and movement). The damage or loss of cells in a particular region results in the failure of that region in carrying out its own functioning, giving rise to one or the other types of dementia-related problems or diseases such as Vascular dementia, Alzheimer's disease, Pick's disease, Parkinson's disease, and Huntington's disease. Among all these dementia-related neurocognitive disorders and diseases, Alzheimer's disease is known to be more pronounced and common among older aged people. Let us, therefore, focus first on its discussion.

To Sum Up

The term dementia stands for a disorder or a disturbed state of one's mind representing the deterioration of one's cognitive abilities to the point that his or her overall functioning gets impaired in a variety of ways including great memory loss.

Dementia and delirium, both falling in the category of neurological disorders in late life, have a number of overlapping features and symptoms. However, where in dementia there is a considerable deterioration of cognitive abilities including great memory loss, in delirium one experiences a clouding of consciousness resulting in a state of utter confusion.

Dementia is caused by damage to or loss (death) of nerve cells and their connections in the brain. This damage or loss of nerve cells may be caused either by (i) a head injury, a stroke, or a brain tumor, or by (ii) a neurodegenerative disease such as vascular disease, Alzheimer's disease, Pick's disease, Parkinson's disease, and Huntington's disease.

Alzheimer's Disease

Alzheimer's disease was first identified in a dementia patient in 1907 by German psychiatrist Alois Alzheimer. It is in his honor that the disease has been named Alzheimer's disease. Alzheimer's disease is known for giving rise to a particular type of dementia, known as "Dementia of the Alzheimer's type,"

Alzheimer Disease

A neurocognitive disorder or disease known for giving rise to a particular type of dementia, known as "Dementia of the Alzheimer's type," characterizing a great loss of memory on the part of affected individuals.

symptomizing a great loss of memory on the part of affected individuals. Let us see what happens in this disease that results in such loss of memory.

As pointed out before, dementia (the deterioration in several cognitive domains) is caused by some particular types of damage or loss of brain cells in different regions of the brain. A particular region of the brain affected by such brain cell damage or loss gives birth to a particular type of cognitive deterioration. In the case of Alzheimer's disease, the region of the brain called the hippocampus (the center of learning and memory) is adversely affected on account of the damage or loss of brain cells belonging to this region.

In terms of its early onset, Alzheimer's disease may appear among some individuals in their late 50s or early 60s, but in the majority of cases, it generally appears in the late 60s or early 70s and then gets increased as they reach their late 70s and early 80s. The time between the onset and death is typically eight to ten years among affected individuals. As a progressive disease, the patients suffering from this disease may demonstrate distinctive symptoms in their behavior, such as:

1. In the first phase or beginning of this disease, patients are found to exhibit mild problems associated with their memory and environmental orientation, such as forgetfulness, lapses of attention, and difficulty in language and communication.
2. In the second phase of this disease, with the notable increase in associated symptoms, patients are found to suffer more deterioration in their memory, resulting in difficulties completing tasks, remembering important appointments, and getting confused in their thinking and judgment day by day.
3. In the later phase, with a further intensification of the disease-associated symptoms, Alzheimer's patients are found to demonstrate abnormal behavior characterized by the following features:

   - Withdrawal behavior reflected in their attitude and actions of remaining aloof and cutting themselves off socially and emotionally from others.
   - A confused state of mind reflected in their attitude and actions, demonstrating a considerable lack of time sense, wandering here and there aimlessly, distortion in their perceptual and judgmental ability, and failure to recognize people (even close relatives and family members) and places (even their homes).
   - Becoming increasingly uncomfortable at night and taking frequent naps during the day.

4. In the latest phase of the disorder, patients are found to become fully dependent on other people, needing constant care for their safety and living.

Identification and Diagnosis of Alzheimer's Disease Disorder

The American Psychiatric Association has provided the following criteria for the identification and diagnosis of Alzheimer's disease disorder in the DSM IV TR, as shown in Table 17.4.

Table 17.4 Diagnostic Criteria for Alzheimer's Disease Disorder

A. The development of multiple cognitive deficits manifested by both
(i) memory impairment (impaired ability to learn new information or to recall previously learned information)
(ii) One (or more) of the following cognitive disturbances:
(a) Aphasia (language disturbance); (b) apraxia (impaired ability to carry out motor activities despite intact motor function; (c) agnosia (failure to recognize or identify objects despite intact sensory function); (d) disturbance in executive functioning (i.e., planning, organizing, sequencing, abstracting)
B. The cognitive deficits in criteria A (i) and A (ii) each cause significant impairment in social or occupational functioning and represent a significant decline from a previous level of functioning.
C. The course is characterized by gradual onset and continuing cognitive decline.

(Continued)

Table 17.4 (Continued)

D. The cognitive deficits in Criteria A (i) and A (ii) are not due to any of the following:
  • Other central nervous system conditions that cause progressive deficits in memory
    and cognition (e.g., cerebrovascular disease, Parkinson's disease, Huntington's disease,
    subdural hematoma, normal pressure hydrocephalus, brain tumor)
  • Systematic conditions that are known to cause dementia (e.g., hypothyroidism, vitamin
    B12 or folic acid deficiency, niacin deficiency, hypercalcemia, neurosyphilis, HIV infection)
  • Substance-induced conditions
E. The deficits do not occur exclusively during the course of a delirium
F. The disturbance is not better accounted for another Axis I disorder (e.g., Major
    depressive disorder, Schizophrenia)

Source: APA (2000) DSM-IV-TR

Factors Responsible for Causing Alzheimer's Disease

Alzheimer's disease is caused by a combination of genetic and environmental factors that affect
the brain over time. Let us look into this.

The Role of Genetic Factors

The hereditary transmission in the form of defective genes plays a great role in the causation of
Alzheimer's disease. In playing their roles in this direction, the different types of genes are said
to be responsible for giving rise to early-onset and late-onset types of Alzheimer's disease in the
way described as follows (Comer, 2015:621):

(i) The early-onset type of Alzheimer's disease can be caused by abnormalities in the genes
responsible for the production of two proteins—the *beta-amyloid precursor protein*
(beta-APP) and the *presenilin* protein. However, in the case of the late-onset type of Alzheimer's disease, a gene called the *apolipoprotein* E (ApoE), located on chromosome 19
(and particularly its ApoE-4 form) is normally responsible for the excessive formation of
beta-amyloid proteins.

(ii) The production of these proteins by their respective genes, in both cases, results in spurring
of the formation of plaques and in turn, the breakdown of the tau protein, the formation of
numerous tangles, and the death of many neurons, leading to the onset of one or the other
types of Alzheimer's disease.

The Role of Environmental Factors

Hereditary or genetic factors alone are not the exclusive factors for the causation and development of Alzheimer's or other similar neurocognitive degenerative disorders of old age. Environmental factors of one or the other nature, listed ahead, may also play significant roles in the
causation and precipitation of these disorders.

1. **Past head trauma:** The trauma caused by an accident, stroke, or head injury may play a great
   part in the damage or loss of brain cells responsible for the causation of Alzheimer's disease.
2. **Acute exposure to and poisoning with heavy metals and pesticides:** Acute exposure and
   poisoning with heavy metals and pesticides, such as the long-term exposure and accumulation of lead and aluminum, has been found responsible for the causation and development of
   Alzheimer's and other neurodegenerative disorders.

3. **Air pollution:** Exposure to polluted air containing a toxic cocktail of organic and non-organic compounds, metals, and gases may also work toward the causation and development of Alzheimer's disease.

4. **Unhealthy lifestyle:** There may be other negative factors in one's lifestyle that may be held responsible for the causation and development of Alzheimer's disease and other related neurodegenerative disorders. These may be named as:

   - Lack of physical activity and exercise
   - Obesity
   - Poor sleep patterns, such as difficulty falling asleep or staying asleep
   - Smoking or substance abuse
   - Poor nutrition and unhealthy dietary intake.

5. **Poor health and fatal diseases:** Poor health conditions and fatal diseases such as high blood pressure, heart disease, poorly controlled type 2 diabetes, chronic infection, and medical conditions including HIV infection, meningitis, and advanced syphilis may work as potent causes for the initiation and perpetuation of Alzheimer's disease.

6. **Psychological Factors:** A number of psychological factors inducing a high level of anxiety, depression, and stress among individuals, particularly among the aged, prove quite fatal to their health and well-being, increasing the probability of them being affected by Alzheimer's disease and other types of neurocognitive disorders.

Treatment of Alzheimer's Disease

Treatment of the patients of Alzheimer's disease and other similar neurocognitive disorders involving dementia may involve a combination of different treatment measures depending on the onset stage, causation, and seriousness of the disorder. In this connection, the treatments in a general way may involve important measures and approaches such as medication or drug therapy, cognitive therapy, behavioral therapy, and sociocultural therapy. Let us look into them in brief.

Medication or Drug Therapy

The initial care and treatment of Alzheimer's patients in the early mild stage of the disease generally begins with the introduction of some useful and well-tested drugs (meant for helping in their difficulties related to memory, cognition, and communication), such as:

(i) tacrine—trade name *cognex*, (ii) donepezil—trade name *aricept*, (iii) rivastigmine—trade name *exelon*, (iv) galantamine—trade name *reminyl*, and (v) memantine—trade name *namenda*.

Clinicians are also seen to prescribe vitamin E tablets or capsules along with prescribed drugs to help slow down further cognitive decline among people suffering from Alzheimer's disease.

Cognitive Therapy

There is a considerable loss of brain cells related to memory, reasoning, and judgment in cases of Alzheimer's patients. The techniques used in cognitive therapy are carried out for dealing with this deficiency. For this purpose, efforts are made to carry on specific cognitive activities, including computer-based cognitive stimulation programs aimed at helping Alzheimer's patients in the rehabilitation of those brain parts linked to memory, reasoning, and judgment.

Behavioral Therapy

The use of behavioral therapy in the case of treating Alzheimer's patients is found to involve a number of useful behavior modification and management techniques, such as modeling, role-playing, operant conditioning, and reinforcing the appropriate behavior of the patients. In their application, each of these techniques alone or in combination are focused on providing the needed behavioral intervention to help improve specific symptoms displayed by Alzheimer's patients, such as wandering at night, loss of bladder control, demands for attention, and inadequate personal care. In addition to providing such behavioral interventions to patients, efforts are also initiated for providing behavioral therapy assistance for family members and caregivers of Alzheimer's patients for helping them to cope with the distress, fatigue, and difficulties resulting on account of their attention, time, and energy taking care of the Alzheimer's patients.

Sociocultural Therapy

Sociocultural environment plays an important role in the care, treatment, and rehabilitation of Alzheimer's patients. Some of the efforts made in this direction can be outlined as follows:

- Establishment of suitable daycare facilities with the objective of providing treatment programs and activities for outpatients during the day and returning them to their homes and families at night.
- Establishment of needed facilities in the form of community centers, boarding and lodging houses, and recreation clubs including the presence of well-trained assistive personnel for helping Alzheimer's patients enjoy a caring environment, receive assistance in their treatment, and take part in various activities that bring joy and stimulation to their lives.
- To establish help centers on call at police stations and NGO offices for locating patients who may wander off, for their security and safe return to their homes. The developed technology may also be utilized for tracking the positions of wandering patients in the form of equipping them with GPS trackers tied to their wrists or kept in their shoes.

After this necessary discussion about the most pronounced disease or disorder associated with dementia, let us now have a brief look into the nature and characteristics of some other similar neurocognitive disorders and diseases faced by older people.

To Sum Up

Alzheimer's disease is known for giving birth to a particular type of dementia, known as "Dementia of the Alzheimer's type," symptomizing a great loss of memory on the part of affected individuals. In the case of Alzheimer's disease, the region of the brain called the hippocampus (the center of learning and memory) is adversely affected on account of the damage or loss of brain cells belonging to this region, resulting in great loss of memory. It is a progressive degenerative disease that develops over the years with more deterioration in the memory and subsequent loss in the overall functioning of the patients. In the latest phase of their disorder, patients are found to become fully dependent on other people, needing constant care for their safety and living.

Hereditary transmission in the form of defective genes plays a great role in the causation of Alzheimer's disease. However, hereditary or genetic factors alone are not the exclusive factors for the causation and development of Alzheimer's disease. Environmental factors such as past head trauma, acute exposure to and poisoning with heavy metals and pesticides, air pollution, unhealthy lifestyle, poor health, fatal diseases, and psychological factors like high levels of anxiety, depression, and stress may also play significant roles in the causation and precipitation of Alzheimer's disease.

Treatment of patients with Alzheimer's disease may involve a combination of different treatment measures and approaches including medication or drug therapy, cognitive therapy, behavioral therapy, and sociocultural therapy.

Vascular Dementia

In terms of its formal definition, Vascular dementia may be considered a general term describing problems with one's cognitive abilities such as reasoning, planning, judgment, memory, and other thought processes caused by brain damage from impaired blood flow to one's specific areas of the brain. This impairment of blood flow is concerned with the process of cutting off the flow of blood to the areas of the brain responsible for carrying out specific cognitive functions, including memory and reasoning, on account of one or the other conditions such as the following:

1. *Blockage or damage of brain artery:* A cerebrovascular accident or stroke may result in blocking or damaging a brain artery responsible for the flow of blood in one or the other specific regions of the brain.
2. *Narrowing or chronic damage to brain blood vessels:* Conditions that narrow or inflict long-term damage on one's brain blood vessels may also lead to vascular dementia. These conditions may be caused by factors like the natural process of aging, abnormal aging of blood vessels (atherosclerosis), high blood pressure, high cholesterol, smoking, diabetes, and brain hemorrhage.

In its effect and outcome, vascular dementia is widely considered the second most common cause of dementia after Alzheimer's disease, accounting for five to ten percent of cases. Like Alzheimer's disease, this disorder is also progressive and is often found to coexist with Alzheimer's disease. However, it differs from Alzheimer's disease in the following manner:

- The symptoms related to vascular dementia begin suddenly rather than gradually.
- The person's cognitive functioning may continue to be normal in areas of the brain that have not been affected by the stroke, in contrast to the broad cognitive deficiencies usually displayed by Alzheimer's patients.

To Sum Up

Vascular dementia may be considered a general term describing problems with one's cognitive abilities including memory and other thought processes resulting on account of (i) blockage or damage of brain arteries from a cerebrovascular accident or stroke or (ii) narrowing or chronic damage of the brain blood vessels due to aging, high blood pressure, high cholesterol, smoking, diabetes, and brain hemorrhage. In its effect and outcome, vascular dementia is widely considered the second most common cause of dementia after Alzheimer's disease.

Pick's Disease

Pick's disease is a rare neurological condition or disorder possessing uniqueness in affecting two important parts or lobes of the brain—frontal and temporal—at the same time. This is why it is also known as *Frontotemporal neurocognitive disorder or disease*. In its medical and physical consequences, it much resembles Alzheimer's disease but can be distinguished from it during autopsy. Some of the well-known distinctive features of Pick's disease can be summarized as follows:

(i)   It results in cortical dementia similar to that of Alzheimer's disease.
(ii) In its scope and dimension, it is found to affect about five percent of the overall population suffering from dementia.
(iii) The course of this disease is believed to last from five to ten years.
(iv) Its cause is still unknown despite collaborated research findings and individual attempts.
(v)   Like Huntington's disease, Pick's disease usually occurs relatively early in life, during a person's 40s or 50s, and is therefore considered an example of pre-senile dementia (Durand and Barlow, 2013:520).

To Sum Up

Pick's Disease, also known as *Frontotemporal neurocognitive disorder or disease*, is a rare neurological condition or disorder that possesses uniqueness in affecting two important parts or lobes of the brain—frontal and temporal—at the same time. Pick's disease usually occurs relatively early in life, during a person's 40s or 50s, and is therefore considered an example of pre-senile dementia.

Parkinson's Disease

Parkinson's disease is a degenerative brain disorder or disease that creates a number of motor and behavioral problems to affected individuals in a slow and progressive way, as characterized here:

• Symptoms begin gradually, often with a barely noticeable tremor in just one hand.
• The progression of symptoms is often a bit different from one person to another due to the diversity of the disease. However, in general, the tremors become common and are followed

by other motor problems such as stooped posture, slow body movements, tremors, jerkiness in walking and gait, balance problems, loss of automatic movements and reflex actions, and slowing down of the voice, resulting in hesitation and speaking in a soft monotone.

Parkinson's Disease

A degenerative neurocognitive disorder or disease that creates a number of motor and behavioral problems to affected individuals in a slow and progressive way.

- In a long run, people affected with Parkinson's disease are generally found to develop sub-cortical dementia. It is estimated that 75% of people who survive more than 10 years with Parkinson's disease develop sub-cortical dementia (Durand and Barlow, 2013:519).
- Parkinson's disease is found to come with a number of complications, such as thinking difficulties, depression and emotional changes, swallowing problems, chewing and eating problems, sleep problems and sleep disorders, bladder problems, constipation, blood pressure changes, and sexual dysfunction.
- Treatment options vary and may include medications and surgery. There is no permanent cure for this disease. However, the course of the disease and treatment varies widely, with some individuals functioning well with treatment.

What happens to Parkinson's patients with regard to their motor problems is said to be the result of the damage to the pathways of a neurotransmitter named dopamine. These can be damaged on account of the adverse impact of Parkinson's disease on the dopamine-producing neurons in a specific area of the brain called *substantia nigra*. Because dopamine is involved in complex movement, a reduction in this neurotransmitter makes affected individuals increasingly unable to control their muscle movements, which leads to tremors and other difficulties and problems related to movement.

To Sum Up

Parkinson's Disease is a slowly progressing degenerative brain disorder or disease that creates a number of motor and behavioral problems to affected individuals, resulting in a lot of difficulties in their motor functioning, including their proper speaking. In the long run, people affected by Parkinson's disease are generally found to develop sub-cortical dementia and a number of complications in their health and cognitive as well as social functioning. Treatment options vary and include medications and surgery. However, there is no permanent cure for this disease.

Huntington's Disease

Huntington's disease (HD) is a fatal genetic disorder that causes the progressive breakdown of nerve cells (neurons) in the brain. Certain neurons appear to be more vulnerable to damage in

HD. In later phases of the disease, other regions of the brain are also affected. Damaging of the brain cells in one or the other areas of the brain is responsible for causing motor, cognitive, and psychological problems among affected individuals. As a progressive disease, these problems increase gradually over many years until the death of the individual.

In its initial stage, Huntington's disease affects one's motor movements,

> **Huntington's Disease**
>
> A fatal dementia-related genetic neurocognitive disorder and disease that causes the progressive damaging of the neurons, resulting in a number of problems associated with motor, cognitive, and psychological functioning of affected individuals.

typically in the form of *chorea*, involuntary limb movements. Later on, the movement problems become very problematic, such as severe twitching and spasms. In the years that follow, cognitive and psychiatric problems may also surface in considerable amounts. Just as with Parkinson's disease, the persons affected with this disease may also display dementia of the subcortical type.

In its full bloom, a person affected by Huntington's disease manifests visible symptoms of a triad of motor, cognitive, and psychiatric disorders mentioned as follows.

Motor or Movement disorders associated with both involuntary movement problems and impairments in voluntary movements, such as (i) involuntary jerking or writhing movements (chorea), (ii) muscle problems, such as rigidity or muscle contracture (dystonia), (iii) slow or abnormal eye movements, (iv) impaired gait, posture, and balance and (v) difficulty with the physical production of speech or swallowing.

Cognitive disorders involving cognitive impairments or difficulties such as (i) difficulty organizing, prioritizing or focusing on tasks, (ii) lack of flexibility or the tendency to get stuck on a thought, behavior or action (perseveration), (iii) lack of impulse control that can result in outbursts, acting without thinking, and sexual promiscuity, (iv) lack of awareness of one's own behaviors and abilities, (v) slowness in processing thoughts or "finding" words, and (vi) difficulty in learning new information.

Psychiatric disorders involving Depression (visible through the symptoms like feelings of sadness, apathy, irritability, social withdrawal, insomnia, fatigue, loss of energy, and frequent thoughts of death or suicide) as a major common disorder accompanied by some other psychiatric disorders like Obsessive-compulsive disorder, Mania and Bipolar disorder.

In addition to the aforementioned symptoms, weight loss is common in people with Huntington's disease, especially as the disease progresses.

Regarding the causation of Huntington's disease, it is said to be caused by an inherited defect in a single exceptional gene belonging to chromosome 4. It has also been well established through ongoing researches that this disease is inherited in an autosomal dominant fashion, so that each child of an affected parent has a 50% chance of developing the disease. Symptoms usually appear between the ages of 30 to 50, and worsen over a 10 to 25-year period, adversely affecting the individual's ability to reason, walk, and speak, and developing serious complications for his or her health and living. Eventually, a person with Huntington's disease requires help with all the activities of daily living and care. Late in the disease, he or she will likely be confined to a bed and unable to speak.

Medications are available to help manage the symptoms of Huntington's disease. It is said to be incurable in the sense that the provided treatments cannot prevent the physical, mental, and behavioral decline associated with the condition.

To Sum Up

Huntington's disease is a fatal genetic disorder that causes the progressive damaging of the nerve cells, resulting in a number of problems associated with motor, cognitive, and psychological functioning of affected individuals. Just as with Parkinson's disease, the persons affected with this disease may also display dementia of the subcortical type. Huntington's disease is said to be inherited in an autosomal dominant fashion, so that each child of an affected parent has a 50% chance of developing the disease. Symptoms usually appear between the ages of 30 to 50, and worsen over a 10 to 25-year period to the extent of the total dependence of the patient on others. It is incurable but proper medication and looking after may help in managing the symptoms and problems of the patients.

Review Questions

1. What are neurocognitive disorders? Name the disorders categorized as neurocognitive disorders in the DSM-5.
2. What is delirium? State its distinguishing features and throw light on its identification and diagnosis in light of the criteria laid down by the APA in its DSM-IV-TR.
3. Discuss the underlying causes and treatment of delirium.
4. What do you understand by the term dementia? Throw light on its characteristic features and describe its diagnosis and identification in light of the criteria laid down by the APA in its DSM-5.
5. What are delirium and dementia? How do they differ from each other? Discuss.
6. What is dementia? Discuss its different types and throw light on its underlying causes.
7. What is Alzheimer's disease? Tell about its distinctive symptoms and diagnosis in light of the criteria laid down by the APA in its DSM-IV-TR.
8. Describe the factors responsible for causing Alzheimer's disease and throw light on its treatment.
9. What is vascular dementia? How is it caused?
10. While differentiating vascular dementia from Alzheimer's disease, describe its effects and outcomes.
11. What is Pick's disease? Throw light on its distinctive features and outcomes.
12. What is Huntington's disease? Tell about its distinctive symptoms.
13. Throw light on the causation and treatment of Huntington's disease.

References

American Psychiatric Association (2000), *The diagnostic and statistical manual of mental disorders, DSM-IV-TR*, Washington, DC: American Psychiatric Association.

American Psychiatric Association (2013), *The diagnostic and statistical manual of mental disorders, DSM-IV-TR*, Washington, DC: American Psychiatric Association

Comer, R. J. (2015), *Abnormal psychology* (9th ed.), New York, NY: Worth Publishers (A Macmillan Education Imprint).

D'Avolio, D. (2018), Case study: Delirium in an older hospitalized woman, *NIDUS, Network for Investigation of Delirium: Unifying Scientists*, retrieved from https://deliriumnetwork.org/case-study-delirium-in-an-older-hospitalized-woman/

Durand, V. M., & Barlow, D. H. (2013), *Essentials of abnormal psychology* (6th ed.), Belmont, CA: Wadsworth.

Knight, B. G. (1996), *Psychology with the older adults* (2nd ed.), Thousand Oaks, CA: SAGE.

Kring, A. M., Johnson, S. L., Davison, G. C., & Neale, J. M. (2012), *Abnormal psychology* (12th ed.), New York, NY: John Wiley & Sons, Inc.

Yoo, H., Choi, W. H., Jung, W. S., Park, Y. H, Lee, C. U, & Lim, H. K (2017), A case report of a 37 year old male patient of the dementia of the Alzheimer's type, *Psychiatry Investigation*, retrieved from www.ncbi.nlm.nih.gov/pmc/articles/PMC5561413/

Clinical Assessment (Non-Testing Devices)

What is Clinical Assessment?

The term clinical assessment stands for a type of assessment carried out for serving clinical purposes—for knowing about or diagnosing a problem. As a clinical psychologist, you will need it to provide assistance for understanding the mental health problem or treating the mental illness or disorder of your client/patient. Whenever a client

Clinical Assessment

The assessment of the strengths and weaknesses of the client and his functioning in cognitive, emotional, and behavioral areas, and the nature of his mental health problem, aimed at planning his treatment and its follow up from time to time.

turns themselves in to the clinic for the treatment of his mental health problem, illness or disorder (i.e., difficulty in remembering, sleeping disorder, or experiencing acute anxiety, stress, or depression), your first requirement will be to conduct the needed assessment of the nature of his problem (in terms of its kind or type and degree of its seriousness), and the nature of the client (in terms of his abilities and capacities, interests and attitudes, personality makeup, and cognitive and behavioral functioning) for planning and initiating the process of treatment. Thinking in this way, we can term the process of clinical assessment as a way of understanding the client and his problem for the purpose of initiating the treatment process. The assessment work carried out by you in this concern, thus, may be needed on your part to help in answering the following questions:

DOI: 10.4324/9781003398325-18

1. What type of problem or difficulty is the client experiencing at present, as reported by him and his companions, and what are the signs or symptoms apparently visible in this concern regarding his body and behavior?
2. What name or classification can be provided to his problem on the basis of what has been reported by him and his companions, along with the symptoms apparently visible and the actual assessment work carried out by you in this concern?
3. What might be the most possible causes lying behind the problem?
4. What type of treatment will be suitable in view of the nature of the problem and the client himself?
5. Is the treatment given to the client working well? Should it be continued or not?

For getting answers to such queries in the interest of fulfilling your responsibilities as a clinical psychologist, you certainly need to engage in the process of clinical assessment—knowing about the client and his mental health problem by making use of one or the other methods and measures of clinical assessment. These may include (i) observation of the signs and symptoms, (ii) case history, (iii) the informal as well as the formal diagnostic interview, (iv) psychological testing with the use of tests like intelligence tests, achievement tests, personality tests, attitude scales, adjustment inventory, anxiety test, self-esteem assessment, and (v) neuropsychological testing.

The methods and measures listed subsequently may be utilized in clinical assessment on the part of clinical psychologists in deriving the needed information.

- *Information about the client:* His level of achievement in academic areas such as mathematics and language, level of performance in skilled areas, abilities and capacities, interests and attitudes, communication and interpersonal skills, personality characteristics, adjustment to self and others, cognitive, emotional, and behavioral functioning, his environmental setup in terms of his family environment, relationships, community and cultural background, ethnicity and language spoken, and so on.
- *Information about the problem:* The visible and non-visible symptoms related to the problem, naming and classification of the problem, and the nature of the problem in terms of its kind, intensity and seriousness.
- *Information about the suitability of the applied treatment*: The assessment or evaluation of the applied treatment is also helpful in furnishing data or information about its appropriateness or weakness. It can be ascertained by making comparison between the two separate assessment measures, one taken at the start of the treatment and the second after some time in the treatment process or at the time when the treatment is over.

In light of what has been said earlier, we may now derive a formal comprehensive definition of the term clinical assessment in the manner as follows:

Clinical assessment refers to an array of methods and measures used by clinical psychologists to make assessment or evaluation of the strengths and weaknesses of the client and his functioning in cognitive, emotional, and behavioral areas, and the nature of his mental health problem in terms of its kind/type and seriousness aimed not only to plan and a treatment process but also to plan its follow up from time to time.

Needs and Purposes Served by Clinical Assessment

The task of clinical assessment performed on the part of clinical psychologists is aimed to provide effective treatment to the client (in its individualized way) suiting him and the nature of his problem. In this sense, it may serve the various needs and purposes of clinical psychologists and other mental health professionals (helping in the treatment task) as well as clients and their well-wishers (benefitted through the treatment) in the manner as detailed below.

1. *Knowing the client in its various aspects of functioning*: It is quite essential to know and understand the client with regard to his strengths and limitations in terms of his cognitive, emotional, and behavioral functioning in his day-to-day life. This can be ascertained through the use of appropriate assessment techniques that can suitably help the clinical psychologist to find appropriate treatment means for dealing with the problem of the client.

2. *Acquainting with the nature of the problem felt by the client:* Any treatment planned for the problem depends on the nature of the problem and it is the assessment or diagnosis that can help a treatment giver in knowing well about the nature of the problem in terms of its classification and degree of seriousness.

3. *Drawing conclusions about the possible causes underlying the problem*: The prevention as well treatment of the problem can be carried out if one knows the possible causes underlying the problem. The conclusions derived from the assessment data may help well in listing out the possible underlying causes leading one to plan the remedy or treatment in tune with the possibility of the emergence of the problem.

4. *Predicting the possibility of improvement:* With the information available on the nature of the client, his problem and the underlying causes with the courtesy of the clinical assessment it become possible to predict the possibility of improvement in the client's condition regarding his cognitive, emotional, or behavioral problem motivating or readying the clinical psychologists for going ahead in the treatment of the client.

5. *Helping in the attainment of insight:* The other useful purpose served through the data available though clinical assessment is helping the concerned persons in the attainment of essential insight. Accordingly, we may see the client gain essential insight in knowing and understanding his self in the context of his felt problem. The cooperation rendered to the therapist in his treatment is more often the positive outcome of such insight gained. Similarly, the clinical psychologists also gain essential insight into the client and his problem through the conclusions derived through the clinical assessment and it helps him well in the planning and implementation of a suitable treatment for his client.

6. *Making decisions about the treatment given to the client:* Assessment of the nature of the client and his problem sets everything regarding the planning and processing of a treatment. The story on this account may begin in the form of making decisions on the part of clinical psychologists in the form of whether some type of treatment is to be planned for the client. While assessing the client and his problem (through his reporting, observation, informal interview, and visible symptoms), they can come to the conclusion that no long-term treatment is needed and the problem can be solved by talking to the client for a while about his felt problem or issue. In case, when the initial assessment findings reveal the necessity of introducing a treatment, they then try to introduce an organized program of clinical assessment for knowing what type of treatment will work best for the client in view of the type and seriousness of his problem. It may help them in adopting one or the other types of

psychotherapies in their single or eclectic ways. For some clients and their problems, here they may sometime require forwarding serious cases to psychiatrists and neurologists for the required medical treatment. The assessment can, thus, help the clinical psychologists to figure out what is suitable for the client in terms of dealing with his problem.

7. *Knowing about whether or not the treatment is working and making decisions about its continuance*: The follow up of a treatment is as essential as its planning and processing. The need for assessing the client, need of further assessing, thus, may be increasingly felt on the part of clinical psychologists for knowing the progress of the treatment given to the client. How he was before the introduction of the treatment, and how he is now at present in terms of the assessment results; findings like these can be availed with the help of the critical assessment. In case there is progress noted in the condition of the client, we may continue the introduced treatment, or otherwise, we may consider some other alternative. In this way, assessment may be termed as a necessary as well as essential condition for the planning, implementation, and follow up of any treatment scheme for dealing with the problem of the client in the form of a continuous ongoing process.

To Sum Up

The term clinical assessment stands for a type of assessment carried out on the part of clinical psychologists for serving the clinical purpose—knowing about the client and his mental health problem by making use of one or the other methods and measures of clinical assessment such as observation of the signs and symptoms, case history, diagnostic interview, and use of various types of psychological tests. It helps the clinicians in deriving the needed information or data for serving purposes such as (i) knowing the client in his various aspects of functioning, (ii) acquainting with the nature of the problem felt by the client, (iii) drawing a conclusion about the possible causes underlying the problem, (iv) predicting the possibility of improvement, (v) planning and implementing a suitable treatment for the client, and (vi) knowing about whether or not the treatment is working and making a decision about its continuance.

Ways and Methods of Clinical Assessment

The task of clinical assessment performed by clinical psychologists for helping their clients in dealing with their mental health problems requires well organized, thoughtful attempts in the forms of adopting a number of assessment methods and measures, broadly categorized as (i) Non-Testing devices and (ii) Testing devices. Whereas in the category of non-testing devices, we can include the devices and means of observation, interview, and case history, the means such as various types of testing devices in the names of psychological tests, achievement tests, and neurological tests are frequently employed for the purpose of clinical assessment on the part of clinical psychologists. In this chapter, we discuss the former while leaving the discussion of the latter for the upcoming Chapter 19. Let us try to do this.

Observation as a Method of Clinical Assessment

For knowing and understanding the nature of the abnormality in one's behavior, including states of mental illness and disorder, the systematic observation of this behavior in its natural setting may prove an effective assessment measure on the part of clinical psychologists. Assessment through behavioral observation in its actual practice, thus, consists of the direct systematic observation of a target behavior (i.e., disruptive or delinquent behavior, obsessive-compulsive behavior, anxiety-ridden or phobic behavior) of the affected individual in their natural environment (at the site or the situation in which it is taking place in day-to-

---

Naturalistic Observation Method

The assessment method in which the clinical psychologists try to observe and record the occurrence of the behavior of the client in its natural setting in a systematic way for having a needed assessment of his problematic target behavior.

---

day life) for taking stock of its nature in terms of its causation, characteristics, intensity, and consequences.

The nature of observation made in the use of the systematic observation method for the clinical assessment of a problem behavior differs a lot from our routine observation in daily life. It is quite systematic as well as objective in its processing and outcomes. We can get valuable quantitative as well as qualitative information about one or the other aspects of the individual's target behavior taking place in its natural, usual way in his routine daily life for its proper clinical assessment. Moreover, the information we get from such direct observation of the target problem behavior can help us in providing a far more accurate assessment of the behavior than that available to us by merely asking the client to recall or summarize it verbally during an interview or on a questionnaire. Besides this, in a situation where for a particular problem behavior, its observation in the natural setting is not possible, clinical psychologists may arrange an analogue observation, in which they attempt to replicate the real-world setting in the clinic and observe the client's responses there (Haynes and Kaholokula, 2008). In this way, we may find the use of observation as a method of behavioral assessment as a quite convenient, plausible, and useful method for the assessment of one or the other problematic or abnormal behaviors of the client.

How to Make Use of Observation as a Method of Behavioral Assessment?

The systematic procedure for this purpose may run as follows.

1. *Be specific about the target behavior:* First, be clear about the target problem or abnormal behavior that is to be assessed. It needs to be properly identified and operationally defined for its appropriate objective observation.
2. *Have a proper observation of the target behavior in a systematic way:* Once the target behavior is identified, it should be subjected to a properly systematic observation of its occurrence in its real-life settings by considering factors such as the following:

   - The client should not have any idea that his behavior is under observation. As far as possible, observation should be made in a naturalistic condition for deriving the sample of the target problem behavior occurring in its most natural and spontaneous way.
   - The recording of information or data needed for the assessment of the target behavior should always be done at the time of the observer making observation of the behavior.

The failure to do so proves quite costly, as the observer may forget or miss some or the other important things or links regarding the observed behavior. It is always better to use recording devices or prepare a checklist for tallying things to be observed in one's behavior during the observation. This process may require on the part of observers tallying the frequency, duration, or intensity of the target behavior across the specified time periods.

- During the observation of the target behavior aimed at its clinical assessment, the observers should try to access "the ABCs of behavior," meaning that they should try to take care of the:

  - Antecedents (what precedes before the occurrence of the target behavior in the form of the environmental events or stimuli triggering the behavior)
  - Behavior (what the client thinks, feels, says, and does in the execution of the target behavior)
  - Consequences (things occurring after the occurrence of the target behavior).

- It is not proper to rely on the results of a single observation of the client's behavior for making decisions about the characteristics of the target behavior. For a desirable objectivity, reliability, and validity, such observation work must be repeated by the same observer for a desirable number of times, or it should be carried out by a number of different observers (including the family members, friends, or the client himself). In addition, help may also be taken from the task done in the form of self-monitoring (measuring and recording one's own ABCs of the target behavior) on the part of the client.

- The observation work must be carried out properly in an effective way on the part of the observers in both the audio and visual modes by making use of effective audio-visual instruments, such as telescopes, cameras, audio-video recording devices, smart phones, laptops, and other technological means helpful not only in the automatic recording of the events but also for proper analysis, interpretation, and conclusions drawn from the recorded information about the target behavior.

To Sum Up

Assessment through the use of the observation method consists of the direct systematic observation of a target behavior (i.e., disruptive, anxiety-ridden or phobic behavior) of the affected individual in their natural environment (at the site or the situation in which it is taking place in day-to-day life) for taking stock of its nature, in terms of its causation, characteristics, intensity, and consequences.

In this observation, care is to be taken for deriving the necessary information about the target behavior occurring in its most natural and spontaneous way (without letting the client know) by making use of the technological means for observing and recording the observed events. In making such observations, observers should try to access the ABCs of behavior, meaning that they should consider the *Antecedents* (what precedes the occurrence of the target behavior), things occurring in the *occurrence of the Behavior*, and *Consequences* (things occurring after the occurrence of the target behavior).

Case History as a Method of Clinical Assessment

In its meaning, the term case history stands for the history of the case. The term case in our real life is used in a variety of senses, such as a case being argued in a court of law, or the disposal of a case by the concerned official of a department. In the world of medicine and clinical psychology, it is used for the patient/client as well as the health problem experienced on the part of a patient/client. The term history, on the other hand, stands for the description of the past and present of a thing in its detailed and comprehensive way. Acquainting well with the history of the case, in all walks of our life, thus may be seen to provide great help in dealing with the case in hand in a proper way.

It is in this context that when you visit a doctor in connection with the treatment of a health problem; he tries to collect information from you and the other available sources about the past and present of your problem along with the necessary background data of yours (by studying you and your problem as a single case) before taking any further steps for the diagnosis and treatment of your problem.

The same is equally true for the visits carried out for mental health problems. Here, it is also quite usual on the part of clinical psychologists to make use of the case history method for collecting information and data for knowing and understanding the past and present of the client and his felt problem in the needed way helpful in the diagnosis and treatment of the target problem behavior.

As a matter of its formal definition, we can, thus, term the case history method as a method of clinical assessment in which we try to have a detailed and in-depth study of the client and his problem as a single case with the help of the necessary data collected in this concern from his past and present in the real life context directed toward introducing necessary interventions and measures for dealing with his felt problem.

How to Make Use of Case History as a Method of Clinical Assessment

Mental health professionals and clinical psychologists can proceed as follows for making use of case history for the needed assessment and diagnosis of a mental health problem of a client aimed at its proper cure and treatment.

1. As a first step, the mental health problem is to be clearly defined in the form of a particular case being studied in terms of its historical aspect (past and present) on the part of clinical psychologists.
2. In compiling the case history related to the client and his problem, the clinical psychologists should try to exploit all the available resources and make use of as many methods and ways (such as direct observation, administration of questionnaire, and conducting interviews with the client, his family members, teachers, the family physicians, friends and other acquaintances, as well as viewing the available records and documents in the form of diaries, personal notes, letters photographs, notes, appraisal and medical reports etc.) for collecting relevant information and data related to the past and present of the client and his problem, of the nature as follows:

   - *Information about the client's background* including his age, gender, work, food habits, sleeping patterns, daily routine, health status, drug and alcohol history, physical, emotional and social development, medical, educational, and vocational history, motivations, goals, aspirations, conflicts, frustrations and depressions, life challenges and difficulties, coping skills and weaknesses related to his past and present.

- *Information on the client's family background* including family physical and mental health history, relationships prevailing in the family, educational, economical and social status of the family, problems and difficulties faced, the coping capabilities or weaknesses supportive or non supportive to the client in reference to their past and present.

- *Information about the client's problem* including the visible and non-visible signs and symptoms, its classification into a specific category per specification of the latest version of the DSM and ICD, history of its emergence and present status, the details about any screening or diagnostic measures taken for knowing about its nature in terms of kinds, intensity and seriousness, and underlying causes and plausible treatment methods or approaches.

- *Information about the present happenings* including what is occurring at present in his everyday life in respect to his own living and adjustment, family, and social relationships, occupational and professional adjustment, and the motivations, aspirations, and levels of anxiety, frustrations or stresses faced by him on one or the other accounts.

3. In the last step, clinical psychologists try to analyze the contents of the information or data collected about the past and present of the client and his felt problem for drawing necessary conclusions helpful in the needed clinical assessment and diagnosis of the problem, and interpreting its underlying causes and plausible treatment measures for effectively dealing with the problem of the client.

To Sum Up

In making use of case history as a method of clinical assessment, clinicians try to have a detailed and in-depth study of the client and his problem as a single case with the help of the necessary data collected in this concern from his past and present in the real-life context directed toward introducing necessary interventions and measures for dealing with his felt problem. For this purpose, clinicians try to exploit all the available resources and make use of many methods and ways for collecting information about the client's personal background, his family background, his problem, and happenings with him at present, and then go for drawing necessary conclusions helpful in the needed clinical assessment and diagnosis of the problem aimed at planning for the treatment of the problem.

Interview as a Method of Clinical Assessment

Interview as a method of clinical assessment represents a way of collecting relevant information on the part of a trained clinical psychologist from the client by putting appropriate questions to him in this regard and then make him feel comfortable to tell freely about himself and the felt problem during one or a series of episodes consisting of face-to-face interactions and dialogue taking place between the clinical psychologist and client.

The success of interview as a method utilized for clinical assessment depends upon factors such as

A. The competency of the clinical psychologist as an interviewer
B. The appropriateness of the format of the interview
C. The appropriateness of the interview setting and way of conducting the interview.

Let us know about them in detail.

A. The Competency of the Clinical Psychologist as an Interviewer

The key component in the success of a clinical interview as a method of clinical assessment is none other than the clinical psychologist himself. Everything in this regard depends on his competency and skill in conducting the clinical interview. The necessary training for this purpose needs to be essentially given to them at the time of their education and preparation as a clinical psychologist. On one's part, a clinical psychologist for this purpose should try to equip themself with the characteristics, skills, and competencies listed ahead.

The Skill of Establishing Rapport with the Client

The establishment of proper rapport in the form of developing a comfortable positive working relationship with clients on the part of the clinical psychologist is quite essential for the successful execution of the clinical interview. When the client feels connected and assured, he tends to disclose more information and feel at home while taking part in the interview process. Therefore, clinical psychologists should try to establish proper rapport with the client at the time of the clinical interview, much in the same way as done on their part while introducing a psychotherapeutic treatment.

The Skill of Being Self-Aware and Making Good Impressions on the Clients

The clinical psychologist as interviewer should try to be equipped with the characteristics of being self-aware of his strengths and limitations for being adequately prepared to maximize this capacity, tend to his affect, and impress others interpersonally for winning their confidence and having useful interactions with them. Accordingly, he is able to maintain an impressive personality and mannerism by caring for his look, voice, gestures, mannerisms, body language, accent, and so on within the framework of his unique traits (Sommers-Flanagan and Sommers-Flanagan, 2009).

The Skill of Questioning and Interacting in the Right Way

The clinical psychologist, as an interviewer, should be equipped with the skill of questioning—putting questions to the client in the interview sessions in an effective way for getting needed responses in realizing the target clinical assessment objectives. This skill on his part equips him with the necessary ability in relation to framing and asking questions best suited for being responded to on the part of clients in a proper way. For this purpose, the clinical psychologist must make use of questions that are easy to grasp on the part of the clients. The contents of the questions and interactions going on between them should be in the language spoken and culture specific of the clients for getting specific answers from them helpful in the task of needed clinical assessment.

The Skill of Active Listening and Paying Attention to the Client

Regarding the client and the problem he is experiencing, information in this regard can be ascertained with the help of the responses given by him during the interview session through his verbal and nonverbal behavior. These responses need to be properly caught and grasped on the part of the interviewer for deriving their proper meaning. For this purpose, the clinical psychologist (interviewer) must be well equipped with the skill of active listening and attending to the verbal and nonverbal responses of the concerned client. The acquisition of such skills is related to the learning and acquisition of the following type of desirable behavior and responses on his part as a good interviewer.

- He should learn the art of quieting his self. For this purpose, he should not only pick up the habit of talking less and listening more, but also try to quiet his internal, self-directed thinking pattern. Instead of getting preoccupied by his own thoughts, he should make himself fully devoted to the listening and attending to his client. He should keep himself receptive by refraining from expressing judgments of approval or disapproval, but maintaining a warm, relaxed, and interested attitude.
- Besides paying full attention to the active listening of what is conveyed by the client through his verbal responses, he should be attentive for catching all that is conveyed by the client through the nonverbal contents of his response and overall behavior demonstrated during the interview session in the form of the language of the eyes, body language, gestures and postures, pitch of the voice, mood and temperament, panicky normal, aggressive, hostile, tolerant and passive behavior, and so on.
- The clinical psychologist in the role of the interviewer should himself demonstrate all that is desirable for positioning him as an active listener to the responses and behavior of the client during the interview session in the form of making appropriate eye contact with the client, taking care of his own body language, postures, gestures, and body movements, the manner in which he interacts with the client, and his voice in terms of its comprehension and qualities such as pitch, tone, volume, and fluctuation.

The Skill of Verbal Tracking

The clinical psychologists (interviewers) should also employ the skill of verbal tracking. For this purpose, he should first try to get skilled in mastering the vocal qualities of the common language being used in the process of the interview. Then, he should concentrate on learning the art of verbal tracking—the ability to repeat key words and phrases back to the client in an indirect way to assure him that he has been properly understood.

The Skill of Drawing Conclusions from the Responses of the Clients

All that is done during the interview session in terms of information gathering from the client for the purpose of clinical assessment has to pass at its end through a process of analysis, interpretation, and conclusion at the hand of the clinical psychologist. It is an important and essential task to be done by him, as the tasting of the fruits of the labor done in conducting interview can be only plausible with its proper execution. Accordingly, in the use of the interview as a method of clinical assessment, the clinical psychologists need to be adept at the skill of interpreting and drawing conclusions in its proper form from the information being gathered from the clients in terms of their responses and behavior demonstrated during the interview session.

B. The Appropriateness of the Format of the Interview

In making use of the interview as a method of clinical assessment, its success depends not only on the competency of the interviewer but also on the appropriateness of the format of the interview regarding its structural organization (the type of questions included and type of responses elicited). In general, an interview schedule for the necessary clinical assessment can be shaped in the formats known as structured and unstructured. Let us look into these two types of interview formats.

Structured Format

In such a format of interview used for clinical assessment, clinical psychologists try to structure it well in advance before using it for getting information from the client as per the need of the clinical assessment. This is done by taking care of the following:

- Selection of appropriate questions, usually direct and close ended in nature, for eliciting definite and short answers from the clients.
- Deciding about the order and sequence of the questions.
- Deciding on the type of answer or responses for an asked question that will be able to provide the required information in light of the objectives of the clinical assessment.

Hence, by making definite decisions about the mode, procedure, and outcomes of the interview, the desired control can be effectively exercised over the total operation of the interview. Such control and effective organization of the interview then automatically makes it more objective, reliable, and valid. The path of the interviewer becomes clear, as he has all the material with him (pre-planned and well structured) for the achievement of the interview objectives. Let us know more about the type of questions asked and responses elicited in this type of interview format.

The questions asked in the structured format are referred to as directive questions targeted toward eliciting specific pieces of information from the client about his self and the problem. The responses drawn through these questions are typically brief, sometimes as brief as consisting of a single word or answer in the form of "yes" or "no." However, the use of this mode of questioning is capable of eliciting crucial data or information that clients may not otherwise choose to discuss or reveal: important information about the genetic component behind the problem (e.g., "Has anyone from your mother's or father's side been a patient of schizophrenia?") and the frequency and duration of the problem (e.g., "How often have you had panic attacks in a month, and for how long have you been experiencing them as such?").

Unstructured Format

In this type of interview format, the clinical psychologists possess neither a pre-prepared set numbers of questions with them for getting the client's response, nor do they have a set of prior decisions about the evaluation of the client's responses in terms of the objectives of the assessment. The nature of the questions set in the format of this interview is open ended, leaving the choice of responding to the client in their own ways. The interviewer here is totally free to ask any type of questions to the client to get the desired information. However, this unstructured and unplanned format of the interview may result in losing control over the systematic schedule of the interview. Thus, this type of interview is regarded as less objective, reliable, and valid in comparison to the structured interview. However, it scores a merit point over the structured interview in its characteristic of providing complete freedom to the clinical psychologist and the client for setting the direction of the interview as per their perceptions and the needs of the situation. The client gets enough opportunity for his self expression through the spontaneously formed questions of the interviewer and here lies a great opportunity for availing important additional information for the proper assessment of the client and his problem. The major weakness of this format lies in its characteristic of providing undue freedom to the client for talking about his self and the problem, and thus there is every possibility of his going off track and choosing to spend a lot of time on some topics and none on others.

The Decision About the Use of a Particular Format

We have seen that both formats have their own merits and demerits in terms of deriving information for the needed clinical assessment of the client and his problem. Each one of them may play an important role in the success of interviewing as a method of clinical assessment in its unique way. It is thus quite beneficial on the part of clinical psychologists to make use of both formats for conducting a clinical interview session. For this purpose, the beginning can be made with the use of an unstructured format by asking a few open-ended questions (e.g., What more can you tell me about your sleeping problems you mentioned on the phone?) for providing opportunity to the clients to talk freely about their problem. It may help in availing a lot of important information for being used in the ongoing clinical assessment task. Later in the session, the focus should be shifted to the use of the organized, structured format in the form of asking well-directed, close-ended questions.

C. The Appropriateness of the Interview Setting and Way of Conducting the Interview

The success of the interview as a method of clinical assessment also depends to a great extent upon the setting of the place of the interview and the professional activities of the interviewer during the course of interview. The following considerations must be attended to by the clinical psychologist in this concern.

- *The interview place or room* where the interview session with the client is planned should be client-friendly and suitable for conducting the clinical interview in an appropriate way. Accordingly, it needs to serve two important purposes—capable of fulfilling all the professional requirements for conducting the interview in a proper way and providing ease, comfort, and friendly feeling to the client. For making decisions in this concern, it is therefore appropriate to follow a general rule that states, "When choosing a room (the place of interview), it is useful to strike a balance between professional formality and casual comfort" (Sommers-Flanagan and Sommers-Flanagan, 2009:31).
- *Establishment of needed rapport and winning the confidence* of the clients is very much essential for smooth and purposeful conduct of the clinical interview. Accordingly, the clinical psychologists here should try to apply the essential professional skills for establishing proper rapport and winning confidence of their clients, enabling them to disclose and respond well to the interview questions. Moreover, their hesitation regarding the disclosure of one or

the other things regarding them and their problem should also be removed by telling them the needed confidentiality in this regard to be essentially maintained by them under the ethical code prescribed for them by their professional bodies to which they belong.

- *The task of noting down or recording the responses of the clients* is an essential activity that should be properly carried out by the clinical psychologist during the interview session. With the available developed technology, formal note-taking has now been completely replaced by the use of recording devices (audio as well as visual) fitted at the interview place; or, more appropriately, the task is now often automatically performed with the use of smart devices available in the form of smart phones, or recording tools available even in the interviewer's watch, spectacles or pen.

The task of taking interview need to be properly performed for the desired success of a clinical interview. Considerations like those below must be taken care of by the clinical psychologist in this concern.

- Introduce yourself with necessary legitimate identification as an interviewer to the respondent and explain to him the purpose of asking questions by clearly emphasizing that it must be done to help him regarding his felt problem.
- Give proper time to the respondent to get ready to be interviewed for your clinical assessment interview.
- Make him feel at home and address him by his name while asking any questions or reacting to his responses.
- Ask the questions (open- or close-ended per requirement of the unstructured and structured format of the interview) very carefully in a simple common language easily graspable for eliciting the needed information about him and his problem.
- Do not dominate or monopolize the conversation during the interview. Do not put words unnecessarily into the mouth of the respondent. Be a patient listener and never feel disappointed, irritated, or surprised by what the respondent says.
- Use the silent probe technique for getting adequate responses. Just pause and wait. It really works by suggesting to the respondent that you are waiting for his response.
- Encourage the respondent by providing direct encouragement. However, this does not imply that, as an interviewer, you approve or disapprove his responses. It may be as simple as saying "OK" or nodding your head.
- Try to get more desired information by asking for elaboration, such as, "Is there anything else you would like to say or add?"
- Ask for desired clarification, if needed, by putting suitable clarification questions (e.g., "I want to make sure I'm understanding this correctly—did you mention that you've been struggling with the night sleepwalking issue for about one year?"). The purpose of asking these questions is to make sure the interviewer has an accurate understanding of the client's comments, besides communicating to the client that the interviewer is actively listening and processing the responses to the client.
- Try to accept the responses and reactions of the respondent in their original form and make their record as adequately as possible.
- Try to make use of confronting questions whenever you notice discrepancies or inconsistencies in a client's comments. These questions, while looking similar to the clarification questions, try to focus on apparently contradictory information provided by the clients. For example, an interviewer might say to a client suffering from binge eating disorder,

"Earlier, you mentioned that you had been happy with your body and weight as a teenager, but then a few minutes ago you mentioned that during high school you felt fat in comparison with many of your friends. I'm a bit confused. Please clarify." (Pomerantz, 2020).

- Ensure optimum realization of the objectives of the clinical interview in terms of availing the needed information (as complete as possible) about the client and his problem.
- In the end, try to derive valid conclusions from the information or data gathered from the interview about the assessment and diagnosis of the problem of the client aimed at planning its treatment.

To Sum Up

Interview as a method of clinical assessment represents a way of collecting relevant information on the part of clinical psychologists from the client through the help of appropriate questions by making him feel comfortable to tell freely about his self and the felt problem during one or a series of discussions consisting of face-to-face interaction and dialogue. The success of its use depends upon factors such as the competency of the clinical psychologist as an interviewer, the appropriateness of the format of the interview, and the appropriateness of the interview setting and way of conducting the interview.

For the required competency as interviewer, the clinical psychologist should employ skills such as: (i) the skill of establishing rapport with the client, (ii) the skill of being self-aware and making a good impression on the client, (iii) the skill of questioning and interacting in a proper way, (iv) the skill of active listening and paying attention to the client, (v) the skill of verbal tracking, and (vi) the skill of drawing conclusions from the responses of the client.

Regarding making use of an appropriate format of the interview, it is quite beneficial to make use of both formats for conducting a clinical interview session. For this purpose, the beginning can be made with the use of an unstructured format by asking a few ope-ended questions for availing important information helpful in the ongoing clinical assessment task. Later in the session, he should ask well-directed, close-ended questions aimed at availing the pinpointed specific information regarding the client and his problem.

Regarding the appropriateness of the interview setting and way of conducting the interview, the clinical psychologists should take care of the things such as (i) the interview place or room, (ii) establishment of needed rapport and winning the confidence of the clients, and (iii) the task of taking interview in an appropriate way, including the noting down or recording of the responses of the client.

Review Questions

1. What is clinical assessment? Throw light on its meaning and discuss the different purposes served by it.
2. Define the term clinical assessment and name the ways and methods of carrying it out on the part of clinical psychologists.
3. Discuss naturalistic observation as a method of clinical assessment.

4. What is case history? Throw light on its use as a method of clinical assessment.
5. Describe in detail how the clinical psychologists should make appropriate use of informal and formal interviewing as methods of clinical assessment.

References

Haynes, S. N., & Kaholokula, J. K. (2008), Behavioural assessment, In M. Hersen & A. M. Gross (Eds.), *Handbook of clinical psychology* (Vol. 1, pp. 495–522), Hoboken, NJ: Wiley.

Pomerantz, A. M. (2020), *Clinical psychology-science, practice and diversity* (5th ed.), London: SAGE.

Sommers-Flanagan, J., & Sommers-Flanagan, R. (2009), *Clinical interviewing* (4th ed.), Hoboken, NJ: Wiley.

Chapter 19

Clinical Assessment—Psychological and Neurological Testing

Learning Objectives

After going through this chapter, you will be able to:

- Describe the use of psychological testing as a method of clinical assessment.
- Discuss the use of achievement testing as a method of clinical assessment.
- Discuss the use of intelligence tests for the purpose of clinical assessment.
- Throw light on personality testing as a method of clinical assessment with the utilization of personality inventories.
- Discuss the use of objective psychological tests for measuring specific single aspects of one's personality, such as adjustment, depression, anxiety, and self-esteem.
- Describe the use of projective personality testing for the purpose of clinical assessment.
- Discuss the use of neuropsychological testing as a method of clinical assessment.

Psychological Testing as a Method of Clinical Assessment

An important method used by clinical psychologists for the clinical assessment of clients and their problems is psychological testing—administration and interpretation of one or the other standardized psychological tests for assessing specific abilities, attributes, and characteristics of one's personality, or measuring specific potential, strengths and weaknesses of one's functioning in one's physical and social environment. A number of psychological tests are available to clinical psychologists for assessing one or the other psychological attributes of the clients, providing a lot of information regarding their functioning—normal as well disruptive or maladaptive in their environment—for use in the diagnosis and treatment of the problem of their clients.

In general, the psychological tests utilized most often on this account by clinical psychologists may be classified into the following categories:

- *Achievement tests:* Used in assessing the achievement potential of the clients (what they have achieved, acquired, or learnt in a particular academic or performance area).
- *Intelligence tests:* Used for assessing the intelligence or level of cognitive functioning of the clients.
- *Personality tests or Inventories:* Used in assessing personal qualities or characteristics referred to as personality traits or overall personality of the clients.

DOI: 10.4324/9781003398325-19

- *Adjustment inventories or tests:* Used in assessing the level of client's adjustment or maladjustment toward the self and environment.
- *Specific clinical tests:* Used to assess specific matters of clinical concerns such as state of mood, happiness or sadness, as well as levels of motivation, anxiety, depression, mental retardation, emotional disturbance, and so on.
- *Neuropsychological tests:* Used in assessing deficits in cognitive functioning (i.e., ability to think, speak, reason) that may result from some sort of brain damage, such as stroke or brain injury.

Competency to be Acquired by Clinical Psychologists for Psychological Testing

Psychological testing is a very skilled and professional task. Therefore, clinical psychologists must have the essential competency and know-how for getting along with the task of making use of psychological tests for clinical assessment, in the manner as briefed ahead.

- First of all, they should be quite specific about the objectives or purposes being served through the psychological testing being done on their part, and decide that they will remain objective, scientific, and ethically fair to all subjects during the course of psychological testing.
- Then, they should search for an appropriate standardized psychological test for assessing the psychological attribute in question, such as achievement, intelligence, personality, adjustment level, level of anxiety, depression, and emotional disturbances.
- The third stage of the use of psychological testing is the test administration. The clinical psychologists must have essential expertise in the administration of psychological tests in a proper way, as needed and provided in the manual of the test developed by the test developer. Here, they should be quite specific and particular about the maintenance of uniformity required in connection with the environmental conditions, seating arrangement, noise levels, ensuring or responding to the structured or unstructured stimuli, time or duration of the test, and so on.
- Next is the task of scoring and interpretation of the responses of the subjects, available separately on their test sheets. The clinical psychologist, as the administrator of the test, should try to acquire the necessary expertise in this technical task of scoring and interpretation. They should strictly follow the procedure laid down in the manual for the scoring of the responses and their interpretation in light of the standardized age, grade, or gender norms given in the manual.
- What is interpreted through the administration and scoring of a psychological test is then recorded in the form of a written psychological report—the formal means of communicating the test results to the clients and their well-wishers, including other mental health professionals. In this regard, it is important that clinical psychologists not only write intelligible, accurate reports that address the reason for referral but that they also "know their audience" in order to customize their reports in terms of readability, selection of relevant information, and recommendations (Goldfinger and Pomerantz, 2010).

To Sum Up

Psychological testing as a method of clinical assessment consists of making use of one or the other standardized psychological tests for assessing psychological attributes of the clients, providing a lot of information regarding their functioning—normal or maladaptive—for use in the diagnosis and treatment of their problem. In general, the psychological tests utilized most often on this account may be classified into categories such as Achievement tests, Intelligence tests, Personality tests or Inventories, Adjustment inventories or tests, Neuropsychological tests, and Specific clinical tests to assess specific matters of clinical concern like state of mood, happiness or sadness, as well as levels of motivation, anxiety, depression, mental retardation, emotional disturbance, and so on. For making use of psychological tests for clinical assessment, clinical psychologists are required to be equipped with essential competency and know-how of their availability, administration, scoring, and interpretation.

Availability and Utilization of the Various Types of Psychological Tests

Let us examine the essentials about the availability and utilization of the previously mentioned various types of psychological tests on the part of clinical psychologists for the needed clinical assessment of clients and their problems.

Achievement Tests as a Method for Clinical Assessment

As the name suggests, achievement tests are the type of tests that are used for assessing or measuring the achievements of an individual in a particular field or area, such as academics, sports, workplaces, and so on. An achievement test helps us in assessing the potential of an individual in a learning area related to school education. In reference to clinical assessment, achievement tests are usually employed by clinical psychologists in the form of academic achievement tests—testing or measuring the academic achievement of the client in language, mathematics, and so on. Achievement tests may be available in two prominent forms—teacher-made tests and standardized achievement tests. While the latter are structured or developed by an outside agency and are readily available for administration, the former are constructed by individual teachers in their respective subjects or areas for assessing the degree of the individual learner's achievement or diagnosing their learning difficulties and disabilities. It is the standardized achievement tests developed for assessing and measuring the achievement of learners in academic areas that are generally used by clinical psychologists for clinical assessment purposes.

As an example of their use on the part of clinical psychologists, we may name the use of the standardized achievement tests in academic areas like language and mathematics for the required clinical assessment of clients suffering from the learning disabilities (termed as learning disorders in the DSM-5 and DSM-5-TR) such as dyslexia and dyscalculia. The comparison between the scores obtained by the clients with the norms provided for their age and grade by the test developer may help in assessing the level of their underachievement, indicating the nature of their learning difficulties in an academic area.

Psychologists and researchers have developed a number of achievement tests in assessing and measuring the learning achievements of individuals in one or the other learning areas. In Table 19.1, we present a few more common specific tests used by clinical psychologists for the assessment and diagnosis of learning difficulties or deficits of clients (by comparing their academic achievements with the norms provided in the test).

Table 19.1 Commonly Used Achievement Tests for Clinical Assessment

Name of the Test	Test Developer Reference
1. Wechsler Individual Achievement Test (III)	Wechsler, (2009), Wechsler Individual Achievement Test (III edition), San Antonio, Tex: Psychological Corp
2. Kaufman Test of Educational Achievement	Kaufman, A. S., & Kaufman, N. G. (1985). Kaufman Test of Individual Achievement, Circle Pines, MN: American Guidance Service.
3. Wide Range Achievement Test 3	Wilkinson, G. S. (1993). Wide Range Achievement Test 3. Wilmington, DE: Jastak Associates.
4. Woodcock-Johnson Tests of Achievement	Woodcock, Richard W. (1989) Woodcock-Johnson Tests of Achievement. Allen, Tex.: DLM Teaching Resources.
5. Woodcock Johnson Psycho-educational Battery-Revised	Woodcock, R. W. (1989), Woodcock Johnson Psycho-educational Battery-Revised: Technical Report. Allen, TX: DLM Teaching Resources.
6. Woodcock Language Proficiency Battery-Revised	Woodcock, R.W. (1991). Woodcock Language Proficiency Battery-Revised. English and Spanish Forms. Chicago: The Riverside Publishing Company.
7. Durrell Analysis of Reading Ability	Durrell, D. D., & Catterson, J. H. (1980). Durrell Analysis of Reading Difficulty (3rd ed.). Cleveland, OH: Psychological Corporation.
8. Woodcock Reading Mastery Tests-Revised	Woodcock, R. W. (1987). Woodcock Reading Mastery Tests-Revised. Circle Pines, MN: American Guidance Service.
9. Keymath Revised	Connolly, A. J. (1988). Keymath Revised. A Diagnostic Inventory of Essential Mathematics. Circle Pines, MN: American Guidance Service.
10. Stanford Diagnostic Mathematics Test	Beatty, L. S., Madden, R., Gardner, E. G., &Karlsen, B. (1976). Stanford Diagnostic Mathematics Test. Cleveland, OH: Psychological Corporation.
11. Test of Mathematical Abilities	Brown, V. L., Cronin, M. E., & Mc Entire, E. (1994). Test of Mathematical Abilities, Second Edition. Austin, TX: PRO-ED.
12. Written Language Assessment Test	Grill, J. J., &Kerwin, M.M. (1989). Written Language Assessment Test. Novato, CA: Academic Therapy Publications.

At this stage, you may be curious to know about the nature, characteristics, and use of the aforementioned achievement tests. To illustrate this, we now embark on a necessary discussion about the test mentioned at the top of the table in the name of the Wechsler Individual Achievement Test—Third Edition.

Wechsler Individual Achievement Test—Third Edition

In its short version, this test is known as the WIAT-III. Associated with the name of the famous psychologist David Wechsler, it was published in its third edition in 2009. The main features of this test are summarized in the manner as follows.

1. During the development of this test, the test developers tried to standardize the test on 3,000 individuals (students and adults) matching the available US Census data in terms of sex, age, race/ethnicity, geographic region, and parent education level.
2. It is a comprehensive test helpful to the clinical psychologists in assessing the achievements of their clients aged 4–50 years in the academic areas of language and mathematics (related to their learning difficulties or disorders known as dyslexia and dyscalculia).
3. Clinical psychologists are required to administer this test on their clients on a one-on-one basis, as paper-and-pencil tests in a face-to-face mode or online.
4. The scores obtained through the administration of this composite test (comprising a number of subtests) provide measures related to four broad areas: oral language, written language, reading, and mathematical abilities. Each of these broad areas is assessed by two to four subtests as per details shown in Table 19.2.
5. The WIAT-III yields standard scores on a scale with a mean of 100 and a standard deviation of 15, much like most of the intelligence test scales. Besides providing overall norms (age- and grade-wise) for the measurement of academic achievement, it also yields age and grade equivalencies for each subtest.
6. In the standardization of WIAT-III, Wechsler included a number of individuals previously used for the standardization of Wechsler's intelligence tests. It can help us in deriving a unique adavantage of establishing the valadity of WAIT-III against them. Otherwise also we can rely on the significance of its use for clinical assessment as overall, the reliability and validity data supporting the WIAT-III are quite strong (Lichtenberger and Breaux, 2010).

Table 19.2 Description Related to Wechsler Individual Achievement Test—Third Edition

Broad Academic Area	The Subtests Used	What the Subtest Contains and Measures
Written Language	Spelling	Measures the ability to spell dictated letters, blends, and words.
	Sentence Composition	Includes sentence combining and sentence building components, which measure sentence formulation skills, including the use of morphology, grammar, syntax, semantics and mechanics.
	Essay Composition	Measures spontaneous written expression in response to a prompt under timed conditions.
	Writing Expression	Includes Alphabet Writing Fluency, Spelling, Sentence Composition, and Essay composition.

Broad Academic Area	The Subtests Used	What the Subtest Contains and Measures
Reading	Early Reading Skills	Measures several skills deemed important for developing reading skills.
	Word Reading	Measure speed and accuracy of reading isolated single words.
	Pseudo-word Decoding	Measures speed and accuracy of decoding skills (using phonetic skills to sound out nonsense words).
	Reading Comprehension	Measures literal and inferential reading comprehension skills using a variety of passage and question types that resemble those used in a school setting.
	Oral Reading Fluency	Measures oral reading fluency of expository and narrative passages.
	Total Reading	Measures word reading, pseudo-word decoding, reading comprehension, and oral reading fluency.
Mathematical Ability	Numerical Operations	Measures written mathematics calculation skills under untimed conditions.
	Math Problem Solving	Measures the ability to problem solve mathematically using both verbal and visual prompts.
	Math Fluency	Measures written mathematics calculation fluency, accuracy, and speed.
	Alphabet Writing Fluency	Measures ability to write alphabet letters within a 30 second time limit.
Oral Language	Listening Comprehension	Contains receptive vocabulary and oral discourse comprehension components and measures listening comprehension at the level of the word, sentence and discourse.
	Oral Expression	Contains expressive vocabulary, oral word fluency, and sentence repetition components and measures.
		Skills and competencies important for effective speaking vocabulary, word retrieval, flexibility of thought process, and oral syntactic knowledge and short-term memory.

To Sum Up

Achievement Tests as a method for Clinical Assessment are usually employed by clinical psychologists for testing or measuring the academic achievement of clients in academic subjects, language, and mathematics. As an example of their use for this purpose, we may name the use of standardized achievement tests in academic areas like language and mathematics for the required clinical assessment of clients with learning disorders, such as dyslexia and dyscalculia. Psychologists and researchers have developed a number of achievement tests (such as the Wechsler Individual Achievement Test-III Edition) for assessing and measuring the learning achievements of individuals in one or the other learning areas.

Intelligence Tests as a Method of Clinical Assessment

Intelligence tests represent those psychological tests that are used for the assessment or measurement of people's intellectual potential or level of cognitive functioning in terms of its both strengths and deficits. The knowledge and information provided by the administration of these tests is found to help clinical psychologists by providing valuable data for the clinical assessment of the clients suffering from a number of mental health problems and disorders, such as learning disorders (formerly known as learning disabilities), intellectual development disorder (formerly known as mental retardation), mood disorders, disruptive behavior, and so on.

Psychologists and researchers have developed a number of intelligence tests classified as verbal and nonverbal intelligence tests (consisting of a series of tasks asking the subjects to use both verbal and nonverbal skills) for the assessment of intellectual abilities on the individual or group basis. Clinical psychologists here may be found typically to limit the use of the verbal and nonverbal intelligence tests for the assessment of the level of intellect or cognitive functioning of their clients on an individual basis (being administered face-to-face with an individual client). Thus, the tests that clinical psychologists use are neither group intelligence tests nor are capable of being administered by the clients themselves. Administration of these tests occurs in a well-structured interpersonal interaction format requiring extensive training, typically received during graduate programs in clinical psychology (Raiford et al., 2010).

You may be interested now in the availability of these tests being developed in our country and abroad. For this purpose, here we list a few popular ones (in their latest edition or version) for your use as clinical psychologists or trainees.

1. *Wechsler Adult Intelligence Scale—Fourth Edition (WAIS-IV):* Associated with the famous psychologist David Wechsler, the fourth edition of this test has been published by Pearson Education Ltd in the year 2008. It can be successfully employed for the clinical assessment of clients of the age range 16–90 years. Administration of this test yields a single full-scale intelligence score (measure of "g"), and four index/factor scores derived from the respective subtest scores (contributing toward the measure of specific "s" of one's intelligence). The items included in the sub-tests are verbal as well as nonverbal in nature. A group of subtest constitutes a specific factor/index of the test. The test scale has four indexes/factors: (i) verbal comprehension index (measuring verbal concept formation and verbal reasoning), (ii) perceptual reasoning index (measuring fluid reasoning, spatial processing, and visual-motor integration), (iii) working memory index (measuring one's capacity to store, transform, and recall incoming information and data in short-term memory, and (iv) processing speed index (measuring one's ability to process simple or rote information rapidly and accurately).
2. *Wechsler Intelligence Scale for Children—Fifth Edition (WISC-V):* Associated with the famous psychologist David Wechsler, the fifth edition of this test was published in 2014 by Pearson Education Ltd. It can be successfully employed for the clinical assessment of the

clients of the age range 6–16 years. Administration of this test, like the WAIS-IV, also yields a single full-scale intelligence score (measure of "g"), and five index/factor scores derived from the respective subtest scores (contributing toward the measure of specific "s" of one's intelligence). Here, also, the items included in the subtests are verbal as well as nonverbal in nature, and a specific number of subtests constitute the respective factors of the test scale. Among the five factors, it contains three that are the same as in the WAIS-IV: verbal comprehension, working memory, and processing speed. The remaining fourth, named as the perceptual reasoning index, is divided into the visual spatial index and the fluid reasoning index.

3. *Wechsler Preschool and Primary Scale of Intelligence—Fourth Edition (WPPSI-IV)*:
Associated with the famous psychologist David Wechsler, the fourth edition of this test was published in 2012 by Pearson Education Ltd. It can be successfully employed for the clinical assessment of clients of the age range 2 years and 6 months to 7 years and 3 months. Administration of this test, also like the WAIS and WISC, yields a single full-scale intelligence score (measure of "g"), and four index/factor scores derived from the respective subtest scores (contributing toward the measure of specific "s" of one's intelligence). Here, also like the WAIS and WISC, the items included in the subtests are verbal as well as nonverbal in nature, and a specific number of subtests constitute the respective factors of the test scale. In terms of its factor composition, it contains five similar factors as present in the WISC.

4. *Stanford-Binet Intelligence Scales—Fifth Edition (SB5)*: Having a long history since its first publication and dominance in the early 1900s, the latest version of this test in the name of the Stanford-Binet Intelligence Scales—Fifth Edition (SB5) was developed in 2003 by Gail H. Roid. It is one of the most popular tests used by clinical psychologists all over the world, other than the Wechsler tests for the assessment and diagnosis of the strengths and limitations of one's intellectual functioning. It is similar to Wechsler's tests in many ways, such as ways of administration, yielding a singular measure of one's intelligence (or "g"), five factor scores, specific subtest scores (helpful in measuring specific ability or "s"), and features the same means (100) and standard deviations (15) as the Wechsler intelligence tests for its full-scale and factor scores. It is as strong as Wechsler's tests in terms of reliability and validity. Like Wechsler's tests it, also makes use of verbal and nonverbal items for providing subtests scores; moreover, it has a strong advantage in its use and applicability by covering the entire life span (ages 2–85+) of clients as a single test, instead of needing a number of separate tests for the different age groups, as happens with the use of Wechsler's intelligence scales. In its composition in terms of the constituent factors/indexes, it has five factors (each of which yields a factor/index score) named as follows:

   (i)   *Knowledge* (how knowledgeable one is in terms of having general information and know-how of the things in his environment)
   (ii) *Working Memory* (ability to hold and transform information in short-term memory)
   (iii) *Quantitative Reasoning* (ability to solve numerical problems)
   (iv) *Visual-Spatial Processing* (ability to analyze visually presented information)
   (v)   *Fluid Reasoning* (ability to solve novel problems).

There is also an appropriate provision in SB 5 for measuring the aforementioned five factors or constituents of one's intelligence both verbally and nonverbally by including both verbal and nonverbal items in the specific subtests designed for the measurement of one's intelligence.

5. Universal Nonverbal Intelligence Test-2 (UNIT-2): In an effort to developing culturally sensitive testing (for avoiding cultural bias in assessing the intelligence of people of other cultures), psychologists tried to develop a completely language-free test of intelligence (requiring no

use of language on the part of the administrator of the test and the client) in the year 1996 in the name of the Universal Nonverbal Intelligence Test (UNIT). It was revised and named as the Nonverbal Intelligence Test-2 (UNIT-2) in 2015. The important things regarding its development, characteristic features, and use are summarized as follows.

- It is meant for assessing and measuring the intellectual functioning of people belonging to the age range 5–21.
- In terms of its standardization and norm drawing, it was administered on a sample of 1,800 people matching the contemporary US Census data in terms of age, sex, race, parent education, community size, geographic region, and ethnicity.
- In terms of its usability and applicability for the assessment of one's intellectual functioning, it provides a fairly accepted level of reliability and validity (Bracken and McCallum, 2015).
- In terms of its administration, it is administered in a face-to-face mode, much like the other intelligence tests used for clinical assessment. However, on account of being a language free test, the administrator here, instead of using verbal instructions, provides instructions via eight specific hand gestures (taught in the test manual and demonstrated in an accompanying video). Similarly, the clients here are also required to respond to the test items either by pointing with their fingers or performing minor manipulation of objects with their hands or fingers.
- The test as a whole is composed of six subtests containing non-language visual items. Out of these six subtests, three are meant for the assessment of the memory-related aspect of one's intelligence and the other three contribute toward the measure of the reasoning-based aspect of one's intellect. The naming and functions of these subtests are briefed in Table 19.3.

6. Raven's Progressive Matrices (RPM): This is a nonverbal test that has been specifically designed for the assessment of one's verbal reasoning, abstract reasoning, and cognitive functioning in terms of assets as well as deficits. In its application in the clinical field, we may find it usefully employed for clinical assessment by clinical psychologists throughout the world. Its characteristic features may be summarized as follows.

- The test, created in 1938, is named after its developer, John C. Raven.
- It is strictly visual in its composition, making it a language- and culture-fair test.

Table 19.3 Six Subtests Comprising the Universal Nonverbal Intelligence Test-2

Memory Related Subtests	Reasoning Related Subtests
Object Memory Test: It contains items in which the client is required to view first a visual assortment of common objects for five seconds and then afterward view a larger array for identifying the objects from the first array.	Cube Design Test: It contains items in which the client is required to arrange colored blocks in a specific three dimensional design.
Spatial Memory Test: It contains items in which the client is required to recall the placement of colored chips on a three-by-three or four-by-four grid.	Maze Test: It contains items in which the client is required to complete traditional maze puzzles.
Symbolic Memory Test: It contains items in which the client is required to recall and recreate sequences of visually presented symbols.	Analogic Reasoning Test: It contains items in which the client is required to solve visually presented analogy problems.

- It can be used to assess the cognitive functioning of individuals ranging from five years old to the elderly.
- The test consists of 60 multiple-choice questions, listed in order of increasing difficulty. All of these questions consist of visual geometric designs (specific patterns presented in the form of a 6×6, 4×4, 3×3, or 2×2 matrix) with one piece missing.
- The matrices are available in three different forms for participants of different ability, namely, (i) Standard Progressive Matrices (RSPM), where items are presented in black ink on a white background, (ii) Colored Progressive Matrices (RCPM), where most items are presented on a colored background to make the test visually stimulating for participants, (iii) Advanced Progressive Matrices (RAPM), where items are presented in black ink on a white background, and become increasingly complex as progress is made through each set.
- In responding to the test items, the client is required to choose the correct diagram from a set of eight answers that completes a pattern in the matrix, thus identifying the missing element completing a pattern.

7. Bhatia's Battery of Performance Tests: This is a popular nonverbal performance test in the Indian subcontinent used for the assessment of the cognitive functioning of clients belonging to the Indian population in the capacity of a language- and culture-fair test. It was developed in 1955 by Chandra Mohan Bhatia, former director of Uttar Pradesh Mano Vigyanshala. As a composition of five different subtests, it is termed as a battery of tests being administered on an individual client at a time by a test administrator in a face-to-face mode. Among the five subtests included in this battery, the first two, named as Koh's Block Design Test and Alexander Passalong test, have been borrowed, and the other three have been developed by the test developer Mr. Bhatia himself. Let us know more about the nature and administration of these five subtests.

(i) Koh's Block Design Test: 10 designs from the original 17 colored designs from Koh's test have been included in the battery. In the administration of this test, the test administrator presents the cards carrying the specific type of designs before the subject one by one, and asks him to reproduce it by using a set of colored blocks. These designs become increasingly more complex, having been simple at the start. The time provided for the subject to respond to the first five designs is two minutes, and for the remaining five, it is three minutes.

(ii) Alexander Passalong Test: The battery includes all the items of the original Passalong Test for its own working. The items of this test are in the form of colored designs and are arranged in order of increasing difficulty. The task of the subject here is to reproduce similar designs by shifting colored pieces in an open box. The time fixed for completing work on the first four is two minutes, and for the remaining four, it is three minutes.

(iii) Pattern Drawing Test: This test consists of eight cards, each having a different specific pattern. For the purpose of responding to the test items, the client is required to reproduce these patterns one by one in one go without lifting the pencil. The time for the first four cards in two minutes and for the rest of the four cards, it is three minutes.

(iv) Immediate Memory Test: It is a test designed for testing the immediate memory capacity of the client. Here, the test administrator recites digits, which are required to be repeated on the part of the client immediately. The time taken in such reproduction as well as the quality of the reproduced stuff in terms of the correctness of the digits reproduced and order in which they have been reproduced becomes the criteria for memory assessment of the client.

(v) Picture Construction Test: In this test, the client is required to construct a particular picture with the help of the given fragmented pieces of that picture. There are five items in this test in the form of five pictures relating to Indian rural life that are to be constructed by the client with the help of the fragmented pieces numbering 2, 4, 6, 8 and 12 pieces, respectively, for items numbered 1, 2, 3, 4, and 5 of the text. The parts are to be meaningfully combined to construct the required picture. The time prescribed for the construction of the first two pictures is two minutes, and for the remaining three pictures, it is three minutes.

In terms of the development of the five subtests, the work was done for over four years in villages and cities (covering a cross-cultural population of Indian subjects). Regarding the interpretation of the earned scores, the battery provides norms for the assessment of the intellectual functioning of children belonging to the age range 11–16 years. In terms of its outcomes, the battery yields the overall Intelligence Quotient (IQ) based on the five subtests, and Performance Quotient (PQ) based on the four performance tests—Koh's block design, Alexander Passalong, Pattern drawing, and Picture construction.

8. Indian Adaptation of Wechsler's Intelligence Tests: In terms of their useful application with clients belonging to the Indian population, attempts have been made by Indian scholars, psychologists, and publishers to develop adapted versions of the Wechsler's intelligence tests in the manner described ahead.

- The beginning in this direction was made by developing an adaptation of Wechsler's Intelligence Scale for Children (WISC) by Dr. Arthur J. Malin of Nagpur in the name of the Intelligence Scale for Indian Children—ISIC or MISIC. In the beginning, it was constructed in the English language for the English-speaking population of Indian children of the age range 6–15 years and 11 months. Later on, it was adapted for the Hindi- and Marathi-speaking populations of Indian children.

  The MISIC as a composite intelligence test is composed of 11 subtests divided into two groups: Verbal and Performance. The Verbal Scale consists of six subtests: the Information Test, General Comprehension Test, Arithmetic Test, Analogy & Similarity test, Vocabulary Test, and Digit Span Test. The Performance Scale consists of five subtests: the Picture Completion Test, Block Design Test, Object Assembly, Coding, and Mazes. In terms of its administration, it is administered on an individual basis in the face-to-face mode and takes about 2 to 2 and 1/2 hours for its completion.

- Another important attempt for a useful, adapted version of the other Wechsler scale—Wechsler's Adult Intelligence Scale (WAIS)—was made in 1974 by Prabha Ramalingaswamy. Named as Wechsler's Adult Performance Intelligence Scale (*WAPIS*), it was adapted for usage with the Indian adult population belonging to the age group 15–44 years.

- In the series of attempts to provide a useful, adapted version of Wechsler's intelligence scales for the clients of the Indian population, Pearson Education India has brought out the following useful publications (in the form of complete sets of adapted intelligence scales).

  (i) From the year 2003, it began with the publication of the adapted Indian version of the WISC, in the name of Wechsler Intelligence Scale for Children—Fourth Edition (WISC-IV) India, for being standardized and used with Indian children in the field of their clinical assessment.

  (ii) From the year 2008, it released the publication of the adapted Indian version of the Wechsler's Adult Intelligence Scale—Fourth Edition (WAIS-IV) in the name

WAIS-IV India. It has been specifically standardized and designed for use with Indian clients of the age range 16 years to 84 years 11 months. According to the publisher, India norms for WAIS-IV India are the most recent set of norms representative of the Indian population across the country. Accordingly, these tests may be effectively used by mental health professionals for clinical assessment and intervention planning of their clients.

9. Indian Adaptation of Simon-Binet Intelligence Tests

Attempts have been made to create an adapted version of the Simon-Binet intelligence test for usage with the population of Indian clients. For this purpose, we are describing two such well-known attempts.

In an earlier attempt to bring an Indian adaptation of the Simon-Binet intelligence scale (known as Stanford Binet Scale after its revision in 1916), Professor Kamat brought out a test in the regional languages of Kannad and Marathi for the Kannad- and Marathi-speaking populations of the Indian subcontinent. It was based on the 1916 Stanford-Binet Intelligence Scale and named the Bombay-Karnatak version of the Binet-Simon Intelligence Scale.It soon became popularized in the name of the Binet Kamat Test, or BKT. It was later modified and standardized in 1934 for suiting more the Kannada- and Marathi- speaking populations of Indian children.

Another mentionable attempt in this direction was made by professor S.K. Kulshreshtha by bringing a Regional adaptation of the Stanford-Binet Intelligence Scale in the Hindi language for measuring the intelligence of the Hindi-speaking population of Indian clients. Its 1960 revision covers an age range of 2 years to 22 years for the measurement of the intelligence of the clients. In its composition, this adaptation includes both verbal and performance tests in the forms of words, objects, and pictures, and requires clients to give responses in the forms of drawing, calculating, writing, and speaking. Its administration yields valid scores for the estimation of mental age (MA) and intelligence quotient (IQ) of the clients.

To Sum Up

The use of Intelligence tests helps clinical psychologists acquire valuable data regarding the clinical assessment of their clients suffering from a number of mental health problems and disorders such as learning disorders, intellectual development disorder (formerly known as mental retardation), mood disorders, and disruptive behavior. For this purpose, psychologists and researchers have developed a number of intelligence tests classified as verbal and nonverbal intelligence tests. For clinical assessment, these tests are administered on one-on-one with an individual client. As examples of these tests, we may cite the names of more widely used tests, such as (i) the Wechsler Adult Intelligence Scale—Fourth Edition (WAIS-IV) for the use with clients of the age range 16–90 years, (ii) the Wechsler Intelligence Scale for Children—Fifth Edition (WISC-V) for the use with clients of the age range 6–16 years, (iii) the Wechsler Preschool and Primary Scale of Intelligence—Fourth Edition (WPPSI-IV) for the use with clients of the age range 2 years and 6 months to 7 years and 3 months, (iv) the Stanford-Binet Intelligence Scales—Fifth Edition (SB5) for use with clients ages 2–85, (v) the Universal Nonverbal Intelligence Test-2 (UNIT-2) for use with the clients ages 5–21, (vi) Raven's Progressive Matrices

(RPM)—a nonverbal test for use with clients ranging from 5-year-olds to the elderly, (vii) Bhatia's battery of performance tests, a nonverbal performance test for use with clients belonging to the Indian population, (viii) the Indian Adaptation of Wechsler's intelligence tests, and (ix) the Indian Adaptation of Simon-Binet intelligence tests.

Personality Tests as a Method of Clinical Assessment

The psychological tests referred to as personality tests are specifically designed to assess one or the other personality traits, characteristics, or attributes of one's personality, including the level of motivation and interests, self-concept and self-esteem, anxiety and depression, mood and emotional states, and levels of adjustment or maladjustment. Personality tests developed on this account may be broadly classified as objective tests and projective tests. In the category of objective tests, we may put the measures in which we try to seek information from the clients themselves about their personality attributes by asking them to respond to printed statements or structured questions of measuring instruments such as personality inventories and question-naires, attitude scales, interests and aptitude tests, temperament and mood scales, anxiety and depression scales, and frustration and adjustment measures. In the second category of personal-ity tests, we may include the various measures based on projective techniques in which the cli-ents are asked to respond in their own ways to the relatively unstructured or ambiguous material of the test. In the pages to follow, we will be discussing the availability and use of some of the important and widely used personality measures on the part of clinical psychologists all over the globe for the task of clinical assessment of the mental health problems of their clients.

The Description of Some Popular Contemporary Personality Inventories Used for Clinical Assessment

Minnesota Multiphasic Personality Inventory-2 (MMPI-2)

The MMPI-2 brought out in 1989 is the most popular inventory at present in use by clinical psychologists all over the globe for the psychometric assessment of the personality of clients. It is the revision of the original MMPI (authored by Starke Hathaway and J.C. McKinley), which was published in 1943.

The characteristic features of MPPP-2 are briefed as follows.

- It aims for the psychometric assessment of the personality of adults (18 years and older).
- There are 567 items in MPPI-2 (in comparison to 37 contained in the original version of MPPI) in the form of self-descriptive sentences (such as "I feel like I am low on energy much of the time") aimed to assess the personality attributes of the individuals covering a wide range of the positive and negative aspects of their feelings, attitudes, likes and dislikes, mood and states of being, and so on.
- The client under assessment is required to respond to them on the given answer sheet by marking each sentence with the pen/pencil as either true or false in the way as he thinks it so for himself.
- Among the 567 items of the inventory, there are a number of factors taking into account undesirable test-taking attitudes shown on the part of clients, in the forms of faking being unwell (appearing more impaired than they really are); faking wellness (appearing healthier

than they really are); or responding randomly without paying needed attention. Responses to these items, when grouped together, constitute the three specific validity scales of MPPI, known as L (Lying), K (Defensiveness), and F (Infrequency). These validity scales warn the clinical psychologists about the client's undesirable test-taking attitude, and thus impact the validity of the assessment arrived at through the MPPI, as well as the type of adjustment needed for the interpretation of scores on clinical scales.

- According to the directions provided in the manual, all 567 items (appearing in a random order in the inventory) for scoring purposes are organized in to 10 specific groups, each representing one or the other specific pathology (symptoms of some mental illness or disorder). Each of these 10 specific groups is referred to as one or the other clinical scales providing assessment or diagnosis of the nature and level of a specific mental illness or disorder of the client.

- Items are scored according to the directions provided in the manual. However, the administration of the inventory provides two types of scores: total score earned on the inventory and the scored earned on each clinical scale. While total scores earned on the inventory indicate the overall state of one's mental health, higher scores earned on a clinical scale demonstrate the presence of psychopathology linked to that particular clinical scale.

At this stage, you may be interested to know more about the nature of the 10 clinical scales used for scoring in the MPPI-2. They are described in Table 19.4.

It is no doubt that the use of the MPPI and its revision, the MPPI-2, has dominated the field of clinical assessment for psychometric purposes since their publications on the part of clinical psychologists all over the world. However, criticism in terms of their limitations, specifically related to their use with adults (18 years and above), and the cumbersome amount of 567 items necessitated the development of their newer version in the name of the MPPI-A and MPPI-2-RF. Let us know about them.

Minnesota Multiphasic Personality Inventory-Adolescent (MMPI-A)

Published in 1992, this inventory has been specifically designed for the psychometric assessment of the personality of clients aged 14 to 18 years. It is quite similar to the MPPI-2 in terms of its composition, format, administration, scoring, and interpretation. There are 478 items in the inventory representing statements (related to teen-specific problems and issues), requiring responses from clients in the form of true/false markings on a given answer sheet. It was standardized on a population of 2,500 adolescents chosen to match the 1980 US Census data on many important demographic variables. In terms of its scoring, it yields a total score as well as separate clinical scores, like the MMPI, for the interpretation of the needed clinical assessment.

The MMPI-2 Restructured Form (MMPI-2-RF)

Available to us since 2003, this personality inventory represents a shorter version of the MMPI-2 used for the psychometric assessment of adult clients. It contains 388 items (in comparison to the 567 items present in the original MMPI and its revised version, the MMPI-2) in the form of statements responded to in a true/false format. Its clinical scales have also been restructured by including fewer items and making them more homogeneous or tighter by reducing their overlap with others. On account of its shortening and ease of interpretation (compared to the MMPI-2), the use of the MMPI-2-RF is now preferred by many practitioners in the clinical world.

Table 19.4 Clinical Scales of the MPPI-2

Name of the Clinical Scale	Abbreviation	Scale Description
1. Hypochondriasis	Hs	Somatic problems, excessive bodily concern, weakness, ailments, complaining and whining
2. Depression	D	Depressed, unhappy, low confidence, pessimistic
3. Hysteria	Hy	Vague medical reactions to stress, somatic symptoms, denial of conflict and anger
4. Psychopathic deviate (Antisocial)	Pd	Antisocial, rebellious, blaming others, poor consideration of consequences of actions
5. Masculinity- Femininity	Mf	Rejection of traditional gender roles, effeminate men, masculine women
6. Paranoia	Pa	Suspicious, guarded, hypersensitive, belief that others intend to harm
7. Psychasthenia (Anxiety)	Pt	Anxious, nervous, tense, worrisome, obsessive
8. Schizophrenia	Sc	Psychotic, disorganized, or bizarre thought process, unconventional, hallucinations, delusions, alienated
9. Mania	Ma	Manic, elevated mood, energetic, overactive, accelerated movement and speech, flight of ideas
10. Social Introversion	Si	Introverted, shy, reserved, more comfortable alone than with others

Source: Adapted from Ben-Porath and Archer, 2008, Archer (1997) and Butcher (2011).

Personality Assessment Inventory (PAI)

Much like the MMPI, this personality inventory is useful for clinical assessment. It was originally devised in 1991 by Leslie Morey (Morey, 2003). Some of its basic features are summarized ahead.

- It is aimed at making clinical assessment of clients belonging to 18–89 years of age. It also has an adolescent version called the PIA-A for assessing clients of the age group 12–18.
- In its composition, it contains 344 items and 11 clinical scales (a few of which match with those of the MMPI) for the assessment and diagnosis of the problems related to the mental retardation, antisocial personality, anxiety disorders, alcoholism, and drug addiction, and so on.
- The clients are required to respond to inventory items in choosing one of the four options available in the form of (i) Totally false, (ii) Slightly true, (iii) Mainly true, and (iv) Very true.
- In addition to its 11 clinical scales, it also possesses validity scales (as possessed by the MMPI) for assessing the test-taking attitude of the client and thus maintaining the needed objectivity and validity in its measurement.

Millon Clinical Multiaxial Inventory-IV (MCMI-IV)

The Millon Clinical Multiaxial Inventory-IV (MCMI-IV) at present stands as a direct competitor of the MMPI-II in the field of the clinical assessment of mental disorders. Its basic features and use may be briefly summarized as follows.

- The MCMI was originally created in 1977 by Theodore Millon. Its second edition was published in 1987 in the name MCMI-II, and the third one as MVMI-III in the year 1994. The current version, MCMI-IV, was published in 2015.
- The MCMI-IV is designed for adults, but there are separate Millon personality inventories for adolescents and children, as well as another designed for use in medical situations in which the health care professional believes that personality may influence physical health (Millon and Millon, 2015).
- The MCMI-IV consists of 195 true/false items (in comparison to 567 in the MPPI-II). Its version meant for adolescents (13–19 years) contains even fewer items, numbering only 160.
- The 195 items, while appearing in the test in random order, provide scores for 24 clinical scales by constituting separate groups for this purpose. These 24 clinical scales are further grouped into four broad categories: (i) clinical personality disorder (11 scales), (ii) severe personality disorder (3 scales), (iii) clinical syndromes (7 scales), and (iv) severe clinical syndromes (3 scales). In this way, the MCMI-IV is distinct in its many scales related to the measurement of a number of personality disorders described in the DSMs.
- In addition to the clinical scales, it also includes "modifier indices" for assessing the test-taking attitude of the clients, similar to the validity scales of the MPPI.
- In this way, while having similarities in various aspects, it differs from the MMPI mainly on its distinction of possessing a number of clinical scales specifically meant for the assessment and diagnosis of a variety of personality disorders commonly visible among mentally disturbed persons. In this way, it is considered a wise choice to make use of the MCMI on the part of clinical psychologists who need a broad assessment of personality with an emphasis on personality disorders (Craig, 2008).

NEO Personality Inventory-3

A personality inventory developed by Paul Costa and Robert McCrae in the name of the NEO Personality Inventory (NEO-PI) is also credited for its role in the assessment and diagnosis of clinical disorders, although in a lesser amount in comparison to the previously discussed personality inventories—the MMPI, PAI, and MCMI. The aspects of its nature and use can be briefed as follows.

- Instead of emphasizing the search of syndromes related to abnormality and pathological aspects of one's personality (as do the MMPI, PAI, and MCMI), its developers looked for a personality measure that assesses "normal" personality characteristics of adult clients.
- In the original version of this inventory, published in 1985, the items of the inventory were grouped into three major dimensions, namely Neuroticism, Extraversion, and Openness. The first letters of these three dimensions were used by the developers of the inventory for its naming as the NEO Personality Inventory or NEO-PI.
- The revised version of this inventory, named the NEO-PI-R, was published in 1992 and had been quite popular in its use with the clients 17 years of age and older. For usage with clients

as young as 12, or older clients whose reading skills may be relatively weak, an improved version of this inventory was developed in 2005 in the name of the NEO-PI-3.

- In terms of format, the NEO-PI-3 is a 240-item, pencil-and-paper, self-report questionnaire. All the items of the inventory are in the form of short statements with multiple-choice responses ranging from "strongly agree" to "strongly disagree."
- Based on a five-factor model of personality, or "Big Five," the NEO-PI-3 (and its predecessor NEO-PI-R, as well) provides a measure of five fundamental traits of personality that characterize everyone in varying degrees. These traits/characteristics are:

  (i)   Neuroticism (aspects of personality related to one's adjustment and emotional stability)
  (ii) Extraversion (aspects of personality related to one's sociability and assertiveness)
  (iii) Openness (aspects of personality related to openness of experience, ideas, and values)
  (iv) Agreeableness (aspects of personality related to interpersonal tendencies such as altruism, sympathy toward others, and the belief that others are similarly inclined)
  (v)   Conscientiousness (aspects of personality related to the active processes of planning, organizing, and following through)

- For scoring purposes, each of these five dimensions of personality is further subdivided into individual traits or facets. In this way, the NEO-PI-3 also produces 30 "facet" scores (six facets within each of the five domains) to offer more specific descriptions of the component traits within each major dimension or factor of one's personality.
- While considered a suitable objective test for the assessment of a client's personality attributes, the major criticism of this test lies in its inability to provide validity scales (well available in the MMPI and MCMI) for the detection of a negative approach of the test-taker in terms of "faking" or inattention.

Eysenck Personality Questionnaire (EPQ-R)

The Eysenck Personality Questionnaire is a personality test in the form of a questionnaire that was devised by Eysenck and Eysenck (1975) as a major revision of their already developed personality inventory known as the Eysenck Personality Inventory (EPI) for assessing the personality traits of a person. Going ahead in the process of further improvement, a revised version of the EPQ was brought out by them in 1985 in the name EPQ-R. Let us briefly examine the nature and use of this test.

- The EPQ-R is available in two formats: full and short scale versions. It has 100 yes/no questions in its full version and 48 yes/no questions in its short version for the assessment of the personality attributes of individuals.
- It measures three pervasive, independent dimensions of personality: Extraversion-Introversion, Neuroticism-Stability, and Psychoticism-Socialization.
- As a measure of personality traits, it has four scales named as the (i) Extraversion scale ("E score" for knowing how much of an extrovert one is), (ii) Neuroticism scale ("N score" for knowing how neurotic one is), (iii) Psychoticism scale ("P score" for knowing how psychotic one is), and Lie scale ("L score" to know how socially desirable one is trying to be in your answer).
- It is regarded as a reliable, objective, and valid tool for the assessment of one's personality. The major weakness of this test, however, lies in its possession of yes/no questions, which sometimes forces inaccurate response, and it can be psychometrically inferior.

To Sum Up

The psychological tests referred to as personality tests are specifically designed by clinical psychologists to assess personality traits, characteristics, or attributes of the client's personality. Among the most commonly used non-projective techniques or personality tests we may name the use of one or the other personality inventory. As examples of popular contemporary personality inventories used for clinical assessment, we have the (i) Minnesota Multiphasic Personality Inventory (MMPI-2) for use with adult clients aged 18 years and above, (ii) Minnesota Multiphasic Personality Inventory-Adolescent (MMPI-A) for use with clients aged 14 to 18 years, (iii) MMPI-2 Restructured Form (MMPI-2-RF) for the use with adult clients, (iv) Personality Assessment Inventory (PAI) for use with clients of 18–89 years of age, and its version PIA-A for clients aged 12–18, (v) Millon Clinical Multiaxial Inventory—IV (MCMI-IV) for use with adolescents (13– 19 years), (vi) NEO Personality Inventory (NEO-PI-R) for use with clients 17 years of age and older, and its version NEO-PI-3 for use with clients 12 years of age and older, and (vii) Eysenck Personality Questionnaire (EPQ) and its revised version EPQ-R for use with adult clients (18 years and above).

The Objective Psychological Tests for Measuring a Specific Single Aspect of One's Personality

With the use of the objective personality tests discussed so far in the form of one or the other personality inventories or questionnaires, clinical psychologists may get an overall comprehensive assessment with the scores available on various traits or variables of a client's personality. Besides having such broader assessment of the client's personality, there are occasions when instead of such comprehensive assessment of one's personality, we may need measures that focus exclusively on one characteristic or trait, such as maladjustment, depression, anxiety, frustration, sleeping or eating disorders, and so on. In the pages to follow, we will discuss the nature and use of a few psychological tests aimed to assess one or the other single aspect of a client's personality.

Measures for the Assessment of the Client's Adjustment

The psychological tests called adjustment inventories are used for assessing the adjustment or maladjustment level of the client with the self and environment. There are a number of good measures available to clinical psychologists for the purpose. As examples, we can name the measures like (i) Bell Adjustment Inventory (a measure for assessing the adjustment of adults in general), (ii) Heston Personal Adjustment Inventory (a measure for assessing the level of one's adjustment to his self), (iii) Sexual Adjustment Inventory (the best available measure available for evaluating sex offenders) (iv) Asthna's Adjustment Inventory and Sinha's Adjustment Inventory (for assessing the Hindi-speaking student population of our country), and Mangal's Teacher Adjustment Inventory (developed by the first author of this text for assessing the adjustment— personal and professional—of school teachers). Among these measures, the Bell Adjustment Inventory is the most popular among clinical psychologists for assessing and diagnosing the symptoms as well as levels of maladjustment prevailing among clients. Let us look into it in brief.

Bell Adjustment Inventory

- This is available in two forms: for students and for adults. In the adult form of the inventory, Bell (1958) provides five separate measures related to one's home, health, social, emotional, and occupational adjustment.
- The items of the inventory are in the format of choosing the answers "yes" or "no" or "?" and are selected on the basis of their capability of assessing the degree of one's adjustment or maladjustment.
- High scores on the inventory signify poor adjustment and low scores, better adjustment, in different areas and also in respect of one's overall adjustment.

Measures for the Assessment of Depression

The diagnosis of symptoms and the assessment of the degree of depression is a common need on the part of clinical psychologists. There are a number of measuring instruments available to them for this purpose. The popularly used among them are: (i) the Beck Depression Inventory-II (BDI-II), (ii) the Children's Depression Inventory (CDS), (iii) the Hamilton Rating Scale for Depression (HRSD), and (iv) the Children's Depression Rating Scale (CDRS).

For knowing about the nature and use of these depression-measuring instruments, let us illustrate it with a brief description of the most widely used clinical measure, the BDI-II.

The Beck Depression Inventory-II (BDI-II)

This is the most widely used instrument for the clinical assessment of depression in terms of its initial screening and detection of the severity of depression. Created in its original version by Aaron Beck in the 1960s, its currently available version in the name of the BDI-II was published in 1996 (Beck et al., 1996). Its basic features and use can be summarized as follows.

- The BDI-II is a self-report, pencil-and-paper test aimed at the clinical assessment of the depressive symptoms of clients within the age range of 13–80.
- The BDI takes approximately 8–10 minutes to complete.
- In its composition, it contains 21 items to be responded to on the part of the clients with the use of multiple-choice response formats, as depicted below through the following example:

I never think about dying.   (0 points)
I occasionally think about dying. (1 point)
I frequently think about dying.   (2 points)
I constantly think about dying.   (3 points)

- For obtaining a total score, the 21 item scores are summed up by the clinical psychologist to determine an overall level of depression of the client.
- The validity and reliability of the BDI has been tested across populations worldwide.

Measures for the Assessment of Anxiety

The clinical psychologists are often required to make a clinical assessment of the anxiety behavior of their clients. There are a number of measures or instruments available to them for this purpose. The mentionable popular ones include: (i) the Beck Anxiety Inventory (BAI), (ii) the seven-item Generalized Anxiety Disorder Scale (GAD-7), (iii) the Hamilton Anxiety Rating Scale (HARS), and (iv) the Overall Anxiety Severity and Impairment Scale (OASIS). For illustration purposes, we present a brief description of The Beck Anxiety Inventory (BAI)—the most popular anxiety measure among clinical psychologists.

The Beck Anxiety Inventory (BAI)

The credit for the development of this inventory goes to Aaron T. Beck and his colleagues (Beck et al., 1988). The aspects of its nature and use can be summed up as follows.

- It is a 21-question multiple-choice self-report inventory that is used for measuring the severity of anxiety in adolescents and adults ages 17 and older.
- The questions used in this inventory ask the client to tell about the common symptoms of anxiety experienced by him during the past week (including the day he is appearing for testing).
- It takes approximately 5 to 10 minutes to answer the questions of the inventory. Each answer given by the client is scored on a scale value of 0 (not at all) to 3 (severely).
- The highest total score may thus be 21 x 3= 63 for a client. The standardized cutoff scores provided in the manual for the measurement of various levels of anxiety are:

    (i) Minimal anxiety (0 to 7), (ii) Mild anxiety (8 to 15), (iii) Moderate anxiety (16 to 25), and (iv) Severe anxiety (30 to 63).

Measures for Assessing Self-Esteem

There exists a strong positive correlation between one's poor mental health and a poor level of one's self-esteem. This is why clinical psychologists often employ tools for the clinical assessment of the self-esteem of their clients. As examples of such self-esteem assessment tools, we may look at the Rosenberg Self-Esteem scale (RSE) and the Coopersmith Self-Esteem Inventory (SEI). For illustration purposes, here we present a brief discussion of the nature and use of the SEI.

Coopersmith Self-Esteem Inventory (SEI): This scale has been developed by S. Coopersmith in 1967. It consists of 50 items and aims to measure attitudes toward the self. Its items require the respondents to report feelings about the self directly and are typically scored using a dichotomous scale ("Like me" vs. "Unlike me"). Thus, a SEI score can range from 0 to 50, with higher scores reflecting higher self-esteem.

To Sum Up

There exist several psychological tests for providing a clinical assessment of a single aspect or attribute of a client's personality, such as maladjustment, depression, anxiety, and self-esteem. In this sequence, the psychological tests known as *adjustment inventories* are used for assessing the adjustment or maladjustment level of the client with the self and environment. As examples, we can name the measures such as the Bell Adjustment

Inventory, (ii) the Heston Personal Adjustment Inventory, (iii) the Sexual Adjustment Inventory, (iv) Asthna's Adjustment Inventory and Sinha's Adjustment Inventory for assessing the Hindi-speaking student population of our country. For the diagnosis of symptoms and assessment of the degree of depression among clients, we have instruments such as the (i) the Beck Depression Inventory-II (BDI-II), (ii) the Children's Depression Inventory (CDS), (iii) the Hamilton Rating Scale for Depression (HRSD), and (iv) the Children's Depression Rating Scale (CDRS). For the clinical assessment of the anxiety levels, we have measures like the (i) the Beck Anxiety Inventory (BAI), (ii) the seven-item Generalized Anxiety Disorder Scale (GAD-7), (iii) the Hamilton Anxiety Rating Scale (HARS), and (iv) the Overall Anxiety Severity and Impairment Scale (OASIS). Similarly, for the clinical assessment of the self-esteem of clients, we have tools such as the Rosenberg Self-Esteem scale (RSE) and Coopersmith Self-Esteem Inventory (SEI).

Projective Personality Tests

So far, we have discussed only those personality tests in the name of objective tests that usually evaluate the overt or conscious behavior or personality of an individual by directly asking him to describe himself. These provide us with an incomplete description or assessment of one's personality. Therefore, there should be other types of personality tests employed to try to assess the total personality of an individual instead of assessing it in fragments. Projective tests are devised to accept this challenge. Let us know about them.

What are Projective Tests?

These tests are based on the phenomenon of projection. In the development and use of these tests, relatively indefinite and unstructured stimuli (like vague pictures, ink blots, incomplete sentences, etc.) are provided to the subject, and he is asked to structure them in any way he likes. In doing so, he unconsciously projects his own desires, hopes, fears, repressed wishes, and so on, and thus not only reveals his inner or private world but also gives a proper clue to estimate his total personality.

The common Projective Techniques are described ahead.

The Rorschach Ink Blot Test

The Rorschach Ink Blot Test, a well-known projection instrument, owes its origin and development to Swiss psychiatrist Harman Rorschach, the son of an art teacher. It was first published in 1921 in a monograph *Psychodiagnostics*, described as a "form-perception test using inkblots." The distinguished features and use of this test are briefed as follows.

- The test material consists of 10 cards on which are ink blots. Five of them are in black and white and five are multi-colored. These ink blots are completely unstructured—the shapes of the blots do not have any specific meaning.
- Administration of the test occurs in two phases, named the (i) Response or Free Association phase, and (ii) the Inquiry phase. In the response phase, the client is presented with one card at a time and is asked to respond to questions like, "What do you see in it? What does it look

like?" He is left free to provide his response in his way. His response is noted down by the test administrator. After the client has responded to all 10 cards, the second phase, "inquiry," begins with the objective of seeking clarification or addition to the original responses given in the first phase.

- For the purpose of scoring, the responses are given specific symbols, which are entered into four columns. These scoring categories are named:

  (i)   Location, (the part of the blot with which the client associates each response)
  (ii) Contents (what is seen by the client irrespective of the way of its perception)
  (iii) Originality (some type of originality visible in the client's response)
  (iv) Determinants (what aspect of the inkblot—its form, color, shading, and so on—caused the client to make a particular response?

- A system known as the Rorschach Comprehensive System (RCS) is the most common method used for the scoring and interpretation of the responses of clients in the Rorschach Inkblot Test across almost their entire lifespan. It was developed in the 1960s by Dr. John E. Exner. However, there has emerged at present an entirely new scoring system, the Rorschach Performance Assessment System (R-PAS), which has stronger norms than the Comprehensive System (Mihura and Meyer, 2015).

TAT or Thematic Apperception Test

The test consisting of the perception of certain pictures in a thematic manner (revealing imaginative themes) is called the TAT or Thematic Apperception Test. This test came into operation in 1935 with a publication by Henry Murray and Christiana Morgan (Morgan and Murray, 1935). The description regarding its nature and use are briefed ahead.

- The TAT includes a total of 31 cards (depicting different scenes or pictures of interpersonal tendencies in human beings), but the clinical psychologists typically select their own subset of cards—often about 10 or so—to administer to a particular client for the clinical assessment of his personality.
- The picture cards are presented one at a time. They are vague and indefinite. The client is required to make up a story for each of the pictures presented to him within a fixed time period by taking care of aspects such as "What is going on in the picture? What has led to this scene? What would likely happen in such a situation?" They are also required to describe what the characters may be thinking and feeling (Bellak, 1993).
- As the client tells stories aloud and the psychologist writes them down, the clinical psychologist may proceed further to gather more information from the client by putting questions during the recitation of the stories by him.
- In making up the stories, the subject unconsciously reveals many characteristics of his personality. Its special value resides in its power to explore the underlying hidden drives, complexes, and conflicts of the client's personality. In addition to its working as a global measure of one's personality, its strength may lie in its ability to measure interpersonal relationship tendencies (Ackerman et al., 2008).
- The success of this test as a method of clinical assessment of one's personality lies much in the interpretation of what has been said by the client in knitting their stories by using an appropriate scoring system. Originally, Morgan and Murray (1935) analyzed the contents of the stories according to needs and pressures (the need of the hero and the environmental

forces to which he is exposed). Today, no formal scoring system is followed by the clinical psychologist for the interpretation. Rather, most clinicians today seem to rely on their own impressionistic inferences for performing this task (Moretti and Rossini, 2004).

- As a result of the non-availability of a well-standardized empirical scoring and interpretation procedure, the validity and reliability of the TAT are less well established than those of other personality tests (Mihura and Meyer, 2015). However, still on account of its strength in the power of its stories furnishing valuable information about one's personality makeup, it continues to be recognized as a significant method of clinical assessment of a client's personality.

CAT (Children Apperception Test)

The TAT works well with adults and adolescents, but for children, it is not suitable. For children between three to ten years, the CAT was developed in 1949 by Leopold Bellak and Sonya Sorel Bellak as an offshoot of the widely used TAT. It is similar to the TAT in many ways regarding its administration, use, and interpretation. The difference lies in the composition of the test material. In contrast to the 31 cards in the TAT, the CAT contains a total of 10 cards and the cards have pictures of animals instead of human characters. All 10 cards are presented one by one and the subject is asked to make up stories from them. The scoring and interpretation of these stories again have no standard method or system, and like the TAT, this test is usually interpreted by clinical psychologists through their own impressionistic inferences. The most recent revision of the CAT was published in 1993.

The Other Picture Story Tests Available for Clinical Assessment

Besides the Rorschach Ink Blot Test, the TAT, and CAT, there are a number of other picture story projective tests available to clinical psychologists for their use in the clinical assessment of clients. A few popular ones are named below.

- *Senior Apperception Test* (Bellak and Bellak, 1973): A picture story test depicting themes relevant to older adults.
- *Picture Story Test* (Symonds, 1949): For use with adolescents, it contains pictures designed to elicit adolescent-related themes such as coming home late and leaving home.
- *Michigan Picture Test* (Andrew et al., 1953): For use with children aged 8–14 years, it contains pictures designed to elicit various themes ranging from conflicts with authority to feelings of personal inadequacy.

Word Association Tests

Word association tests used for the clinical assessment of clients represent a type of projective tests in which the client is presented with a list of simulated words (uttered by the clinical psychologist one by one) for being responded to by the client verbally or in writing with whatever comes to mind first upon hearing the word. The contents of the responses, along with other related things (such as reaction time and any unusual speech or behavior manifestation accompanying a given response) are then analyzed for deriving conclusions about the clinical diagnosis of the personality of the client. There are a number of standardized word association tests available for clinical assessment. We are here naming the two popular ones.

- *Menninger Word Association Test:* Consisting of 60 words, this test was developed by Rapaport et al. (1946) at the Menninger clinic with the sole objective of helping clinicians in detecting impairment of thought processes and revealing areas of significant internal conflicts.
- *Kent-Rosanoff Free Association Test:* Developed by Kent and Rosanoff (1910), this test consists of a set of 100 stimuli of commonly used words appropriate for evoking responses from the client for arriving at the clinical assessment of psychopathology.

Sentence-Completion Tests

Sentence completion tests represent those projective tests in which a series of incomplete sentences (in their beginning form) are presented before the client for their completion as quickly as possible (without giving a second thought to his answers). As an example, such a test may have the items like: "I am worried over . . ." The contents of the responses given by the clients to the test items are then analyzed by the clinical psychologists for deriving conclusions about the clinical assessment of the personality of the clients. As a result of ongoing development in the construction of the needed tests in this field, we at present have a number of sentence completion tests for the use of clinical psychologists. Some of the widely used standardized sentence completion tests in this concern are: (i) the Rotter Incomplete Sentence Blank, (ii) the Minor Sentence Completion Test, and (iii) the Washington University Sentence Completion Test.

For illustration purposes, here we are providing a brief introduction to the most widely used standardized test, the Rotter Incomplete Sentence Blank (RISB).

- Developed and standardized by Rotter and Raffery, it was published in its original form in 1950. Its most recent revision was carried out on in 1992. It can usefully serve the assessment purpose of the population from grade 9 through adulthood and is available in its three versions: High school (grades 9 through 12), College (grades 13 through 16), and Adult.
- The RISB tests include 40 written incomplete sentences, followed by blank spaces in which the client is required to provide his response for completing the sentence.
- For interpretation of the client's responses, the manual of the test provides a number of categories: Family attitudes, Social and Sexual attitudes, General attitudes, and Character traits, and asks to evaluate each response on a seven-point scale that ranges from a need for therapy to extremely good adjustment.

Figure Drawing Tests

Figure drawing tests represent a category of projective tests in which clients are required to produce a drawing for being used on the part of clinical psychologists as important clues for the needed clinical assessment. The popular figure drawing tests available at present for this purpose are:

(i) *Goodenough's draw-a-man test* or *Goodenough-Harris Drawing Test* (asking the client to complete three individual drawings on separate pieces of paper by drawing a man, a woman, and himself)
(ii) *Machover's draw-a-person test* (asking the client to draw a figure of a person of his choice in the first phase and then to draw the figure of a person of the sex opposite to the first in the

second phase, and after that putting inquiry questions about the first and second drawings in the third phase)

(iii) *The house-tree-person test:* (asking the client to draw a picture of the "house" of his choice in the first phase and then draw the pictures of a "tree" and a "person" as well as possible in the second and third phases)

(iv) *Kinetic family drawing test*: (asking the client to draw a picture of everyone in his family, including him doing something).

To Sum Up

Unlike the personality tests (available in the form of personality inventories and objective tests), which evaluate the overt or conscious behavior or personality of an individual, projective tests help clinical psychologists with the assessment of the total personality of their clients in a more appropriate way. In the development and use of these tests, relatively indefinite and unstructured stimuli (like vague pictures, ink blots, incomplete sentences, etc.) are provided to the subject and he is asked to structure them in any way he likes. In doing so, he unconsciously projects his own desires, hopes, fears, repressed wishes, and so on, and thus not only reveals his inner or private world but also gives a proper clue to estimate his total personality. The popular and widely used projective tests used for the clinical assessment may be named as (i) the Rorschach Ink Blot Test, (ii) the Thematic Apperception Test (TAT), (iii) the Children Apperception Test (CAT), (iv) other Picture story tests known as (a) the Senior Apperception Test for use with older adults, (b) the Picture Story Test for use with adolescents, and (iii) the Michigan Picture Test for use with 8–14-year-old children, (v) the Word Association Tests such as the Menninger Word Association Test and Kent-Rosanoff Free Association Test, (vi) Sentence completion tests such as the Rotter Incomplete Sentence Blank, the Minor Sentence Completion Test, and the Washington University Sentence Completion Test, (vii) Figure drawing tests such as Goodenough's draw-a-man test, Machover's draw-a-person test, the house-tree-person test, and the Kinetic family drawing test.

Neuropsychological Testing as a Method of Clinical Assessment

The task of conducting medical tests such as computed tomography (CT), magnetic resonance imaging (MRI), and positron emission tomography (PET) scans for detecting brain abnormalities is the task of Neurologists. On the other hand, the main task of neuropsychological testing is to assess problems that might result from a head injury, prolonged alcohol or drug use, or a degenerative brain illness.

There are two types of neuropsychological tests available for the use of clinical psychologists. The first type are neuropsychological batteries of tests (helpful in knowing about the specific cognitive weaknesses of the clients) and the other type are briefer single tests, typically used for screening neuropsychological impairment rather than working as full-fledged neuropsychological assessment tools. Let us discuss the popular tests belonging to these two categories.

1. *The Halstead-Reitan Neuropsychological Battery (HRNB)*

- The HRNB was first constructed by Ward C. Halstead of Chicago University, together with his doctoral student, Ralph Reitan.

- It is a comprehensive battery consisting of eight standardized neuropsychological tests that must be administered as a whole. A few of these eight tests involve sight, whereas others involve hearing, touch, motor skills, and pencil-and-paper tasks.
- It is suitable for clients of age 15 and older, but alternate versions are available for younger clients.
- Essentially, its primary purpose is to identify people with brain damage and to furnish detailed information about the consequential specific cognitive impairments. The findings of the HRNB are thus helpful in the diagnosis and treatment of problems related to brain malfunction (Broshek and Barth, 2000).
- The main difficulty in the use of the HNRB lies in the excessive time required for its administration (up to three hours or more in some brain-injured patients).

2. Luria-Nebraska Neuropsychological Battery (LNNB)

- Based on the previous work done on this account by Alexander Luria, the LNRB was created by Charles Golden in 1981.
- It is available in its two versions; its original version is for use with ages fifteen and over, and the other version in the name of the *Luria-Nebraska Neuropsychological Battery for Children (LNNB-C)* can be used with child clients of ages eight to twelve. The administration time for both these tests is two to three hours in general.
- The LNNB is similar to the HNRB in that it is a wide-ranging test of neuropsychological functioning. It consists of 269 items divided among 14 scales helpful in identifying damage occurring in particular regions of the brain.
- It differs from the HNRB in two aspects: (i) it tends to be slightly briefer than HNRB, and (ii) in comparison to the HNRB, it provides greater emphasis on qualitative/written comments of the test administrator about the behavior of the client at the time of test-taking.
- It has been found to be more reliable and valid than the other available neuropsychological tests in its ability to differentiate between brain damage and mental illness.

3. The Bender-Gestalt test

- As a brief neuropsychological measure, this test was originally developed in 1938 by child psychiatrist Lauretta Bender and is now available in the name of the *Bender Visual-Motor Gestalt Test—Second Edition (Bender-Gestalt-II)*.
- It is the most commonly used neuropsychological screening among clinical psychologists for assessing the visual-motor functioning, developmental disorders, and neurological impairments in children ages three and older, as well as in adults.
- The test consists of nine index cards picturing different geometric designs (primarily made of combinations of circles, dots, lines, angles, and basic shapes). The cards are presented individually to the clients and they are asked to copy the design as accurately as possible before the next card is shown. Test performance of the client is scored on the quality of the accuracy and organization of the reproductions.
- The results arrived at through the administration of this test suffer from the limitation of not being capable of specifying locations of brain damage or providing details of the suspected neuropsychological problem. However, the test can serve a useful primary screening purpose and, as such, can alert the clinical psychologist to the general presence of neuropsychological problems for being confirmed and investigated thoroughly by an advanced testing program.

4. Rey-Osterrieth Complex Figure Test (ROCF)

- This test owes its name on account of the men who were behind its creation and the material involved in the test. This test was was first proposed by the Swiss psychologist André Rey in 1941 and then got its standardization in 1944 at the hands of Paul-Alexandre Osterrieth. The test material and task done in the test involve the drawing/copying of a single complex figure.
- In its composition and administration, it is a brief pencil-and-paper drawing neuropsychological test in which the client is asked to reproduce a complicated line drawing, first by copying it freehand and then drawing it from memory.
- Since a number of cognitive abilities (such as visuo-spatial abilities, memory, attention, planning, working memory, and task execution ability) are involved in performing the assigned task, the performance of the client helps in the evaluation of the cognitive functioning of all these abilities.
- As an effective clinical assessment device, the test may be properly used to further explain any secondary effect of brain injury in neurological patients, to test for the presence of dementia, or to study the degree of cognitive impairment or improvement in children.

5. Wechsler Memory Scale—Fourth Edition (WMS-IV)

Belonging to the family of tests designed by David Wechsler for assessing the intellectual abilities and functions of individuals, the Wechsler Memory Scale (WMS) represents the type of neuropsychological test aimed at measuring different memory-related functions of the clients. Its current version, available in the name of the *Wechsler Memory Scale—Fourth Edition (WMS-IV)*, was published in 2009. Its main features are briefed as follows.

- WMS-IV is basically a memory test, designed to assess the memorization abilities of the clients in their varying aspects, such as visual and auditory memory, visual working memory, and immediate and delayed recall.
- The task of carrying out such broader memorization assessment is executed by the WMS-IV through the analysis of the client's responses to the items included in its subtests.
- The client's performance in the different subtests is reported through five Index Scores, named as: Auditory Memory, Visual Memory, Visual Working Memory, Immediate Memory, and Delayed Memory.
- As a clinical assessment device, it can be used with clients aged 16 to 90 who are suspected of having memory problems due to brain injury, dementia, substance abuse, or other factors.
- The research evidences have established the validity of the WMS-IV in differentiating clinical groups (such as those with dementias or neurological disorders) from those with normal memory functioning.

To Sum Up

Neuropsychological testing as a method of clinical assessment aims to assess problems that might result from head injury, substance abuse, or a degenerative brain illness. There are two types of neuropsychological tests available for this purpose to clinical psychologists. The first type are in the form of neuropsychological batteries of tests (helpful in knowing about the specific cognitive weaknesses of the clients) and the other are in the form of briefer single tests typically used for screening neuropsychological impairment. The popular testing devices available on this account may be named as (i) the Halstead-Reitan Neuropsychological Battery (HRNB), (ii) the Luria-Nebraska Neuropsychological Battery (LNNB), (iii) the Bender-Gestalt test, (iv) the Rey-Osterrieth Complex Figure Test (ROCF), and (v) the Wechsler Memory Scale—Fourth Edition (WMS-IV).

Review Questions

1. What is psychological testing? How can it be used as a method of clinical assessment on the part of clinical psychologists?
2. What are achievement tests? Name five achievement tests available for clinical assessment and discuss the use of any one of them for illustration purposes.
3. What are intelligence tests? Name any five intelligence tests used by clinical psychologists for the clinical assessment of their clients and discuss the use of any two in detail.
4. Throw light on personality testing as a method of clinical assessment by illustrating the use of a personality inventory or a projective test.
5. Discuss the use of objective psychological tests for measuring specific single aspects of one's personality by illustrating the measurement of the client's adjustment, depression, anxiety, and self-esteem with the help of a suitable measurement device.
6. What are projective tests? Name the different types of projective tests used for the clinical assessment and illustrate their use with the help of a suitable projective technique.
7. What do you understand by the term neuropsychological testing as a method of clinical assessment? Name the different types of tests used for this purpose and discuss the use of any one for illustration purposes.
8. Discuss in brief the use of any three of the following psychological testing devices for the purpose of clinical assessment: (i) the Wechsler Adult Intelligence Scale—Fourth Edition (WAIS-IV), (ii) the Stanford-Binet Intelligence Scales—Fifth Edition (SB5), (iii) the Wechsler Individual Achievement Test-III Edition, (iv) the Minnesota Multiphasic Personality Inventory (MMPI-2), (v) the Bell Adjustment Inventory, (vi) the Beck Depression Inventory-II (BDI-II), (vii) the Beck Anxiety Inventory (BAI), and (viii) the Coopersmith Self-Esteem Inventory (SEI).

References

Ackerman, S. J., Fowler, J. C., & Clemence, A. J. (2008), TAT and other performance-based assessment techniques, In R. P. Archer & S. R. Smith (Eds.), *Personality assessment* (pp. 337–378), New York, NY: Routledge.

Andrew, G., Hartwell, S. W., Hutt, M. L., & Walton, R. E. (1953), *The Michigan Picture test*, Chicago, IL: Science and Research Association.

Archer, R. P. (1997). *MMPI-A: Assessing adolescent psychopathology* (2nd ed.). Mahwah, NJ: Erlbaum.

Beck, A. T., Epstein, N., Brown, G., & Steer, R. A. (1988). An inventory for measuring clinical anxiety: Psychometric properties, *Journal of Consulting and Clinical Psychology*, 56: 893–897.

Beck, A. T., Steer, R. A., & Brown, G. K. (1996), *Manual for the Beck Depression Inventory-II*, San Antonio, CA: Psychological Corporation.

Bellak, L. (1993). *The TAT, CAT, and SAT in clinical use* (5th ed.), Needham Heights, MA: Allyn & Bacon.

Bellak, L., & Bellak, S.S. (1973), *Senior apperception technique*, New York, NY: C.P.S.

Ben-Porath, Y. S., & Archer, R. P. (2008), The MMPI-2 and MMPI-A, In R. P. Archer & S. R. Smith (Eds.), *Personality assessment* (pp. 81–131), New York, NY: Routledge.

Bracken, B. A., & McCallum, S. (2015), *The Universal Nonverbal Intelligence Test2 (UNIT)*, Austin, TX: PRO-ED.

Broshek, D. K., & Barth, J. T. (2000), The Halstead-Reitan neuropsychological battery, In G. Groth-Marnat (Ed.), *Neuropsychological assessment in clinical practice* (pp. 223–262), New York, NY: Wiley.

Butcher, J. N. (2011), *A beginner's guide to the MMPI-2* (3rd ed.), Washington, DC: American Psychological Association.

Craig, R. J. (2008), Millon Clinical Multiaxial Inventory-III, In R. P. Archer & S. R. Smith (Eds.), *Personality assessment* (pp. 133–165), New York, NY: Routledge.

Eysenck, H. J., & Eysenck, S. B. J. (1975), *Manual of the Eysenck Personality Questionnaire*, London: Hodder and Stoughton.

Goldfinger, K., & Pomerantz, A. M. (2010), *Psychological assessment and report writing*, Thousand Oaks, CA: SAGE.

Kent, G. H., & Rosanoff, A. J. (1910), A study of association in insanity, *American Journal of Insanity*, 67: 37–76; 317–390.

Lichtenberger, E. O., & Breaux, K. C. (2010), *Essentials of WIAT-III and KTEA-II assessment*, Hoboken, NJ: Wiley.

Mihura, J. L., & Meyer, G. J. (2015), Thematic apperception test, In R. L. Cautin & S. O. Lilienfeld (Eds.), *The encyclopedia of clinical psychology* (pp. 2813–2818), Chichester: Wiley Blackwell.

Millon, T., & Millon, C. (2015), Millon inventories (MCMI, MACI, M-PACI, MBMD), In R. L. Cautin & S. O. Lilienfeld (Eds.), *The encyclopedia of clinical psychology* (pp. 1820–1830), Chichester: Wiley Blackwell.

Moretti, R. J., & Rossini, E. D. (2004), The Thematic Apperception Test (TAT), In M. J. Hilsenroth & D. L. Segal (Eds.), *Comprehensive handbook of psychological assessment: Personality assessment* (Vol. 2, pp. 356–371), Hoboken, NJ: Wiley.

Morey, L. C. (2003), *Essentials of PAI assessment*, Hoboken, NJ: Wiley.

Morgan, C. D., & Murray, H. A. (1935), A method for investigating fantasies: The thematic apperception test, *Archives of Neurology and Psychiatry*, 34: 289–306.

Raiford, S. E., Coalson, D. L., Saklofske, D. H., & Weiss, L. G. (2010), Practical issues in WAIS-IV administration and scoring, In L. G. Weiss, D. H. Saklofske, D. Coalson, & S. E. Raiford (Eds.), *WAIS-IV clinical use and interpretation: Scientist-practitioner perspectives* (pp. 25–60), London: Elsevier.

Rapaport, D., Gill, M. M., & Shaffer, R. (1946), *Diagnostic psychological testing* (Vol.2), Chicago, IL: Year Book.

Symonds, P. M. (1949), Review of the software Symonds picture-Story test, *Journal of Consulting Psychology*, 13(1), 67–68.

Chapter 20

Clinical Intervention or Therapeutic Approaches

Learning Objectives

After going through this chapter, you will be able to:

*   Discuss the various medical or somatic therapies named as Drug or Chemotherapy, Shock Therapy, and Psychosurgery.
*   Differentiate between the nature and use of the medical and psychological therapies.
*   Explain the use of Psychoanalytic or Psychodynamic therapy.
*   State about the use of Client-Centered Psychotherapy.
*   Discuss the use of various types of behavior therapies known as (i) Counter Conditioning, (ii) Desensitization Method, (iii) Aversive Conditioning, (iv) Modelling, and (v) Method of Positive Reinforcement.
*   Throw light on the nature and use of various types of cognitive therapies designated as (i) Rational Emotive Therapy (RET), (ii) Beck's Cognitive Therapy (CT), and (iii) Cognitive Behavior Therapy (CBT).
*   Explain the nature and use of Humanistic-Existential Therapy.
*   Throw light on the nature and use of other alternative therapies designated as (i) Group Therapy, (ii) Family Therapy, (iii) Dramatic Therapy, and (iv) Meditation Therapy.
*   Discuss the rehabilitation of the mentally ill.

Introduction

The mental disorders or abnormalities in one's behavior discussed in the previous chapters of this text are undesirable and harmful to the individual, as well as to society in their various ways. Every care, therefore, needs to be taken to avoid their occurrence by adopting one or the other preventive measures. However, we cannot eliminate the possibilities of their occurrence. They are bound to occur and therefore, suitable treatment measures need to be taken for helping maladjusted and sick individuals. However, a mental disorder or abnormality in behavior is an individual phenomenon and situational problem, and thereby, it is not possible to lay down a general treatment plan for all such ailments and disorders. Moreover, the disorder needs to be treated in terms of superficial symptoms as well as its root causes. Therefore, the problem of the treatment of mental illness or disorder should include medical, psychological, and sociological procedures managed by three types of professionals: (i) medical professionals (especially

DOI: 10.4324/9781003398325-20

psychiatrists and neurosurgeons), (ii) clinical psychologists (trained in psychotherapeutic treatment), and (iii) social psychologists, counselors, and social workers. Thus, as far as the role of clinical psychologists is concerned, it is very much limited to the psychotherapeutic treatment given by them to mentally ill or disturbed people. As a text of clinical psychology, therefore, we focus only on the discussion related to the use of various psychotherapies for the treatment of one or the other behavioral and mental disorders. But it should also be noted that professionally, clinical psychologists need to be reasonably aware about the mode and effectiveness of available medical treatments for the treatment of one or the other types of mental illness and behavioral problems, especially the serious ones. Moreover, in some states and countries, clinical psychologists are authorized to prescribe medicines, and they are often needed by psychiatrists and neurologists to work along with them for the treatment of the patients. Thus, there remains a general requirement on the part of clinical psychologists to be equipped with the necessary working knowledge of the medical means utilized for the treatment of mental illness and behavioral disorders. Let us therefore discuss them in brief.

Use of Somatic or Medical Therapies

Somatic or Medical therapy concerns the physiological treatment of mental illnesses and behavioral disorders. Some of the main measures included in this category are drug or chemotherapy, shock therapy, and brain surgery.

Drug or Chemotherapy

There has been a widespread use of psychotherapeutic drugs derived from chemical substances in the treatment of mental illness. These drugs can be grouped into the categories: (i) major tranquilizers, (ii) minor tranquilizers, (iii) anti-depressives, (iv) sedatives, and (v) hallucinogenic.
    Let us know about the uses and importance of such drugs.

- Major tranquilizers are used with psychotic patients but may also be found useful in cases of alcoholic and senile patients. They diminish anxiety, agitation, aggressive behavior, hallucinations, and delusions, and thus help to control various psychotic symptoms without impairing intelligence or clarity of consciousness. Chlorpromazine, a drug derived from phenothiazine and reserpine, a crystalline alkaloid extracted from *Rauwolfia serpentina*, are the two notable tranquillizers which have been found effective.
- Minor tranquilizers like meprobamate and chlordiazepoxide reduce anxiety, apprehension, and tension. Usually, they elicit no psychotic symptoms, and are widely used with neurotic and psychosomatic patients.
- Anti-depressive drugs like phenelzine, isocarboxazid, imipramine, and amitriptyline diminish apathy and lethargy and are therefore widely used in controlling depressive reactions.
- Sedative drugs like phenobarbital reduce anxiety, over-activity, and insomnia. Sedatives carry side effects such as interference with clarity of consciousness and causing drowsiness, and therefore, in many cases, the use of tranquilizers is widely recommended in place of sedatives.
- Depressants like lithium carbonate are mainly used in the treatment of agitated depression.
- Anticonvulsant drugs like trimethadione and sodium diphenylhydantoinate are found to be effective in controlling several types of epilepsy.
- Hallucinogenic drugs such as LSD and mescaline are useful in the treatment of schizophrenic patients, particularly children.

- The use of drugs has been effective in reducing the severity of symptoms and making the management of patients convenient in the hospital or at home. It has made possible for many patients to function in the community instead of remaining in the hospital. The drugs make many more patients accessible to psychological and sociological treatment.

However, the use of drugs has many limitations and drawbacks. The drugs and the dosage vary for different illnesses and patients. Therefore, matching drug and dosage to meet the needs of a given patient in a particular situation is an uphill task. Moreover, the drugs may also carry side effects. The advantages also may not be enduring, as the drugs tend to "mask" symptoms rather than help the patient come to grips with the actual causes of their abnormal behavior and mental health problem. Hence, drug therapy cannot be taken as a complete treatment for an abnormal behavior or mental disorder, and has to be supplemented with other physical or psychological measures.

Shock Therapy

This involves an artificial induction of deep comas, convulsions, or both by shock-inducing drugs or electric current. This therapy is recommended to patients who are difficult to control or do not benefit from drug therapy.

With *Insulin Shock Therapy (IST) or Insulin Coma Therapy (ICT),* the patient is given an insulin injection intramuscularly early in the morning, causing a decrease in the blood sugar level. As a result, he passes through the stages of restlessness, unconsciousness, convulsions, and eventually goes into a coma, in which he does not respond even to a pinprick or other painful stimulation. He remains in this stage of coma for about an hour and then his blood sugar level is raised through his own body chemistry or by giving sugar contents resulting in the end of the insulin shock episode. Although insulin shock therapy was formerly used extensively in the treatment of schizophrenia, it has been largely replaced by newer drug therapies and electroconvulsive therapy.

In Electroconvulsive Therapy (ECT), also referred to as Electro Shock therapy (EST), convulsion is produced by passing an electric current through the brain of the patient. For this purpose, he is placed on a comfortable bed and electrodes are placed on each side of his head and an alternating current, usually between 100 and 200 volts, is passed between them for a period of about two seconds. Patients are generally given muscle relaxant before administering ECT. While inducing a current, the shoulders and limbs of the patient are held lightly by nurses and attendants and a rubber gag is placed between his teeth to prevent injury during the convulsion. About five to ten ECTs are given two to three times a week depending upon the requirement of the situation. There is confusion and loss of memory during the period immediately before and after treatment, but it gradually returns in a few weeks.

ECT has been found helpful for depression, involutional melancholia, mania, schizophrenia, and other psychotic reactions. It is quite popular for controlling cases of agitated depression and schizophrenia and is found useful for patients who do not respond well to drug therapy.

Psychosurgery

This involves surgical operation of the patient's brain and aims to destroy or isolate certain mal-adaptive cell complexes in the frontal areas of the brain responsible for undesirable emotional responses and mental disorders. This is done in one of the following ways:

- Some of the nerve connections are severed between the frontal lobes and the thalamus. This technique is known as lobectomy or prefrontal lobectomy (leucotomy).

- Certain parts of the frontal lobes are actually removed. This technique is known as topectomy.
- Certain nerve tracts in the thalamus are severed by the insertion of a surgical electric needle. This technique is known as thalectomy.

The removal of maladaptive cell complexes in the frontal lobes or the cutting of nerve pathways between the prefrontal lobes of the brain and the thalamus or hypothalamus by the surgical operations described above results in reducing the emotional torment of disturbing thoughts, apathy, delusions, and hallucinations. Consequently, psychosurgery may be found useful with a wide range of mental patients, including schizophrenics, involutional melancholics, antisocial personalities, alcoholics, manic depressives and patients suffering from stubborn obsessive and other severe neurotic reactions.

Psychosurgery as a method of treatment of mental patients involves considerable risk and negative consequences. It may reduce or even impair the patient's intellectual abilities. There may be temporary or permanent organic complications, including convulsions, aphasia, increased appetite, and rectal or vesical incontinence. In some cases, brain surgery may lead to death. Therefore, in all cases, psychosurgery should be the last resort, and its use restricted to patients with whom everything else has been tried and failed, so that any improvement at all may be considered a great gain.

To Sum Up

The treatment of mental illness and behavioral disorders may be classified into two broad categories, namely somatic or medical therapies and psychological or psychotherapies.

Somatic or medical therapies are concerned with the physiological or medical treatment of affected individuals. Some of the main measures belonging to this category are drug or chemotherapy, shock therapy, and brain surgery. In the use of drug therapy, it may be seen that various drugs prove effective in reducing the severity of symptoms and make the management of the patient convenient in the hospital or at home. But the drugs also carry severe side effects and the treatment docs not remove the actual causes of the abnormality or disorder. Drug therapy has therefore to be supplemented by other measures.

The therapy known as shock therapy involves an artificial induction of deep comas, convulsions, or both by shock-inducing drugs or electric current. The popular therapy for this purpose is Electro Shock therapy (EST), in which convulsion is produced by passing electric current through the brain of the patient. It is quite popular for controlling cases of agitated depression and schizophrenia, and is found useful for patients who do not respond well to drug therapy.

Psychosurgery involves the surgical operation of the patient's brain to reduce the emotional torment of disturbing thoughts, apathy, delusions, and hallucinations. However, it involves considerable risk and negative consequence and should be taken as a method of last resort.

Use of Psychotherapies

The majority of cases of mental disorders or illnesses may be adjudged as products of severe maladjustment caused by psychological factors. Physical or medical treatment in such cases does not prove very useful. Such patients need psychological treatment for solving their psychological difficulties and achieving better personality adjustment. This form of psychological treatment is known as psychotherapy.

Psychotherapy is a difficult term to define. However, it may be understood as a method of treatment of a psychological problem or disorder of an individual by a therapist through a behavioral approach in the form of establishing a psychological relationship with the patient for the purpose of solving the patient's emotional difficulties and promoting adequate personality growth and adjustment.

> *Psychotherapy:* A method of treatment of a psychological problem or disorder used by a therapist through a behavioral approach in the form of establishing a psychological relationship with the patient with the purpose of solving his emotional difficulties for achieving adequate adjustment and mental health.

The main objective in psychotherapy is to bring about changes in the patient's perception of himself and of his environment, thus resulting in positive, enduring changes in his behavior for achieving adequate adjustment and regaining better mental health. For the realization of this objective, a number of systematic approaches to psychotherapy, differing in goals and procedures, have been evolved. In this chapter, we focus our discussion on the use of various psychotherapies on the part of clinical psychologists and practitioners worldwide.

Psychoanalytical or Psychodynamic Therapy

The founder of psychoanalytical or psychodynamic therapy was Sigmund Freud, who developed the theory and technique of psychoanalysis for the treatment of abnormality and mental disorders. Freud believed that early conflicts, desires, painful or anxiety-arousing experiences, though repressed and unconscious, are responsible for the present abnormal behavior or mental disorder of an individual. With the use of psychoanalysis technique, he tried to help clients become aware of their thoughts, feelings, and other mental activities. Once they become aware of the underlying unconscious processes, they can make efforts to control them deliberately, rather than being controlled by them. In this way, the psychoanalytic or psychodynamic method invented by him for the treatment of mentally ill was primarily aimed at making one's unconscious conscious (Cabaniss et al., 2011; Karon and Widener, 1995).

Assessing or Uncovering One's Unconscious

Freud recommended the use of the techniques of *free association* and *dream analysis* for uncovering one's unconscious, with the objective of tracing the real causes of one's present problem.

Free association is a technique in which the therapist simply asks the client to say whatever comes to his mind without censoring themselves at all. In practicing this technique, the client is made to lie on a couch, with the therapist sitting out of his range of sight. The client is then asked to "free associate," that is, to speak freely about whatever comes into his mind, no matter what it is, and to go on talking about his thoughts and feelings as subsequent associations reveal themselves. He is expected to speak frankly. He must not hold back past or present events, attitudes toward the therapist or fantasies, no matter how unpleasant or embarrassing they may be. In case the patient remains silent or claims that "nothing comes to mind," it may indicate his resistance to treatment. He is told that all thoughts and feelings are important to the treatment process. If he insists that he is really trying, it may be postulated that the resistance is caused by unconscious parts of his mind. Such resistances themselves provide clues to the patient's conflicts.

Dream analysis is another major technique used in psychoanalytical therapy for uncovering unconscious motivation and repressed conflicts. During sleep, the defenses of the ego are lowered, allowing repressed material to reach the conscious. For this reason, dreams, to some extent, may be taken as the "royal road" to the unconscious. Expressing his views in this concern, Freud asserts that one's dreams are loaded with repressed material, although in symbolic form. The manifest content of the dream is the actual dream and its events, but the latent content is the hidden, symbolic meaning of those events that would, if correctly interpreted, reveal the unconscious conflicts creating the nervous disorder (Freud, 1900).

Consequently, through the analysis of material produced by means of free association and patient's dreams, the therapist begins to gather clues about the possible underlying causes of the behavioral disorder of his patient. For the most part, the analyst has to on the verbal responses based on the memories of the patient. Later on, more direct evidences become available. The patient's personality is reflected in the way he behaves during the analytic period. His habitual patterns of behavior, his way of looking at things, his likes and dislikes, his prejudices and biases, may all affect the way in which he deals with his analyst. His total behavior is to be analyzed by the therapist for going deep into his problem.

Many times, on account of the *phenomenon of transference*, the patient's attitudes and behavior toward his therapist are unrealistic. During the interaction in the process of psychoanalytical therapy, the patient and therapist develop a complex emotionally charged relationship. As a result, the patient usually transfers his deepest emotions to the analyst, the analyst becoming the love object or the hate object, depending upon the early experiences of the patient with his parents or other important persons. For example, a female patient may view the analyst as an ideal husband and lover, or may exhibit feelings she had as a child toward her father. The mechanism of transference is important in effecting the cure of the patient, as it allows the release of repressed feelings toward persons resembling husband, lover, or father figures. The analyst intelligently establishes rapport and relationships for the uncovering of the unresolved conflicts and repressed feelings, and tries to make interpretations based on the emotional attitude and behavior shown by the patient toward the analyst.

In brief, psychoanalytical therapy rests on the following assumptions and techniques:

(i) The abnormal behavior or mental illness of the patient is the result of repressed desires or conflicts experienced earlier in one's life.

(ii) Through free association and recalling day-to-day dreams, the patient is given an opportunity to uncover his unconscious desires and repressed conflicts.

(iii) The mechanism of transference helps in the task of uncovering the conflict, as it is once again made into an interpersonal one, this time between the patient and the therapist.

(iv) The analysis of free association, dreams, transference, and overall behavior of the patient helps in knowing the abnormal behavior of the patient.

(v) The therapist tries to show the patient how some early experiences affected his emotional life and helps him to achieve new and more adaptive modes of adjustment in order to lead a normal life.

(vi) Finally, the therapist tries to break the bond of interpersonal relationship between himself and his patient in order to make the patient face the realities of life and solve his problems independently (after developing an impressive insight into his problem) without any emotional support from the therapist.

The prevalent mode of psychoanalytical therapy has been modified in many ways from orthodox psychoanalysis propagated by Freud and his followers in the manners such as the following:

- The couch is gone, and the client (the term used now in place of the Freud's term "patient" for the individual seeking therapy) may sit face to face with the therapist and he or she may also stand or walk about.
- Rather than remaining quiet until the client says something revealing, the modern psychoanalyst is far more directive, asking questions, suggesting helpful behavior, and giving opinions and interpretations earlier in the relationship, which helps speed up the therapeutic process.
- The treatment session now may go on two to four times a week for two or more years. These sessions are more likely to be focused on current situations, interpersonal relationships, and other sources of conflict. The therapist may also take advantage of adjunct treatments such as play therapy, art therapy, group therapy, and hypnosis, instead of being dependent upon free association and dream analysis only.
- Today's psychoanalysts also focus less on the "id" as the motivator of behavior, instead looking more at the "ego" or sense of "self" as the motivating force behind all actions. Some psychoanalysts also focus on the process of transference more than on other typical aspects of traditional psychoanalysis, leading to the more general method called psychodynamic therapy. Psychodynamic therapy is typically shorter in duration than traditional psychoanalysis.
- Even so, all the psychodynamic techniques require the client to be fairly intelligent and verbally able to express his or her ideas, feelings, and thoughts effectively. People who are extremely withdrawn or who suffer from the more psychotic disorders are not good candidates for this form of psychotherapy. People who have non-psychotic adjustment disorders, such as anxiety, somatoform, or dissociative disorders, are more likely to benefit from psychodynamic therapy (Ciccarelli and White, 2012).

> ## Psychoanalytical therapy
>
> *Psychoanalytical therapy* assumes that repressed desires or conflicts experienced earlier in one's life are the real source of mental illnesses and behavioral disorders. The analysis of material produced by means of free association, dreams, and other measures helps in getting clues for the underlying causes of mental or behavioral disorder. The therapist then tries to acquaint the patient with the effect of his early experiences and helps him to achieve new and more adaptive modes of adjustment.

Client-Centered Psychotherapy

This is also known as non-directive therapy and is the outcome of the philosophy and experiences of American psychologist Carl Rogers (1902–1987), who, as a strong humanitarian, had full faith in the worth and competencies of the human individual. His assumption was that people are innately good and effective. They have an innate tendency for self-actualization, that is, to realize their potentials. As the self has an innate tendency toward self-actualization, the most important evaluation should come from the self. In the case where a person accepts evaluation from others and if these evaluations are negative or conditionally positive, the result is a conflict between self-evaluation and the evaluation of others. This type of conflict may give rise to undue anxiety and tension, and thus, in due course, cause abnormalities. For example, a newly married girl may fall victim to mental health problems by considering herself worthless after being repeatedly criticized by her mother-in-law or husband.

Consequently, as asserted by Rogers (1961), his therapy, known as Rogers therapy, demands the individual return to his basic nature of evaluating himself positively. It believes that the client (the term used for a patient) is quite competent to resolve his conflict as he has within himself resources for self-actualization and healthy adjustment. He needs only a deep, affectionate relationship with the therapist to learn how to use his resources. Rogers therapy involves very strong conviction about the client's worth and his basic urge for self-actualization. The therapist is there not to direct but merely to help the client direct himself for his healthy adjustment. On account of this non-directive role of the therapist, Rogers therapy is known as non-directive therapy. It is known as client-centered therapy (and more recently as person-centered therapy) because it revolves totally around the client or the person seeking therapy, as may be seen in some of the following steps associated with this therapy.

1. In Rogers therapy, the client himself approaches the therapist for help in order to get rid of some psychological stress. During the first interview, the therapist assures him of his help in working out the client's own solutions.
2. In the next interview, the client is encouraged *to talk about his most deeply felt emotions as freely as possible*. In this way, the negative feelings that have been bottled up inside the client come out into the open. Here, the therapist does not intervene but creates suitable therapeutic conditions which facilitate the client to talk in a more honest and emotional way about himself and his problem.
3. The next move is concerned with helping the client *to gain insight* into his emotional conflicts. It involves acceptance, recognition, and clarification of the feelings of the client by the therapist. Here, attention is paid to the emotional aspect, rather than to what the client says. The therapist tries to provide an environment for removing the emotional conflicts that are blocking self-actualization by selecting and focusing on statements and feelings expressed by the client. It is a sort of help rendered by the therapist to the client for learning suitable ways to evaluate himself and his environment in a true perspective. As a result, the client gains insight by (i) understanding the causes behind his behavior, (ii) recognizing and accepting his self in its real position, and (iii) working toward his positive self-growth and better adjustment.
4. After gaining insight into his problem, the client is helped in seeking minor positive actions for the solution to his problem. Here, also, the therapist is not to direct or lead but to recognize and render clarification about the possible courses of action. The minor positive actions bring satisfaction and develop self-confidence, paving the way for more positive action and thus helping the client in his self-actualization.
5. Finally, there comes a stage when the client, after gaining confidence in his self, feels that he does not need further therapeutic interviews. As such, the decision to end the therapeutic relationship comes from the client. At this stage, he is known to acquire his original drive for self-actualization by learning positive ways of understanding and promoting his self.

In this way, evidently, from beginning to end, Rogers therapy is centered round the client. He is the main actor who plays the leading role. The therapist encourages and sets the therapeutic environment to help him discover ways of self-actualization by gaining insight into his problem, removing the discrepancy between his real self and his idealized self-image, and developing confidence in his self for healthy adjustment. Unlike other psychotherapy, Rogers therapy does not

demand special intellectual and professional knowledge of human behavior
from the therapist. Rogers asserts that
it is only the ability to establish good
interpersonal relationships that counts
in being a good therapist. For this purpose, he emphasizes the following therapeutic traits:

(i) The therapist must be genuine and
     not superficial in relationship with
     his client. He should be what he is.
     Anything going on in him that is

> ### Client-centered psychotherapy
>
> *Client-centered psychotherapy* is centered
> around the client. It creates a proper therapeutic
> environment for helping him to discover ways
> of self-actualization by gaining insight into his
> problem, removing the discrepancy between
> his real self and his idealized self-image, and
> developing confidence in his self for his healthy
> adjustment.

relevant to the relationship can be seen by his client. He should be able to bring a direct
personal encounter with his client, meeting him on a person-to-person basis.

(ii) The therapist should have the capacity for empathy. To sense the client's inner world
      of private meanings as if it were his own, without losing the "as if" quality, is empathy.
      He should also be able to communicate some of the significant fragments of that under-
      standing. By showing *empathy*, by sensing and reflecting their clients' feelings, therapists
      can help clients experience a deeper self-understanding and self-acceptance. As Rogers
      (1980:10) explained:

> Hearing (active listening) has consequences. When I truly hear a person and the meanings
> that are important to him at that moment, hearing not simply his words, but him, and when
> I let him know that I have heard his own private personal meanings, many things happen.
> There is first of all a grateful look. He feels released. He wants to tell me more about his
> world. He surges forth in a new sense of freedom. He becomes more open to the process
> of change. I have often noticed that the more deeply I hear the meanings of the person, the
> more there is that happens. Almost always, when a person realizes that he has been deeply
> heard, his eyes moisten. I think in some real sense he is weeping for joy. It is as though he
> were saying, "Thank God, somebody heard me. Someone knows what it is like to be me."

(iii) The therapist must experience a warm, positive acceptance toward what is in the client. He
      must praise and respect his client as a person and thus pay a positive regard. As far as pos-
      sible, this positive regard should be unconditional.

Thus, the therapist acts in such a way that his client may perceive the genuineness of the acceptance and empathy that the therapist experiences for him. The perception of such a psychological climate in the relationship by the client results in the constructive personality growth and
desirable changes in the behavior of the client. Thus, Rogers therapy heavily depends upon the
attitudes of the therapist.

The acceptance, positive regard, and clarification of the feelings of the client by the therapist
is properly reciprocated, resulting in the removal of the discrepancy between his ideal self and
present self, and thus paving the way to his healthy adjustment and self-actualization.

As far as the suitability of the therapy is concerned, Rogers therapy may not, in fact, be
appropriate for a severe psychological disorder. It may, however, work well with mildly disturbed people if handled properly by a therapist in an appropriate environment of interpersonal
relationship.

Humanistic-Existential Therapy

Humanistic-existential therapy represents a blend of two types of therapies known as humanistic therapy and existential therapy. Humanistic therapy is governed and guided through the key ideas and principles inherent in the humanistic perspective postulated by the humanists like Abraham Maslow and Karl Rogers. The humanistic perspective views human nature as basically good, with an inherent potential to maintain healthy, meaningful relationships, and to make choices that are in the interest of one self and others. These choices help one to satisfy his basic needs, including the need for self-actualization—striving for a goal true to one's nature or becoming his true self (e.g., becoming musician, dancer, technician, etc). Whenever there is a hurdle in their realization, it results in one's maladjustment and abnormalities in one's behavior. Actually, the humanistic perspective mainly emphasizes that "not being one's true self" is the main source of problems, and the therapist should try to help the client in getting out of this mess for living a meaningful life.

Existential therapy is directed and shaped on the basis of ideas and principles inherent in the philosophy and perspective of existentialism. Existentialism advocates the need for exercising free will on the part of individuals to make choices in life for making their life meaningful. For this purpose, it assumes that people should live peacefully with no incalculable loss in their life by having love and respect for themselves and others. They should also own responsibility and show creativity in performing the tasks of their own choices. Failure in one or the other such aspects may breed anxiety, despair, and frustration in one's life. Moreover, these may also be caused on account of one or the other ill happenings in one's life, such as the death of a dear one, accidental and incidental losses, or fear of eventualities such as death. In this way, in the view of existential therapists, the central problems people face are embedded in anxiety over loneliness, isolation, despair, and, ultimately, death. In dealing with such aroused anxiety and depression, therapists are needed to provide the client opportunity for their free expression, creativity, love, and authenticity for making his life meaningful.

In adopting a synthesis of both the humanistic and existential therapies a therapist is found to help the clients in overcoming their problems through a well planned and organized therapeutic program with the assumption mentioned below.

Clients must be helped to perceive and remove the obstacles in the path of the satisfaction of their basic needs, as well as the important need related to their self-actualization (becoming true to their self). Similarly, they may also be helped in identifying the nature of their anxiety or frustration and the things responsible for its eruption, and then dealing with it successfully by adopting suitable means. In attaining both these objectives, the therapists attempt to help clients first by creating a therapeutic relationship that is warm and accepting and that trusts that they are capable of identifying and dealing with their problems, and then helping them in the manner as follows:

(i)   To help them in freeing themselves from disabling assumptions and attitudes responsible for their problems so that they can live fuller lives.

(ii)   To emphasize growth and self-actualization rather than curing diseases or alleviating disorders.

(iii) To help them not to see anxiety nor despair as a symptom of a disorder, but view them as a normal part of life, accept them, and use their energy to help them make authentic or genuine choices about their life and to take responsibility for their future experiences rather than just reacting to circumstances.

(iv)   To provide opportunities for exercising creativity, love, authenticity, and free will on the part of the clients for helping them to come out from states of acute anxiety, stress, frustration, and despair, and enabling them to live meaningful lives in the face of uncertainty and suffering.

(v)   To help clients achieve a dimension of self-respect, self-motivation, and self-growth to facilitate their early and meaningful recovery.

To Sum Up

Humanistic-existential therapy, while adopting a synthesis of the humanistic and existential therapies, helps clients in overcoming their problems through a well-planned and organized therapeutic program focusing on (i) their perceiving and realization of their basic needs, including the need related to their self actualization, and (ii) identifying the nature and cause of their anxiety or frustration and then dealing it with successfully by adopting suitable means.

Behavior Therapies

The psychotherapies discussed so far represent therapies that cannot be termed as sufficiently empirical and scientific in their processing and implications. In spite of their valuable contribution toward revealing one's unconscious, and their capability of understanding one's motives and actions, the procedures adopted by them cannot be precisely defined, directly observed, or scientifically tested. In this concern, the rise of the behavioral therapies provided a suitable alternative for overcoming this weakness.

The basic assumption underlying the technique of behavior therapy is the belief that behavior in its all forms and shapes is learned. Accordingly, maladaptive behavior related to one's mental health problems or disorders grows out of improper or defective learning. Therapy, in turn, becomes an attempt to provide corrective learning experiences through the use of the same kinds of learning techniques that people (and animals) used to learn any new responses.

As a term, behavior therapy denotes the use of experimentally established principles of learning for the purpose of changing maladaptive or problematic behavior. As far as the origin of maladaptive or defective learning is concerned, it is traced either in classical conditioning, as advocated by Pavlov, or in operant conditioning, as explained by Skinner. Based on these two approaches, various methods of behavior therapy (discussed ahead) have come into existence.

1. *Counter-conditioning:* One may learn maladaptive or abnormal behavior through conditioning. As a result, a person may show fear responses in the presence of certain normally neutral stimulus objects and events. When that happens, we say that he has developed an unrealistic fear or phobia. Fear of animals, height, water, darkness, closed or open places—all such phobias may be seen as a result of defective learning or improper conditioning. The treatment of such behavior lies in its counter-conditioning.

   For illustration, let us take the case of a child who has developed a generalized fear of rabbits through conditioned fear responses. In this case, the treatment may be worked out by associating some pleasant or favorable responses with the presence of a rabbit. The child may be given his favorite food or allowed to listen to his favorite song or play a game in the presence of a rabbit. The rabbit may be kept at some distance and then gradually moved closer on successive occasions. The fear responses can thus be gradually eliminated.

   Sexual dysfunctions like frigidity, impotence, and early ejaculation may also be treated by the process of counter-conditioning. Most often, such dysfunctions are the result of anxiety that causes sexual inhibition. Thus, the treatment process involves conditioning as follows:

   - To attempt sexual relations only when there is a minimum of anxiety, for example, in situations in which there is a clear desire,
   - To attempt sex relations only when desirable support, cooperation, or assistance is available from the sex partner.

Gradually, the reaction of anxiety to sexual experiences may be eliminated because they will now not be permitted to happen, and adequate sexual responses may in time be strengthened, resulting in the treatment of a particular sexual dysfunction.

2. **Desensitization methods:** Conditioned anxiety responses are the root causes for the development of many abnormalities in the behaviors of individuals. The treatment of such abnormalities may involve a variety of techniques designed to increase the individual's capacity to tolerate an anxiety-provoking situation. Two such techniques are described ahead:

(i) *Systematic desensitization:* This technique was developed by Joseph Wolpe, an American psychologist. It aims to reduce levels of anxiety related to an anxiety-provoking situation progressively through well-planned systematic steps such as relaxation, outlining a hierarchy of the individual's anxieties, and desensitization.

In this initial stage, attempts are made to develop an anxiety hierarchy. For this purpose, the patient's anxieties are studied and ranked according to the intensity of anxiety to the different stimuli, ranging from most to least frightening. Side by side, in an early session of therapy, the patient is made to learn the art of relaxation of the muscles of the body.

When the patient has mastered the relaxation technique, the desensitization process begins. The patient is made to relax completely in a comfortable chair or on a couch with his eyes closed, and asked to imagine and experience the scene in the hierarchy that is the least anxiety-provoking, progressively reaching the scene highest in the hierarchy. The motor relaxation is viewed by Wolpe as antagonistic to anxiety. The patient imagines and experiences the scene with little or no anxiety, and thus, his sensitivity to the imagining of such experiences is de-conditioned. Treatment is terminated when the patient reaches a stage of complete relaxation, and is able to imagine vividly and without any anxiety the scenes that evoked the greatest anxiety in him before the commencement of the treatment.

There may be certain variations of the desensitization procedure. Instead of imagining a situation, the patient may be exposed to the real stimuli which evoke anxiety. This is termed as desensitization in vivo. In such a procedure, a patient who has a fear of humiliation at making mistakes may be made to commit minor errors and then progressively more serious ones in the presence of the therapist in each instance until all feelings of anxiety disappear. In another variation, desensitization may be done using a tape-recorder or video film eliciting anxiety-provoking situations.

(ii) *Flooding or implosive therapy:* In this method of desensitization, the patient is exposed immediately to the greatest anxiety-provoking situation. He is not gradually introduced to the anxiety-provoking situations but is encouraged to face the frightening or distressing situation and remain there, regardless of how much anxiety is generated, until a spontaneous decrease in anxiety takes place. A child who fears rabbits may be confronted with a rabbit through a videotape or by way of a real-life situation. It may be seen that his peak anxiety does not last very long, and he eventually gets used to it and feels that his fear was irrational.

3. **Aversive conditioning:** Aversive conditioning involves the modification of behavior patterns through pain or punishment. This treatment has proved effective in overcoming obsessional thinking, compulsive acts, sexual deviations, alcoholism, overeating, smoking, drug dependence, gambling, and so on. The method consists of administering a noxious stimulus (resulting in an unpleasant response) to the patient in an appropriate time relation to the stimulus to which aversive conditioning is desired. The assumption of such treatment is that the patient will gradually learn to avoid the abnormal pattern of behavior and prefer a more desirable and normal one.

Similarly, in the treatment of chronic alcoholism aversion, conditioning may be achieved with the help of a drug *Antabuse*. The person who is a chronic alcoholic is persuaded to take the drug. A drink of alcoholic beverages, after taking the drug, results in strong unpleasant and uncomfortable physical reactions like increased pulse rate, difficulty breathing, severe headache, and nausea. The repetition of such unpleasant experiences results in the avoidance of alcoholic beverages.

4. *Modeling:* Modeling is a therapy technique in which the client's behavior is modified as a result of observing appropriate and normal behavior of other people used as models. One may use modeling therapy for eliminating a child's fear of rabbits by making him observe that the other children are playing with the rabbits without fear. Similarly, one's phobia of snakes may also be overcome through modeling therapy. Such patients may be made to observe both real and filmed incidents of people (models) and snakes in which people (models) may be seen approaching the snakes gradually, with no signs of anxiety and fear.

   Modeling as a technique may also be used for learning more adaptable and desirable ways of personal and social adjustment. People may also be helped in the treatment of sexual dysfunctions by means of films or live models depicting practical techniques and normal sex behavior.

5. *Method of positive reinforcement:* In this method, carefully selected rewards and schedules of reinforcement are used to modify a patient's behavior in the direction of socially desirable, adaptive behavior. Anorexia nervosa, a condition in which the person affected refuses to eat, has been found to be successfully treated by arranging for eating to be followed by a proper schedule of positive reinforcement or rewards, such as to be allowed to go to a movie, play a favorable game, use a smart phone, or enjoy the provision of a good company.

A technique known as "token economy" is also used as a method for treating problem behavior. It is based on the principle of positive reinforcement. In this method, plastic or metal tokens are used as rewards for reinforcing the positive and desirable behavior shown by the patients. These tokens may later be exchanged for special privileges such as television viewing, single room accommodation, and obtaining special food, magazines, or novels. Token economy as a behavior modification technique has been found most effective in improving and modifying the behavior of people in institutions or hospitals.

To Sum Up

Behavior therapy denotes the use of experimentally established principles of learning for the purpose of changing maladaptive or abnormal behavior. Based on classical conditioning or operant conditioning, it involves important methods like counter-conditioning, desensitization, flooding, aversive conditioning, modeling, and the method of positive reinforcement. In *counter-conditioning*, the maladaptive or undesirable behavior learned through conditioning is de-learned and replaced through desirable behavior. In the use of *desensitization*, attempts are made to employ a variety of techniques (such as systematic desensitization and flooding or implosive therapy) designed to increase the individual's capacity to tolerate an anxiety-provoking situation. In *aversive conditioning*, the employed technique involves the modification of behavior patterns through pain or punishment. In the use of the technique of *modeling*, the patient's behavior is modified as a result of observing the appropriate and normal behavior of other people used as models. The use of the *method of positive reinforcement* involves the employment of rewards and schedules of reinforcement to modify a patient's behavior in the direction of socially desirable, well-adaptive behavior.

Cognitive Therapies

The growing reaction against the prevailing popular psychotherapies- psychodynamic and behavioral gave birth to a new approach in the treatment of mental illness and problem in the name of cognitive therapies. True to their naming, cognitive therapies focus on one's cognition- the ways of thinking, reasoning and drawing conclusions for identifying and treating abnormality and mental illnesses.

The Basic Assumptions Lying Behind Cognitive Therapy

The process carried out in cognitive therapy aims to make the problem-ridden client think in a reasonable, logical way. The use of this therapy is fundamentally based on assumptions, such as:

- The way we think about events determines the way we respond (Onken, 2015).
- The "individuals' interpretations and perceptions of current situations, events, and problems influence how they react" (J. S. Beck, 2002).
- Psychological problems arise from illogical cognitions (i.e., an irrational or unrealistic interpretation of a life event such as a relationship breakup or failure in examination may cause severe depression and acute state of anxiety).
- Psychological wellness stems from logical cognitions. Therefore, the role of the cognitive therapist is to fix faulty thinking (A. T. Beck and Haigh, 2014).

The Types of Popular Cognitive Therapies Used by Clinical Psychologists

At the present juncture, we may find that in general, the following three types of cognitive therapies are popular among clinical psychologists:

(i)   Rational Emotive Behavior Therapy (REBT) developed by Albert Ellis
(ii) Beck's Cognitive Therapy (CT) brought out by Aaron Beck
(iii) Cognitive Behavior Therapy (CBT), a blend of cognitive and behavioral approaches.

Let us know about them.

Rational Emotive Behavior Therapy (REBT)

The first among the cognitive therapies used for the treatment of abnormality and mental illness was a therapy named Rational Emotive Therapy, developed by Albert Ellis in the 1950s. Later on in his career, Albert Elis changed its name by calling it Rational Emotive Behavior Therapy (REBT). We will make use of this later name in our discussion of his approach.

While proposing his approach to psychotherapy (REBT), Albert Ellis (1962:36) writes:

> The central theme of [REBT] is that man is a uniquely rational, as well as uniquely irrational animal; that his emotional or psychological disturbances are largely a result of his thinking illogically or irrationally; and that he can rid himself of most of his emotional or mental unhappiness, ineffectuality, and disturbance if he learns to maximize his rational and minimize his irrational thinking.

The Main Assumptions Underlying the Use of REBT

The cognitive approach to therapy adopted by Albert Ellis is based on assumptions, such as:

- Our cognition refers to the thought process that determines our feelings and behavior. The abnormality of behavior and mental illness is the outcome of faulty cognitions about the self, others, and the things lying in the environment.
- What makes our cognition—the way of our thinking, reasoning, and interpreting—defective and erroneous is thus the root cause of the abnormality in our behavior and mental illness. According to Ellis, it is one's irrational ways of perceiving and interpreting the things that puts him into trouble of getting entrapped in the vicious cycle of distress and related problems. Take the cases of a perfectionist and a pessimist. Both of them may be attributed to irrational thinking and beliefs. When they face a small failure, they might perceive it to be a bigger one, as if the sky has fallen down on them. They become distressed, and begin to think and believe one or the other negative things about themself, others, and the things in their environment, leading to more distress and creating more problems for them.
- The treatment of the abnormality of behavior and mental illness thus lies in taking care of the irrational and erroneous thinking and beliefs that are responsible for arousing them emotionally in negative and undesirable ways. For this, it is necessary to help them in bringing necessary changes in their thought process and belief system, leading them to the emotional balance. In this way, we may see that this form of cognitive therapy is an opportunity for the patient to learn of his current distortions and successfully eliminate them.

The Procedure and Steps Adopted for Treatment in REBT

The cognitive approach emphasized by Albert Ellis for the treatment of the clients asks for the adoption of a model named as the ABCDE Model. The letters of this model represent different terms related to identifying and treating psychological problems, in the manner sequenced as follows:

A stands for *Antecedent or Activating Event;* B for *Belief;* C for *Emotional Consequence;* D for *Dispute,* and E stands for *Effective New Belief.*

While the functions represented through the first three letters, A, B, and C, are concerned with the execution of Step 1—analyzing and identifying the problem of the patient. The other two, D and E, are concerned with Step 2—seeking the needed treatment for the diagnosed problem. Let us look into what happens in these steps.

Step 1: Employment of ABC (Antecedent-Belief-Consequence) Analysis

- The task begins with the activities covered by the first letter A (*Antecedent* or *Activating events*). By the term Antecedent or activating events, we mean the events or happenings that caused a psychological problem or distress to the patient. The therapist tries to know about them through a variety of means and information collected from the patient, family members, and other possible sources.

- The term *belief* here stands for the irrational beliefs held by the individual through his erroneous thinking about his self, others, and things in his environment. These beliefs are quite far from reality and cannot be supported by empirical evidence. As examples of such beliefs, we may cite the erroneous assumptions held by individuals, such as:

(i)   Feeling excessively upset over other people's mistakes or misconduct
(ii) Believing that you must be perfectly competent and successful in everything to be valued and worthwhile
(iii) Believing that one should be loved and liked by everybody all the time
(iv) Believing that it is catastrophic when things are not the way you want them to be
(v)   Believing that one will be happier if one avoids life's difficulties or challenges.

The holding of one or the other types of such beliefs or outlooks is associated with the evaluation of the role of one or the other antecedent events in causing the felt distress or problem. These irrational beliefs are assessed through a variety of means, such as interviews, questionnaires, inventories, and attitude scales.

- The term *consequence* here stands for the eruption of negative feelings, emotions, and behaviors resulting from the distorted perception of the antecedent event on account of one's erroneous and irrational beliefs having no connection with reality.

Step 2: Providing Therapeutic Treatment

Ellis believes that it is not the antecedent or activating event (**A**) that causes negative emotional and behavioral consequences (**C**), but rather it is the distorted and unrealistic interpretation of these events on the part of an individual resulting in the formation of his irrational belief system (**B**) that leads to problematic consequences (**C**).

According to Ellis, the eradication of the problem lies in adopting measures for bringing necessary changes to one's belief system. Therefore, after identification of irrational beliefs, attempts are made by the therapist to work with the patient/client in the task signified through the last two letters D (Dispute) and E (Effective New Belief) of the model, aimed at taking measures for the eradication of the diagnosed problem.

- Accordingly, in the second step, the task begins with disputing (challenging and refuting) the negative thoughts responsible for causing the problem. For this purpose, although both direct and non-directive questioning in a Socratic dialogue mode may be used, most therapists prefer to make use of the latter for better results. Non-directive questioning provides a gentle, non-probing, and non-threatening mode for the required disputation of the client's irrational beliefs and thoughts. For example, a therapist may ask the client (depressed on account of the irrational belief that he/should be loved or cared by everyone in all situations): Why should everybody always do this for you? Why do you feel you need this? It helps the clients/patients to think and ponder deep into their unrealistic beliefs and illogical way of thinking and emotive responding.
- Regardless of the form of the dispute, if it is effective, it affords the client the opportunity to replace the original, irrational belief with an effective new belief (E) that is more rational and leads to less troubling feelings (Dryden, 2009; A. Ellis, 2008). In this way, on the basis of

the needed support in the form of realistic evidences available to the client with the help of disputing his irrational beliefs and negative thoughts, now there arises the need of translating into action the things represented through the last letter—E (*Effective New Belief*)—of the model. Accordingly, the client now begins to re-interpret the things in a more realistic light. Eventually, it helps him to develop more rational beliefs and healthy coping strategies for leading a meaningful, emotionally balanced, normal life.

Beck's Cognitive Therapy

As a cognitive approach for addressing the behavioral problems and psychological distress especially related to depression and acute anxiety among the individuals, the psychologist Aaron Beck developed a therapy named Cognitive therapy (CT) through his work conducted in the 1960s. His approach in this regard, while resembling in a number of ways the earlier discussed Rational Emotive Behavior Therapy (REBT), differed significantly in terms of attribution of the causes and treatment of mental health problems.

Causation of Mental Health Problems

In adopting a cognitive approach for explaining the distortions in the ways clients/patients look at the things, while Ellis (1957) suggested that it happens on account of irrational and unrealistic thinking, Beck (1967) proposed the *cognitive triad* for this purpose. The cognitive triad, quite typical of people with depression, is visible among them in its three forms of particular cognitions—thoughts about the self, the external world, and the future. Beck theorized that when all three of these beliefs are negative, they produce depression (J. S. Beck, 1995).

These thoughts, occurring in a stream-like fashion, tend to be automatic in depressed people, as they occur spontaneously, one after another—thoughts such as "I am quite poor in my studies; my parents and teachers hate me; I can't finish any task on time; it seems that I am a worthless person; I have no friends to share my concern." Quite often, these negative thoughts persist even in the face of contrary evidence or assurance to the individual, and work as a strong attribute for leading one to utter depression.

In addition to the presence of the aforementioned triad of irrational automatic negative thoughts, there are two other mechanisms that may contribute significantly toward the causation of depression, namely (i) Negative self schemas, and (ii) Errors in Logic (i.e., faulty information processing). Let us look into them.

- The term *Negative Self-Schemas* refers to a set of negative beliefs and pessimistic expectations about oneself, possessed particularly by depression-prone individuals, and learned and acquired by them through their earlier experiences mostly related to their childhood, and often traumatic in nature. These may include (i) parental rejection, neglect or abuse, (ii) public ridiculed in school or community, (iv) being a victim of bullying, exclusion from the peer group, or sexual assault, (iii) occurrence of sad events, such as death of a parent or sibling.
- The possession of a thought pattern in the form of unrealistic negative thinking coupled with negative self-schemas and self-image lowers the self-esteem and self-confidence to such an extent that they are bound to make logical errors in their thinking by focusing selectively on certain aspects of a situation while ignoring equally relevant information in this regard. Beck named it a process of cognitive distortion in which one is found to suffer from the problem of carrying out his thinking in a quite distorted and illogical way for arriving at some conclusion

about his self, others, and the world quite erroneously and far from the reality. It leads to the formation of a *dysfunctional cognitive structure* in depression- or anxiety-prone individuals, making them the victims of depression or anxiety disorders, especially when more precipitating factors appear in their day-to-day life.

Treatment of Mental Health Problems

The treatment of mentally ill persons in Beck's cognitive therapy consists of first identifying the nature of the problem and the possible causes attached to it. It then calls for the adoption of the indirect questioning technique for the soft, non-threatening disputation (challenging) of the client's dysfunctional cognitive structure composed of the distorted, irrational thinking and beliefs. The responding to questions—such as, in the previous example, "Why should everyone care about you?"—may help the client in doing away with his cognitive distorted structure erected through his erroneous belief that "he should be always cared and looked after by others."

Cognitive-Behavioral Therapy

This is aimed to bring needed changes to one's cognitive behavior for feeling and acting in a desirable way. Cognitive-behavioral therapy takes a double-barrel approach for dealing with behavioral problems and disorders. Where, on one hand, it aims to bring desirable change in people's way of thinking, side by side, on the other it also works toward altering the way they act.

In this way, this treatment approach helps in deriving two-sided benefits of both the cognitive as well as behavioral approaches for treating abnormal behavior by (i) making people aware of their irrational negative thinking and replacing it with new ways of thinking, and (ii) training them to practice a more positive approach and way of living their life.

1. The beginning of the application of this approach aims to bring needed changes to the irrational negative attitude and thought processes of the problem-ridden individual. In general, people suffering from depression, anxiety, and mood disorders are found to grapple with pessimistic and negative thinking, and overgeneralized self-blaming behavior, such as "I am worthless, I will not be able to face the interview board, the other candidates are far better than me, they are looking so relaxed and confident, I will get surely nervous in answering the questions, so on and so forth."
2. To change such self-defeating, over-blaming, and pessimistic behaviors into desirable ones, therapists now try to teach affected people to restructure their thinking and behavior positively in stressful situations. The first task in this concern is to replace negative self-talk with positive, confident, and assuring self-talk. This can help them in restructuring their thought process. It can then be followed to train them to act in a desirable way, guided through their restructured thinking.

In practice, the use of cognitive-behavioral therapy has been found quite encouraging and helpful for a number of people suffering from anxiety, depression, and mood disorders. While going through such treatment, the affected people get valuable opportunity to replace their negative thinking and self-defeating pessimistic behavior with more realistic appraisals of themselves, and practice behavior that helps them in overcoming their problems. How cognitive-behavioral therapy is practiced and what gains are available with the use of this therapy may be made clear by going through the following description provided by Myers, David G. (2014:556).

In one study, people with obsessive-compulsive behaviors learned to re-label their compulsive thoughts. Feeling the urge to wash their hands again and again, they would tell themselves, "I'm having a compulsive urge." They would explain to themselves that the hand-washing urge was a result of their brain's abnormal activity, which they had previously viewed in PET scans. Then, instead of giving in, they would spend 15 minutes in an enjoyable, alternative behavior, such as practicing an instrument, taking a walk, or gardening. This helped "unstuck" the brain by shifting attention and engaging other brain areas. For two or three months, the weekly therapy sessions continued, with re-labeling and refocusing practice at home. By the study's end, most participants' symptoms had diminished, and their PET scans revealed normalized brain activity. Many other studies confirm cognitive-behavioral therapy's effectiveness for those with anxiety, depression, or anorexia nervosa.

To Sum Up

The primary goal of cognitive therapy is to promote logical thinking. Cognitive therapists accomplish this goal by helping clients recognize and revise cognitions that are illogical or irrational. There are three types of cognitive therapies used most often by clinical psychologists for this purpose, named Rational Emotive Behavior Therapy, Beck's Cognitive Therapy, and Cognitive-Behavioral Therapy. In Rational Emotive Behavior Therapy, efforts are made to help patients bring necessary changes to their irrational and erroneous thoughts and beliefs, leading them to live an emotionally balanced, normal life. In Beck's cognitive therapy, work begins with the identification of the nature of the problem and its probable causes. It is then followed by the adoption of the indirect questioning technique for the soft, non-threatening disputation (challenging) of the client's dysfunctional cognitive structure composed of the distorted, irrational thinking and beliefs. *Cognitive-behavioral therapy* helps in deriving two sided benefits of both the cognitive as well as behavioral approaches for treating abnormal behavior by (a) making people aware of their irrational negative thinking and replacing it with new ways of thinking and (b) training them to practice a more positive approach and way of living in their life.

Other Alternative Therapies

All these treatment methods discussed so far in this chapter involve a one-to-one relationship, with one helping person (the therapist) and one person coming for help (the patient). There are other behavioral approaches, such as group therapy, family therapy, and dramatic therapy, that involve two or more persons in seeking and providing treatment help. In addition, there are some good approaches available on this account from the ancient civilization, such as Yogic meditation therapy in Indian Culture. Let us know about them.

Group Therapy

In contrast to establishing a one-on-one relationship, group therapy demands the involvement of a group (two or more persons) at a time with a single or several therapists. According to Kisker (1964:388), "Group therapy is a method of treatment in which a number of people are treated at one time or in which group dynamics are used in the treatment of one person." The foundation and functioning of any scheme or form of group therapy is based on the assumption that the group can provide valuable opportunities to the problem-ridden clients for finding the solution to their problems through useful interpersonal interactions available to them in the group. This is why most group therapies strongly emphasize interpersonal interaction, and group therapists' interventions often highlight the way group members feel, communicate, and form relationships with one another. More than any other component, it is this accent on interpersonal interaction that distinguishes group therapy from individual therapy (Burlingame and Baldwin, 2011).

Whereas individual therapy is limited to a two-person interaction between client and therapist, group therapy allows for a far more complex network of relationships to develop among the members of a group. In the usual format of group therapy, a group usually consists of six to 12 members who meet one or more times a week. This group is often homogeneous with respect to age, sex, and type of disorder. Usually, the group is led by a therapist. The different therapeutic measures like psychoanalytical therapy, client-centered therapy, and behavior therapy used in individual therapy may also be successfully used in group therapy, which may take several forms. There are differences in objectives, approaches, and techniques. Some groups are conducted in the format of individual therapy, others are essentially educational, featuring the presentation of certain materials that the members discuss and apply to themselves. A few groups are largely inspirational; others seek to promote insight to release experiences or problems, pent-up emotions, or unconscious impulses to facilitate self-discovery or to teach social skills.

Irvin Yalom has emerged as a leading figure in the interpersonal approach to group therapy and his writings have influenced group therapists of all kinds. According to Yalom (2005), although it may be possible to conduct group therapy as a series of one-on-one interactions between the therapist and clients, such an approach fails to "reap the full therapeutic harvest" (p. xv) that group therapy can offer. In fact, as Yalom (2005) further observes, an individual's behavioral problem or disorder is a byproduct of that individual's disturbed way of getting along with other people. If interpersonal relationship problems are the core of all psychopathology, it follows that a primary focus of group therapy would be the strengthening of interpersonal relationship skills.

Accordingly, group therapists should always try to recognize the unique opportunity that group therapy presents: the display of clients' problematic interpersonal tendencies in the group itself.

Inspired and guided by the path shown by Irvin Yalom and others, in the modern system of group therapy, a group situation known as an "encounter group" is used for the treatment of maladaptive and problem behavior. In such a group, the patients are encouraged to behave in an unguarded fashion. They get immediate and open feedback from fellow members and the therapist or the group leader. In some encounter groups, the members engage in group activities like singing, games, physical exercises, physical intimacy, dance, dramas, and other entertainment programs. The idea behind such group activities is to induce fatigue or pleasure in order to break resistances for closer group interaction and proper catharsis or sublimation of their unconscious, improper motives.

Group therapy has many advantages over individual therapy, the foremost being the economy in terms of time, labor, and financial resources, as the treatment may be given to a number of patients in a group affected with the same disorder. Beyond this, group therapy provides an environment for the learning of desirable social skills and the unlearning of maladaptive behavior through the use of group dynamics. It also permits persons with common problems to support and help one another.

However, group therapy does not necessarily work well with all types of disorders and patients. For example, some people find it impossible to talk about themselves and their problems in a group. In some cases of agitated depression or psychotic disturbances, the group encounter may prove dangerous. As a result, there is a need for considerable skill on the part of the therapist who deals with a group of patients. It is his competency, art of group dynamics, and understanding between him and his patients that prove helpful in generating positive results in group therapy.

Family Therapy

Family therapy is a variation of group therapy in which two or more members of a family are treated together as a unit. The family group in this therapy may consist of a troubled married couple, or it may be a set of parents and one or more of their children. Sometimes it is the whole family being treated in a clinic or in its natural habitat—the home.

Family therapy has grown out of the realization that psychological problems are not absolutely caused through one's irrational and illogical thinking, but in many cases they are a byproduct of the dysfunctional families in which clients lives (F. W. Kaslow, 2011). Unhealthy intrafamilial relationships are often responsible for the maladaptive abnormal behavior of an individual. Since in families each member of the family is influenced by each other member, an abnormal or mentally disturbed member may prove a potent factor in turning the family environment uncongenial, and thus paving the way for making other members maladjusted and abnormal. With such simple yet profound assumptions, the pioneers of family therapy have provided us a fundamentally different mode of treatment in which family members work together with a therapist to improve their interactions, which in turn strengthens the mental health of each member.

Accordingly, the adoption of the technique of family therapy demands that a proper treatment procedure practiced by a therapist must give priority to caring for the related factors in one's family, along with concentrating on to what is wrong with the client under treatment. In other words, in order to bring about a desirable modification in the behavior of an individual, we have to take care of the intrafamilial relationships within his family. If we attempt to change the patient/client without changing the others in the family, we may find family circumstances conspiring to keep him as he is. This is why many patients who improve in the hospital or clinic are found to manifest a reappearance of symptoms when they return to their families.

In this way, we may see that adoption of family therapy for the treatment of a problem behavior or mental disorder is a challenging and promising approach. It requires family members to discuss their attitudes with each other and acquire insight into the intrafamilial relationship. It asks for desirable changes in the interaction pattern of the whole family, ensuring that changes in one person will not be counteracted by the behavior of others. In adopting this approach, therapists have to bring all or a large portion of the family under study, work for the maintenance of the family's equilibrium, and make the family to work with each other to solve adjustment problems as they occur.

Treatment through family therapy often reveals that the patient who first seeks help or is referred for help is not necessarily the most maladjusted. He may be the victim of the maladjustment or defective interpersonal relationship of his parents or other members of the family. For example, difficulties in the marital relationship of the parents may cause difficulties in parenting, and it may, in turn, cause behavioral abnormalities in the children. In such cases, improvement in the marital relationship of the parents through well-planned family therapy brings desirable improvement in the behavior of a child client.

Dramatic Therapy

Dramatic therapy uses the enactment of roles and incidents, where problems are acted out instead of being talked about. Role playing and psychodrama are examples of such therapy.

In role playing, the patient acts out the behavior of an individual in a certain situation. In doing so, he either repeats his own previous behavior or gives an indication of his possible behavior in that situation. In this way, the role play gives the patient and therapist an opportunity to gain insight into the patient's behavior. It also provides an opportunity and stage to achieve catharsis and to practice more adaptive ways of one's behavior. Psychodrama involves a more elaborate procedure than role play for acting out behavior. It generally involves five elements in a dramatic setting: a stage, the therapist in the role of director, the patient as a hero, helping characters (other persons or therapists), and the audience. The patient is made to act out his problems. All concerned persons are made to participate in the spontaneous acting out of problem situations related to the patient's life.

Meditation Therapy

Mediation, as a term, refers to a process of meditating—focusing attention on something so vital as on one's breath or on one's thoughts, recited mantras, or a particular object lying in one's environment, aimed at attaining relaxation and control over one's thoughts. Historically, the practice of meditation is known for its origin in eastern cultures more than four thousand years ago. Our all great Rishies and even the general public had adopted the meditation practice in their regular daily routine. In Patanjali's yoga system, meditation was the highest stage of one's concentration and yogic sadhna. However, in the present modern days, the credit for popularization and export to the western cultures goes to one of our meditation practitioners, Maharishi Mahesh Yogi. Referred to as transcendental meditation, Mahesh Yogi's brand of meditation has been widely accepted in Europe, the United States, and throughout the world. As far as transcendental meditation is concerned, the most common mental device used in this meditation is the repetition of a mantra. The mantra is a simple sound selected by the instructor as a mental concentration device. One such sound, "om" or "ahhom," has been popular. Other mental devices that have been used in meditation include the *mandala* (a geometrical figure), *nadam* (imagined sounds), and *pranayama* (breathing). A general procedure for making use of transcendental meditation is laid down ahead.

Procedural Steps

- Choose a calm and pollution-free environment and place for doing meditation.
- Sit in a comfortable position with eyes closed on a mat or chair (the standing position is also acceptable).
- Concentrate on deep breathing while at the same time repeating the mantra.
- Soon, you will feel that the sound of the mantra is disappearing and your mind is experiencing more subtle thought levels and finally arriving at the source of the thought; when this happens, you are in deep meditation.

Apart from the previously described transcendental meditation, other forms of meditation practices originated from the Patanjali's Yoga system include Vipasana meditation, Chakra Yoga, Mudra yoga, Kundalini Yoga, and SudarshanKriya Yoga (SKY).

All these forms of yogic meditation have been experimentally proven quite effective as an appropriate therapy or method of treatment for abnormalities, mental disorders, and illnesses particularly associated with acute anxiety, depression, stress, frustration, aggression, social deviance, and substance abuse.

To Sum Up

There exist quite useful therapies in the name of group therapy, family therapy, dramatic therapy, and meditation therapy. *Group therapy* stands for a method of treatment in which a number of people are treated simultaneously or in which group dynamics are used in the treatment of one person. In modern group therapy, a group situation—encounter group—has proved effective in treating behavioral disorders. *Family therapy* is a variation of group therapy in which two or more members of a family are treated as a unit. In *Dramatic therapy*, the method of treatment involves enactment of roles and incidents. Here, the problems are acted out instead of merely talked about. Role playing and psychodrama are examples of such therapy. In meditation therapy, the attention of an otherwise agitated, depressed, or anxiety-ridden patient is focused on something so vital as on one's breath or on one's thought, recited mantra, or a particular object in one's environment, aimed to attain relaxation and control over one's thoughts. The two most common meditation practices employed in this therapy are known as transcendental meditation (popularized by Mahesh Yogi) and the therapies based on Patanjali's Yoga system.

Rehabilitation of the Mentally Ill

Dealing with a client's problems of behavioral abnormality, mental disorder or illness does not end with their treatment; It needs to be supplemented with the adoption of suitable rehabilitation measures for helping them in reaching their optimal level of independent functioning in society and for improving their quality of life. The needs of helping them on this account may be varied and multi-dimensional, depending on the nature of their ailments or problems. Accordingly, the rehabilitation measures adopted for patients of severe problems, such as schizophrenia, bipolar disorder, acute anxiety disorder, and depression, need to be somewhat different from cases of milder ailments, such as generalized anxiety, phobia, socially deviant behavior, substance abuse, intellectual disability, and so on. However, one thing is common and sure for all types of cases: all of them need to be helped in getting enabled for living an independent and happy life. For this purpose, they need to be trained and oriented for becoming satisfactorily independent in terms of their physical, economic, and social living. Therefore, the rehabilitation measures or means employed for their welfare may include:

1. They should be oriented about the adoption of *appropriate health habits* in terms of doing regular physical exercise and yoga activities, being careful about their food, and cultivating sleeping habits in proper tune with the type of problem they experience.
2. For their proper socio-psychological adjustment, they should be provided opportunities to acquire necessary skills such as *communication skills, life saving skills,* and *emotional management skills.* There should also be due attempts for getting them accepted and integrated into their familiar sociocultural environment by educating the family and community for the needed awareness and positive attitude toward them through means like family therapy and community awareness.
3. For seeking economic independence they should be trained in acquiring the needed *occupational and vocational skills* for helping them to earn their livelihood by seeking self-employment or jobs in one or the other sectors.

For exercising of all the aforementioned responsibilities regarding the necessary rehabilitation of cured patients, clinical psychologists may also enlist the services of trained social workers. With their assistance, they can perform the needed actions for the rehabilitation and aftercare of treated patients. He can ask them to pay periodic visits, take up their reports, accompany them for follow-ups, and provide help in adjusting satisfactorily in the home, family, community, and world of work, thus minimizing the chances of their relapse and dependence on hospitalization. Besides, by seeking cooperation from the community, government, or some voluntary agencies, he may also help the patient to find employment. Moreover, in cases where patients return to their previous job, the clinical psychologists with the assistance of social psychologists and social workers may help them in their occupational adjustment by advising the employer to understand the patient's illness and recovery.

To Sum Up

Rehabilitation of the mentally ill refers primarily to modification of the environment in order to provide a life situation in which the patient has a reasonable chance of making a successful adjustment. Various sociotherapeutic measures carried out by psychiatric social workers with the help of voluntary and non-voluntary social welfare agencies help a patient in his overall adjustment by bringing desirable changes in his physical, social, educational, professional, and therapeutic environments. Moreover, these measures prove effective in providing systematic care to the patients after their discharge from the hospital in terms of follow-up treatment and proper rehabilitation.

Assessment Questions

1. What is medical or somatic therapy? Discuss in detail the various methods used for medical or somatic therapy for the treatments of mental disorders or abnormalities in behavior.
2. Discuss any two of the following medical or somatic therapy in detail.

   (i) Drug or chemotherapy, (ii) Shock therapy, (iii) Psychosurgery

3. What are psychological therapies? Discuss any two of the various types of therapies designated as psychological therapies used for providing treatment to affected individuals.
4. Discuss in detail the psychoanalytic or psychodynamic therapy used for the treatment of abnormality or mental disorders.
5. What is client-centered psychotherapy? Describe in detail.
6. What is Humanistic-Existential therapy? Discuss its employment for treating abnormality and mental disorders.
7. What is behavior therapy? Discuss any two of the following behavioral therapies in detail.

   (i) Counter conditioning, (ii) Systematic desensitization, (iii) Flooding or impulsive therapy, (iv) Aversive conditioning, (v) Modeling, (vi) Method of providing positive reinforcement

8. What is cognitive therapy? Discuss in detail any one of the cognitive therapies used for the treatment of abnormality or mental disorders.
   (i) Rational Emotive Behavior Therapy (REBT), (ii) Beck's Cognitive Therapy (CT), (iii) Cognitive behavior Therapy (CBT)

9. Discuss in brief the use of the following therapies.
   (i) Group therapy, (ii) Family therapy, (iii) Dramatic therapy, (iv) Meditation therapy
10. Throw light on the rehabilitation of the mentally ill.

References

Beck, A. T. (1967), *Depression: Causes and treatment*, Philadelphia, PA: University of Pennsylvania Press.

Beck, A. T., & Haigh, E. A. (2014), Advances in cognitive theory and therapy: The generic cognitive model, *Annual Review of Clinical Psychology*, 10: 1–24.

Beck, J. S. (1995), *Cognitive therapy: Basics and beyond*, New York, NY: Guilford Press.

Beck, J. S. (2002). Beck therapy approach. In M. Hersen & W. Sledge (Eds.), *Encyclopedia of psychotherapy* (Vol. 1, pp. 155–163). San Diego, CA: Academic Press.

Burlingame, G. M., & Baldwin, S. (2011). Treatment modalities: Group therapy. In J. C. Norcross, G. R. VandenBos, & D. K. Freedheim (Eds.), *History of psychotherapy: Continuity and change* (2nd ed., pp. 505–515). Washington, DC: American Psychological Association.

Cabaniss, D. L., Cherry, S., Douglas, C. J., & Schwartz, A. R. (2011), *Psychodynamic psychotherapy: A clinical manual*, New York, NY: Wiley.

Ciccarelli, S. K., & White, J. N. (2012), *Psychology*, New York, NY: Pearson Prentice Hall.

Dryden, W. (2009), *Understanding emotional problems: The REBT perspective*, New York, NY: Routledge.

Ellis, A. (1957), Rational psychotherapy and individual psychology, *Journal of Individual Psychology*, 13: 38–44.

Ellis, A. (1962), *Reason and emotion in psychotherapy*, New York, NY: Lyle Stuart.

Ellis, A. (2008), Cognitive restructuring of the disputing of irrational beliefs, In W. T. O'Donohue & J. E. Fisher (Eds.), *Cognitive behavior therapy: Applying empirically supported techniques in your practice* (2nd ed., pp. 91–95), Hoboken, NJ: Wiley.

Freud, S. (1900). The interpretation of dreams, In Strachey, J. Trans. & Ed., *The standard edition of the complete psychological works of Sigmund Freud* (Vols. 4–5, pp. 1–28), London: Hogarth Press/Institute of Psychoanalysis. (Original work published 1886–1939).

Karon, B. P., & Widener, A. J. (1995), Psychodynamic therapies in historical perspective: "Nothing human do I consider alien to me." In B. Bongar & L. E. Beutler (Eds.), *Comprehensive textbook of psychotherapy: Theory and practice* (pp. 24–47). New York, NY: Oxford University Press.

Kaslow, F. W. (2011), Treatment modalities: Family therapy, In J. C. Norcross, G. R. VandenBos, & D. K. Freedheim (Eds.), *History of psychotherapy: Continuity and change* (2nd ed., pp. 497–504), Washington, DC: American Psychological Association.

Kisker, G. W. (1964), *The disorganized personality* (3rd International Students ed.), New York, NY: McGraw-Hill.

Myers, D. G. (2014), *Exploring psychology*, New York, NY: Wordsworth.

Onken, L. S. (2015), Cognitive training targeting cognitive processes in the development of behavioral interventions, *Clinical Psychological Science*, 3(1): 39–44.

Rogers, C. R. (1961), *On becoming a person: A therapist's view of psychotherapy*, Boston, MA: Houghton/Mifflin.

Rogers, C. R. (1980), *A way of being*, Boston, MA: Houghton Mifflin.

Yalom, I. D. (2005), *The theory and practice of group psychotherapy* (5th ed.), New York, NY: Basic Books.

Bibliography

Ackerman, S. J., Fowler, J. C., & Clemence, A. J. (2008), TAT and other performance-based assessment techniques, In R. P. Archer & S. R. Smith (Eds.), *Personality assessment* (pp. 337–378), New York, NY: Routledge.

Acosta, M., Haller, D., & Schnoll, S. (2011), Cocaine and stimulants. In R. J. Frances, A. H. Mack, & S. I. Miller (Eds.), *Clinical textbook of addictive disorders* (3rd ed. pp. 183-218), New York, NY: Guilford Press.

Adams, H. E. (1972), *Psychology of adjustment*, New York: Ronald Press.

Advani, L., & Chadha, A. (2003), *You and your special child*, New Delhi: UBS Publishers, Distributors Pvt. Ltd.

American Heritage Publishing Company (2016), American Heritage Dictionary of the English Language—Fifth Edition, New York, NY: Houghton Mifflin Harcourt Publishing Company.

American Psychiatric Association (1952), *Diagnostic and statistical manual of mental disorders*, Washington, DC: American Psychiatric Association.

American Psychiatric Association (1968), *Diagnostic and statistical manual of mental disorders, DSM-II* (2nd ed.), Washington, DC: American Psychiatric Association.

American Psychiatric Association (1980), *Diagnostic and statistical manual of mental disorders, DSM-III* (3rd ed.), Washington, DC: American Psychiatric Association.

American Psychiatric Association (1994), *Diagnostic and statistical manual of mental disorders, DSM-IV* (4th ed.), Washington, DC: American Psychiatric Association.

American Psychiatric Association (2000), *The diagnostic and statistical manual of mental disorders, DSM IV-TR*, Washington, DC: American Psychiatric Association.

American Psychiatric Association (2013), *Diagnostic and statistical manual of mental disorders* (5th ed.), Washington, DC: American Psychiatric Association.

American Psychiatric Association (2022), *Diagnostic and statistical manual of mental disorders: DSM-5-TR*, Washington, DC: American Psychiatric Association.

American Psychological Association (1993), Guidelines for providers of psychological services to ethnic, linguistic, and culturally diverse population, *American Psychologist*, 48: 45–48.

American Psychological Association (2002), Ethical principles of psychologists and code of conduct, *American Psychologist*, 57: 1060–1073.

Andrew, G., Hartwell, S. W., Hutt, M. L., & Walton, R. E. (1953), *The Michigan Picture test*, Chicago, IL: Science and Research Association.

Archer, R. P. (1997). *MMPI-A: Assessing adolescent psychopathology* (2nd ed.). Mahwah, NJ: Erlbaum.

Arkoff, A. (1968), *Adjustment and mental health*, New York: McGraw-Hill.

Autism Society of America Quoted by Sturmey, P., & Servin J. A. (1994), Defining and assessing autism, In J. L. Matson (Ed.) *Autism in Children and Adults: Etiology, assessment and intervention* (pp. 33–36), Pacific Grove, CA: Brooks/Cole.

Avasthi, A., Grover, S., & Kate, N. (2013), Indianization of psychiatry utilizing Indian mental concepts, *Indian Journal of Psychiatry*, 55: 136–144.

Barkley, R. A. (1988), *ADHD and the nature of Self-control*, New York: Wiley.

Barkley, R. A. (2000), *Taking charge of ADHD: The complete authoritative guide for parents*, New York, NY: The Guilford Press.

Beck, A. T. (1967), *Depression: Causes and treatment*, Philadelphia, PA: University of Pennsylvania Press.

Beck, A. T., Epstein, N., Brown, G., & Steer, R. A. (1988). An inventory for measuring clinical anxiety: Psychometric properties, *Journal of Consulting and Clinical Psychology*, 56: 893–897.

Beck, A. T., & Haigh, E. A. (2014), Advances in cognitive theory and therapy: The generic cognitive model, *Annual Review of Clinical Psychology*, 10: 1–24.

Beck, A. T., Steer, R. A., & Brown, G. K. (1996), *Manual for the Beck Depression Inventory-II*, San Antonio, CA: Psychological Corporation.

Beck, J. S. (1995), *Cognitive therapy: Basics and beyond*, New York, NY: Guilford Press.

Beck, J. S. (2002), Beck therapy approach, In M. Hersen & W. Sledge (Eds.), *Encyclopedia of psychotherapy* (Vol. 1, pp. 155–163), San Diego, CA: Academic Press.

Bellak, L. (1993). *The TAT, CAT, and SAT in clinical use* (5th ed.), Needham Heights, MA: Allyn & Bacon.

Bellak, L., & Bellak, S.S. (1973), *Senior apperception technique*, New York, NY: C.P.S.

Ben-Porath, Y. S., & Archer, R. P. (2008), The MMPI-2 and MMPI-A, In R. P. Archer & S. R. Smith (Eds.), *Personality assessment* (pp. 81–131), New York, NY: Routledge.

Best, J. W., & Kahn, J. V. (2006), *Research in education* (10th ed.), New Delhi: Prentice Hall of India.

Bhardwaj, R. and Kumar, S. (2007), Somnambulism: Diagnosis and treatment, *Indian Journal of Psychiatry*, 49(2): 123–125.

Bracken, B. A., & McCallum, S. (2015), *The Universal Nonverbal Intelligence Test2 (UNIT)*, Austin, TX: PRO-ED.

British Mental Deficiency Act (1929), *Quoted in Shanmugam, T.E., Abnormal psychology*, New Delhi: Tata McGraw Hill, 1981.

Broshek, D. K., & Barth, J. T. (2000), The Halstead-Reitan neuropsychological battery, In G. Groth-Marnat (Ed.), *Neuropsychological assessment in clinical practice* (pp. 223–262), New York, NY: Wiley.

Bruch, H. (1973), *Eating disorders: Obesity; anorexia nervosa and the person within*, New York, NY: Basic Books.

Bruch, H. (2001), *The golden age: The enigma of anorexia nervosa*, Cambridge, MA: Harvard University Press.

Burlingame, G. M., & Baldwin, S. (2011). Treatment modalities: Group therapy. In J. C. Norcross, G. R. VandenBos, & D. K. Freedheim (Eds.), *History of psychotherapy: Continuity and change* (2nd ed., pp. 505–515). Washington, DC: American Psychological Association.

Burlingame, G. M., McClendon, D. T., & Alonso, J. (2011), Cohesion in group therapy, In J. C. Norcross (Ed.), *Psychotherapy relationships that work: Evidence-based responsiveness* (2nd ed., pp. 110–131), New York, NY: Oxford University Press.

Butcher, J. N. (2011), *A beginner's guide to the MMPI-2* (3rd ed.), Washington, DC: American Psychological Association.

Cabaniss, D. L., Cherry, S., Douglas, C. J., & Schwartz, A. R. (2011), *Psychodynamic psychotherapy: A clinical manual*, New York, NY: Wiley.

Campbell, D. T., & Stanley, J. C. (1963), *Experimental and quasi-experimental designs for research*, Chicago, IL: Rand McNally.

Carrol, H. A. (1967), *Mental hygiene—the dynamics of adjustment*, Hoboken, NJ: Prentice-Hall.

Ciccarelli, S. K., & White, J. N. (2012), *Psychology*, New York, NY: Pearson Prentice Hall.

Cohen, L., Lawrence, M., & Morrison, K. (2000), *Research methods in education*, London: Routledge.

Cohen, D. J., Donnellian, A. M., & Paul, R. (Eds.) (1987), *Handbook on autism and pervasive developmental disorders*, Silvers Springs, MD: V.H. Winston & Sons.

Coleman, J. C. (1970), *Abnormal psychology and modern life*, Bombay: D.B. Taraporewala & Sons.

Comer, R. J. (2015), *Abnormal psychology* (9th ed.), New York, NY: Worth Publishers (A Macmillan Education Imprint).

Cooper, P., & Bilton, K. M. (2002), *Attention deficit/hyperactivity disorder: A practical guide for teachers* (2nd ed.), London: David, Fulton Publishers.

Craig, R. J. (2008), Millon Clinical Multiaxial Inventory-III, In R. P. Archer & S. R. Smith (Eds.), *Personality assessment* (pp. 133–165), New York, NY: Routledge.

Crow, L. D., & Crow, A. (1951), *Mental hygiene*, New York, NY: McGraw-Hill Inc.

Crow, L. D., & Crow, A. (1969), *Child psychology*, New York, NY: Barnes & Noble, Inc.

Cutts, N. F., & Moslay, P. (1941), *Practical school discipline and mental hygiene*, Boston, MA: Houghton Mifflin.

Davison, G. C., & Neale, J. M. (1978), *Abnormal psychology* (2nd ed.), New York, NY: John Wiley & Sons.

Department of Education USA (1994), *Individuals with Disabilities Education Act (IDEP)*, Washington, DC: Department of Education.

Drever, J. (1952), *A dictionary of psychology*, Middlesex: Penguin Books.

Dryden, W. (2009), *Understanding emotional problems: The REBT perspective*, New York, NY: Routledge.

Durand, V., & Barlow, D. (2013), *Essentials of abnormal psychology* (6th ed.), Wadsworth: Cengage Learning.

Durlak, J. A. (2003), Basic principles of meta-analysis, In M. C. Roberts & S. S. Ilardi (Eds.), *Handbook of research methods in clinical psychology* (pp. 196–209), Malden, MA: Blackwell.

Ellis, A. (1957), Rational psychotherapy and individual psychology, *Journal of Individual Psychology*, 13: 38–44.

Ellis, A. (1962), *Reason and emotion in psychotherapy*, New York, NY: Lyle Stuart.

Ellis, A. (2008), Cognitive restructuring of the disputing of irrational beliefs, In W. T. O'Donohue & J. E. Fisher (Eds.), *Cognitive behavior therapy: Applying empirically supported techniques in your practice* (2nd ed., pp. 91–95), Hoboken, NJ: Wiley.

Eysenck, H. J. (1960), *Handbook of abnormal psychology*, Oxford: Isaac Pitman & Sons Ltd.

Eysenck, H. J., & Eysenck, S. B. J. (1975), *Manual of the Eysenck Personality Questionnaire*, London: Hodder and Stoughton.

Federal Register (1977), *Report of the USA national advisory committee to the education for the handicapped, 1969*, Washington, DC: US Government Printing Office.

Field, A. P. (2013), Meta-analysis in clinical psychology research, In J. S. Comer & P. C. Kendall (Eds.), *The Oxford handbook of research strategies for clinical psychology* (pp. 317–335), New York, NY: Oxford University Press.

Fossum, T. A., Logeais, M. E., & Robiner, W. N. (2016), Related mental health professions, In J. C. Norcross, G. R. VandenBos, D. K. Freedheim, & L. F. Campbell (Eds.), *APA handbook of clinical psychology: Education and profession* (pp. 455–468), Washington, DC: American Psychological Association.

Freud, S. (1900). The interpretation of dreams, In Strachey, J. Trans. & Ed., *The standard edition of the complete psychological works of Sigmund Freud* (Vols. 4–5, pp. 1–28), London: Hogarth Press/Institute of Psychoanalysis. (Original work published 1886–1939).

Goldfinger, K., & Pomerantz, A. M. (2010), *Psychological assessment and report writing*, Thousand Oaks, CA: SAGE.

Goldstein, S. (1999), The facts about ADHD: An overview of attention deficit hyperactivity disorder, retrieved from http://www.samgoldste4in.com/articles/ 9907.html

Good, C. V. (1959), *Dictionary of education*, New York, NY: McGraw-Hill.

Gove, P. B. (Ed.), (1966), *Webster's Seventh New Collegiate Dictionary (1966)*, Springfield, MA: G&C Merriam Company Publishers.

Gravetter, N. E., & Forzano, L.-A. B. (2003), *Research methods for the behavioural sciences*, Belmont, CA: Thomson.

Grossman, H. G. (Ed.) (1983), *Classification in mental retardation*, Washington, DC: American Association on Mental Retardation.

Guzman, C. S., & Wang, Y. P. (2008), Sleep terror disorder: A case report, *Brazilian Journal of Psychiatry*, 30(2)

Hadfield, J. A. (1952), *Mental health and the psychoneurosis*, London: George Allen & Unwin.

Hanrahan, F., Field, A. P., Jones, F. W., & Davey, G. C. (2013), A meta-analysis of cognitive therapy for worry in generalized anxiety disorder, *Clinical Psychology Review*, 33(1), 120–132.

Haynes, S. N., & Kaholokula, J. K. (2008), Behavioural assessment, In M. Hersen & A. M. Gross (Eds.), *Handbook of clinical psychology* (Vol. 1, pp. 495–522), Hoboken, NJ: Wiley.

Hedges, L. V., & Citkowicz, M. (2015), Metaanalysis, In R. L. Cautin & S. O. Lilienfeld (Eds.), *The encyclopedia of clinical psychology* (pp. 1803–1809), Chichester: Wiley Blackwell.

Hitchcock, G., & Hughes, D. (1995), *Research and the teacher* (2nd ed.), London: Routledge.

Hornby, A. S. (1952), The *advanced learner's dictionary of current English (1952)*, London: Oxford University Press.

Hyun Kook Lim (2017), A case report of a 37 year old male patient of the dementia of the Alzheimer's type, Psychiatry Investigation, retrieved from www.ncbi.nlm.nih.gov/pmc/articles/PMC5561413/

Jellinek, E. M. (Ed.) (1942), *Alcohol addiction and chronic alcoholism*, New Haven, CT: Yale University Press.

John, D. J., Manoharan, A., & Varghese, R. (2007), A case of primary hypersomnia, *Annals of Indian Academy of Neurology*, 10: 58–60.

Karon, B. P., & Widener, A. J. (1995), Psychodynamic therapies in historical perspective: "Nothing human do I consider alien to me." In B. Bongar & L. E. Beutler (Eds.), *Comprehensive textbook of psychotherapy: Theory and practice* (pp. 24–47). New York, NY: Oxford University Press.

Kartz, B., & Lehner, G. F. (1997), *Mental hygiene in modern living*, New York: Ronald Press.

Kaslow, F. W. (2011), Treatment modalities: Family therapy, In J. C. Norcross, G. R. VandenBos, & D. K. Freedheim (Eds.), *History of psychotherapy: Continuity and change* (2nd ed., pp. 497–504), Washington, DC: American Psychological Association.

Kavale, K. A., & Forness, S.R. (1985), *The science of learning disabilities*, San Diego, CA: College Hill.

Kent, G. H., & Rosanoff, A. J. (1910), A study of association in insanity, *American Journal of Insanity*, 67: 37–76; 317–390.

Kirk, S. A, Gallagher, J. J., & Anastasiow, N. J. (1993), *Educating exceptional children*, Boston, MA: Houghton Mifflin Company.

Kirk, S. A., & Kirk, W. D. (1971), *Psycho-linguistic learning disabilities; Diagnosis and remediation*, Urbana, IL: University of Illinois Press.

Kisker, G. W. (1964), *The disorganized personality* (3rd International Students ed.), New York, NY: McGraw-Hill.

Kisker, G. W. (1977), *The disorganized personality*, (3rd ed.) New York, NY: McGraw –Hill.

Klein, D. B. (1965), *Mental hygiene* (Revised ed.), New York, NY: Henry Holt.

Knight, B. G. (1996), *Psychology with the older adults* (2nd ed.), Thousand Oaks, CA: SAGE.

Korchin, S. J. (1986), *Modern clinical psychology: Principles of intervention in the clinic and community*, New Delhi: CBS Publishers & Distributors.

Kothari, C. R. (1990), *Research methodology: Methods and techniques* (2nd ed.), New Delhi: Vishwa Prakashan.

Kring, A. M., Johnson, S. L., Davison, G. C., & Neale, J. M. (2012), *Abnormal psychology* (12th ed.), New York, NY: John Wiley & Sons.

Lawkan, P. B. (1949), *Mental hygiene in public health*, New York, NY: McGraw-Hill.

Lazarus, R. S. (1976), *Patterns of adjustment* (International Student Edition), Tokyo: McGraw-Hill, Kogakusha.

Lehner, G., & Kubo, E. (1964), *The dynamics of personal adjustment*, New York, NY: Prentice-Hall.

Levin, M. J. (1978), *Psychology—a geographical approach*, New York, NY: McGraw-Hill.

Lichtenberger, E. O., & Breaux, K. C. (2010), *Essentials of WIAT-III and KTEA-II assessment*, Hoboken, NJ: Wiley.

Lovaas, I. (1994), *Quoted in Heward, William L. (2000), Exceptional children: An introduction to special education* (6th ed.), Upper Saddle River, NJ: Merrill.

Mahoney, M. J. (1980), *Abnormal psychology*, San Francisco, CA: Harper & Row.

Malot, R. W., & Whaley, D. L. (1983), *Psychology*, Holmes Beach, FL: Learning Publications.

Marks, I. M. (1987), *Fears, phobias and rituals: Panic, anxiety, and their disorders*. Oxford: Oxford University Press.

McFall, R. M. (1991), Manifesto for a science of clinical psychology, *Clinical Psychologist*, 44: 75–88.

McFall, R. M. (2006), Doctoral training in clinical psychology, *Annual Review of Clinical Psychology*, 2: 21–49.

McReynolds, P. (1997), *Lightner Witmer: His life and times*, Washington, DC: American Psychological Association.

Menninger, K. A. (1930), *Human mind*, New York, NY: The Literary Guild of America.

Mignon, S. (2014), *Substance abuse treatment: Options, challenges, and effectiveness*, New York, NY: Springer Publishing.

Mihura, J. L., & Meyer, G. J. (2015), Thematic apperception test, In R. L. Cautin & S. O. Lilienfeld (Eds.), *The encyclopedia of clinical psychology* (pp. 2813–2818), Chichester: Wiley Blackwell.

Millon, T., & Millon, C. (2015), Millon inventories (MCMI, MACI, M-PACI, MBMD), In R. L. Cautin & S. O. Lilienfeld (Eds.), *The encyclopedia of clinical psychology* (pp. 1820–1830), Chichester: Wiley Blackwell.

Ministry of Law and Justice (2021), *The Juvenile Justice (Care and Protection of Children) Amendment Act, 2021*, New Delhi: Govt. of India Press.

Moretti, R. J., & Rossini, E. D. (2004), The Thematic Apperception Test (TAT), In M. J. Hilsenroth & D. L. Segal (Eds.), *Comprehensive handbook of psychological assessment: Personality assessment* (Vol. 2, pp. 356–371), Hoboken, NJ: Wiley.

Morey, L. C. (2003), *Essentials of PAI assessment*, Hoboken, NJ: Wiley.

Morgan, C. D., & Murray, H. A. (1935), A method for investigating fantasies: The thematic apperception test, *Archives of Neurology and Psychiatry*, 34: 289–306.

Morgan, C. T. (1961), *Introduction to psychology* (2nd ed.), New York, NY: McGraw-Hill.

Munn, N. L. (1968), *The fundamentals of human adjustment*, London: Georg G. Harrap.

Murthy, S. (2010), From local to global contributions of Indian Psychiatry to International Psychiatry, *Indian Journal of Psychiatry*, 52: 30–37.

Myers, D. G. (2013), *Psychology* (10th ed.), New York, NY: Worth.

Myers, D. G. (2014), *Exploring psychology*, New York, NY: Wordsworth.

Onken, L. S. (2015), Cognitive training targeting cognitive processes in the development of behavioral interventions, *Clinical Psychological Science*, 3(1): 39–44.

Page, J. D. (1976), *Abnormal psychology*, New Delhi: Tata McGraw-Hill.

Pandurangi, A., Keshavan, M., Ganapathy, V., & Gangadhar, B. (2017), Yoga: Past and present, *American Journal of Psychiatry*, 174: 16–17.

Park, C. C. (1998a), Existing Nirvana, *The American Scholar*, 67: 2.

Park, C. C. (1998b), *Quoted in Hunt Nancy, and Marshall Kathleen, Exceptional Children and Youth (2002), An Introduction to Special Education*, Boston, MA: Houghton Mifflin Company, 30.

Pomerantz, A. M. (2020), *Clinical psychology-science, practice and diversity* (5th ed.), London: SAGE.

Prasadarao, P. S. D. V., & Sudhir, P. M. (2001), Clinical psychology in India, *Journal of Clinical Psychology in Medical Settings*, 8(1): 31–38.

Price, J. H. (1972), *Psychiatric investigations*, London: Butterworths.

Raiford, S. E., Coalson, D. L., Saklofske, D. H., & Weiss, L. G. (2010), Practical issues in WAIS-IV administration and scoring, In L. G. Weiss, D. H. Saklofske, D. Coalson, & S. E. Raiford (Eds.), *WAIS-IV clinical use and interpretation: Scientist-practitioner perspectives* (pp. 25–60), London: Elsevier.

Rapaport, D., Gill, M. M., & Shaffer, R. (1946), *Diagnostic psychological testing* (Vol.2), Chicago, IL: Year Book.

Reisman, J. M. (1991), *A history of clinical psychology* (2nd ed.), New York, NY: Hemisphere.

Rogers, C. R. (1961), *On becoming a person: A therapist's view of psychotherapy*, Boston, MA: Houghton/Mifflin.

Rogers, C. R. (1980), *A way of being*, Boston, MA: Houghton Mifflin.

Rosen, E., Fox, R., & Gregory, I. (1972), *Abnormal psychology* (2nd International Student ed.), Philadelphia, PA: Saunders.

SAMHSA (Substance Abuse and Mental Health Services Administration) (2014), *Results from the 2013 national survey on drug use and health: Summary of national findings*, NSDUH Series H-48, HSS Publication No. (SMA) 14–4863, Rockville, MD: SAMHSA.

Schwartz, R., Brooner, R., Montoya, I., Currens, M., & Hayes, M. (2010), A 12-year follow-up of a methadone medical maintenance program, *The American Journal on Addictions*, 8: 293–299.

Scognamiglio, C., & Houenou, J. (2014), A meta-analysis of fMRI studies in healthy relatives of patients with schizophrenia, *Australian and New Zealand Journal of Psychiatry*, 48(10): 907–916.

Sexton, V. S., & Hogan, J. D. (Eds.), (1992), *International psychology: Views from around the world*, Lincoln, NE: University of Nebraska Press.

Shanker, U. (1958), *Problem children*, Delhi: Atma Ram & Sons.

Shin, Y. -K., Hong, S. C., Cho, Y. J., Jeong Jinhyun, Han. J. H., & Lee. S. P. (2007), Case study of a narcoleptic patient with a family history of narcolepsy, Department of Neuropsychiatry, St. Vincent's Hospital, Korea, *Psychiatry Investigation*, 4: 121–123.

Simsek, Z., &Veiga, Z. F. (2001), A primer on internet organized surveys, *Organizational Research Methods*, 4: 218–235.

Sommers-Flanagan, J., & Sommers-Flanagan, R. (2009), *Clinical interviewing* (4th ed.), Hoboken, NJ: Wiley.

Storr, A. (1964), *Sexual deviation*, London: Penguin Books.

Symonds, P. M. (1949), Review of the software Symonds picture-Story test, *Journal of Consulting Psychology*, 13(1), 67–68.

Thorpe, L. P., & Katz, B. (1948), *The psychology of abnormal behaviour*, New York, NY: The Ronald Press Company.

Truax, P. (2002), Behavioral case conceptualization for adults, In M. Hersen (Ed.), *Clinical behavior therapy: Adults and children* (pp. 3–36), New York, NY: John Wiley & Sons Inc.

Wallace, G., & McLoughlin, J. A. (1979), *Learning disabilities: Concepts and characteristics* (2nd ed.), Columbus, OH: Merrill.

Waltin, J. E. W. (1951), *Personality, maladjustment and mental hygiene* (3rd ed.), New York, NY: McGraw Hill.

Wampold, B. E., Mondin, G. W., Moody, M., Stich, I., Benson, K., & Ahn, H. (1997), A meta-analysis of outcome studies comparing bona fide psychotherapies: Empirically "all must have prizes", *Psychological Bulletin*, 122: 203–215.

Wechsler, D. (1979), *Quoted by N.K. psychological foundations of education*, Delhi: Doaba House.

WHO (1965), *International classification of diseases* (8th revision, ICD-8), Geneva: World Health Organization.

WHO (1977), *International classification of diseases* (9th revision, ICD-9), Geneva: World Health Organization.

WHO (1992), *International statistical classification of diseases and related health problems* (10th revision, ICD-10), Geneva: World Health Organization.

WHO (2010), *The ICD-10 classification of mental and behavioural disorders: clinical descriptions and diagnostic guidelines* (10th ed.), Geneva: World Health Organization.

Wig, N. (1989), Indian concepts of mental health and their impact on care of the mentally ill, *International Journal of Mental Health*, 18: 71–80.

Wootton, B. M. (2016), Remote cognitive-behavior therapy for obsessive compulsive symptoms: A meta-analysis, *Clinical Psychology Review*, 43, 103–113.

World Health Organization (1990), *The international classification of diseases* (10th ed.), Geneva: WHO.

Yalom, I. D. (2005), *The theory and practice of group psychotherapy* (5th ed.), New York, NY: Basic Books.

Young, P. V. (1966), *Scientific social surveys and research*, Hoboken, NJ: Prentice Hall.

Zerbe, K. J. (2008), *Integrated treatment of eating disorders beyond the body betrayed*, New York, NY: W.W. Norton.

On line Resources

American Psychological Association (2012), About clinical psychology, retrieved from www.apa.org/divi-sions/div12/aboutcp. html

American Psychological Association (2022), Definition of mental hygiene, *APA Dictionary of Psychology*, retrieved from dictionary, apa.org/mental-hygiene

American Psychological Association, Definition of clinical psychology, retrieved from www.apa.org/ed/graduate/specialize/clinical

APA (2017), Ethical principles of psychologists and code of conduct, retrieved from www.apa.org›code›ethics-code-2017

Canadian Psychological Association, Definition of clinical psychology, retrieved from https://cpa.ca/docs/File/Sections/Clinical%20section/What%20is%20Clinical%20Psychology.pd

D'Avolio, D. (2018), Case study: Delirium in an older hospitalized woman, *NIDUS, Network for Investigation of Delirium: Unifying Scientists*, retrieved from https://deliriumnetwork.org/case-study-delirium-in-an-older-hospitalized-woman/

Dictionary, definition of clinical psychology, retrieved from www.collinsdictionary.com/dictionary/english/clinical-psychology

Encyclopedia, Britannica, Definition of clinical psychology, retrieved from www.britannica.com/science/clinical-psychology

Merriam-Webster, Merriam-Webster.Com Dictionary, definition of clinical psychologist, retrieved from www.merriam-webster.com/dictionary/clinical%20psychologist

Merriam-Webster.Com Dictionary, Merriam-Webster, Definition of clinical psychologist, retrieved from www.merriam-webster.com/dictionary/clinical%20psychologist

N., Sam M. S., Definition of clinical psychology, retrieved from https://psychologydictionary.org/clinical-psychology/

Topp, J. (2009), Case study-disturbed sleep and vivid nightmares, retrieved from www.gponline.com/case-study-disturbed-sleep-vivid-nightmares/neurology/article/965128

What are eating disorders?, retrieved from www.psychiatry.org/patients-families/eating-disorders/what-are-eating-disorders

World Health Organization (WHO) (2022), *ICD-11 for Mortality and Morbidity Statistics* (version: 02/2022), retrieved from https://icd.who.int/browse11/l-m/en

Yoo, H., et al. (2017), A case report of a 37 year old male patient of the dementia of the Alzheimer's type, *Psychiatry Investigation*, retrieved from www.ncbi.nlm.nih.gov/pmc/articles/PMC5561413/

Zee, P. C. (2011), Case histories in circadian rhythm sleep disorders, *MedScape*, retrieved from www.medscape.org/viewarticle/745357

Additional Suggested Readings

Achenbach, T. M. (2015), Achenbach System of Empirically Based Assessment (ASEBA), In R. L. Cautin & S. O. Lilienfeld (Eds.), *The encyclopedia of clinical psychology* (pp. 25–32), Chichester: Wiley Blackwell.

American Psychological Association (2002), Ethical principles of psychologists and code of conduct, *American Psychologist*, 57: 1060–1073.

Barlow, D. (2012), *Abnormal psychology: An integrative approach*. Belmont, CA: Wadsworth Cengage Learning.

Boss, G. (1939), Progress of psychology in India during the past twenty five years, In B. Prasad (Ed.), *The progress of science in India during the past twenty five years*, Calcutta: Indian Science Congress Association.

Carr, A. (2014), The evidence base for family therapy and systemic interventions for child-focused problems, *Journal of Family Therapy:* 153-213, DOI: 10.1111/1467–6427.12032

Cohen, D. P. (2011), Encopresis: A medical and family approach, *Pediatric Nursing,* 37: 107–112.

Compas, B., & Gotlib, I. (2002), *Introduction to clinical psychology*, New York, NY: McGraw-Hill Higher Education.

Dalal, A. K. (2002), Psychology in India: A historical introduction, In G. Misra, A. K. Hansell, James, & L. Damour (Ed.), *Abnormal Psychology*, Hoboken, NJ: John Wiley and Sons.

Herrnsteen, R. J., & Boring, E. G. (1965), A source book on the history of psychology, Cambridge, MA: Harvard University Press.

Klyko, W. M., & Kay, J. (Ed.) (2012), *Clinical child psychiatry* (3rd ed.), Oxford: Wiley Blackwell.

Kring, A. M., Johnson, S. L., Davison, G. C., & Neale, J. M. (2012), *Abnormal psychology* (12th ed.), New York, NY: John Wiley & Sons.

Manickam, L. S. S. (2009), Enabling the disabled, *Indian Journal of Clinical Psychology*, 36: 7–10.

Medhekar, D., & Gupta, N. (2010), Use of sertraline in childhood retentive encopresis, *The Annals of Pharmacotherapy*, 44: 395.

Mohanty, A. K. (Eds.), *Perspectives on indigenous psychology*, New Delhi: Concept Norton.

Nolen-Hoeksema, S. (2013), *Abnormal psychology* (6th ed.), Boston, MA: McGraw-Hill.

Shorter, E. (1997), *A history of psychiatry from the era of the asylum to the age of prozac*, New York: Wiley.

Vahia, N., Vinekar, S., & Doongaji, D. (1966), Some ancient Indian concepts in the treatment of psychiatric disorders, *British Journal of Psychiatry*, 112, 1089–1096.

Wallace, E. R. IV, & Gach, J. (Eds.), (2008), *History of psychiatry and medical psychology*, New York: Springer.

Index

Note: numbers in **bold** indicate a table